COUNTY COLLEGE OF MORRIS LIBRARY

FUNDAMENTAL MATHEMATICS for HEALTH CAREERS

2nd EDITION

Jerome D. Hayden
Howard T. Davis

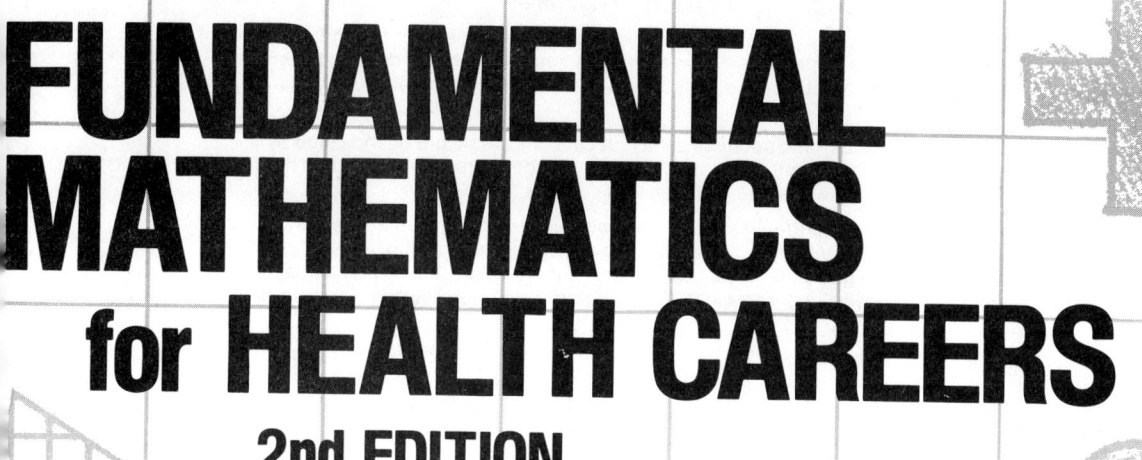

Delmar Publishers Inc.®

NOTICE TO THE READER

Publisher does not warrant or guarantee any of the products described herein or perform any independent analysis in connection with any of the product information contained herein. Publisher does not assume, and expressly disclaims, any obligation to obtain and include information other than that provided to it by the manufacturer.

The reader is expressly warned to consider and adopt all safety precautions that might be indicated by the activities described herein and to avoid all potential hazards. By following the instructions contained herein, the reader willingly assumes all risks in connection with such instructions.

The publisher makes no representations or warranties of any kind, including but not limited to, the warranties of fitness for particular purpose or merchantability, nor are any such representations implied with respect to the material set forth herein, and the publisher takes no responsibility with respect to such material. The publisher shall not be liable for any special, consequential or exemplary damages resulting, in whole or in part, from the readers' use of, or reliance upon, this material.

Cover design by Deborah Shawky-Pedlow

Delmar Staff
Executive Editor: Leslie F. Boyer
Project Editor: Eleanor Isenhart
Production Coordinator: Larry Main
Design Coordinator: Susan C. Mathews

For information, address Delmar Publishers Inc.,
2 Computer Drive West, Box 15-015,
Albany, New York 12212

COPYRIGHT © 1990
BY DELMAR PUBLISHERS INC.

All rights reserved. Certain portions of this work copyright © 1982. No part of this work covered by the copyright hereon may be reproduced or used in any form or by any means—graphic, electronic, or mechanical, including photocopying, recording, taping, or information storage and retrieval systems—without written permission of the publisher.

Printed in the United States of America
Published simultaneously in Canada
by Nelson Canada
A Division of The Thomson Corporation

10 9 8 7 6 5 4 3 2

Library of Congress Cataloging in Publication Data

Hayden, Jerome D.
  Fundamental mathematics for health careers / Jerome D. Hayden, Howard T. Davis. — 2nd ed.

  Rev. ed. of: Mathematics for health careers. ©1980.
  Includes index.
  ISBN 0-8273-3792-2 (pbk.) — ISBN 0-8273-3793-0 (instructor's guide).
  1. Mathematics. 2. Medicine—Mathematics. I. Davis, Howard T. II. Hayden, Jerome D. Mathematics for health careers. III. Title.
QA39.2.H37 1990
513—dc20   89-11856
                                                                                CIP

CONTENTS

SECTION 1 COMMON FRACTIONS
- Unit 1 Introduction to the Mathematical System.................. 1
- Unit 2 Introduction to Common Fractions and Mixed Numbers 7
- Unit 3 Addition and Subtraction of Common Fractions and Mixed Numbers 20
- Unit 4 Multiplication and Division of Common Fractions and Mixed Numbers 30
- Unit 5 Section One Applications to Health Work................. 42

SECTION 2 DECIMAL FRACTIONS
- Unit 6 Introduction to Decimal Fractions 49
- Unit 7 Rounding Decimal Numbers and Finding Equivalents........ 53
- Unit 8 Basic Operations With Decimal Fractions 61
- Unit 9 Exponents and Scientific Notation 71
- Unit 10 Estimation and Significant Digits 81
- Unit 11 Section Two Applications to Health Work 89

SECTION 3 METRIC MEASURE
- Unit 12 Introduction to Metric Measure......................... 95
- Unit 13 Metric Length Measure 101
- Unit 14 Metric Area Measure 109
- Unit 15 Metric Volume Measure................................. 119
- Unit 16 Metric Mass and Temperature Measures.................. 133
- Unit 17 Section Three Applications to Health Work 146

SECTION 4 RATIO, PROPORTION, AND PERCENTS
- Unit 18 Introduction to Ratio and Proportion.................. 151
- Unit 19 Computations With Proportions 156
- Unit 20 Introduction to Percents.............................. 166
- Unit 21 Equations Involving Percents.......................... 175
- Unit 22 Computations With Percents............................ 184
- Unit 23 Section Four Applications to Health Work 196

iii

SECTION 5 SYSTEMS OF MEASURE

- Unit 24 The Apothecaries' System of Weight 207
- Unit 25 The Apothecaries' System of Volume 216
- Unit 26 Household — Apothecaries' Systems of Measure 225
- Unit 27 Household — Metric Systems of Measure 234

SECTION 6 ORGANIZING AND REPORTING DATA

- Unit 28 Interpreting Charts and Graphs 243
- Unit 29 Computers—Tools of the 21st Century 264

Appendix 271
Glossary 280
Health Occupation Information 282
Index 286

PREFACE

Mathematics is a tool for use in our everyday work. Basic computations and the application of these computational skills in problem solving activities allow us to compare data, measure results, and predict outcomes. *Fundamental Mathematics for Health Careers, Second Edition* reviews and teaches skills in mathematics and applies these skills to the solution of practical problems in the health care field.

This is a comprehensive text which follows a developmental sequence of mathematical topics. For some students it is almost a self-teaching text. Both drill and practice exercises reinforce basic principles, concepts and skills. Instructors can identify sections of this text to support an individualized mathematics learning plan for students.

Applications as found at the end of each unit. Most sections also have one entire unit devoted to applications. These applications are diversified and generic to the health care field. It is not the intent of this text to deal with specific medicinal formulations that may vary from clinic to clinic or with the passage of time.

The fields of study that are dealt with include biology, chemistry, physiology, microbiology, technology, and administration. The applications include giving meaningful practice in doses and dosages; solutions; microorganisms, laboratory tests and results, and normal ranges and levels; and the making of administrative decisions. There is also an introduction to medical vocabulary and information relating to the health related fields.

A glossary is included to extend the medical vocabulary. The appendix includes mathematical and health care formulas, equivalences between the systems of measure, and other reference material. Occupation information and a section on denominate numbers also appear in the appendix.

Fundamental Mathematics for Health Careers, Second Edition has been expanded. Computers have become a valuable tool in dealing with mathematical problems. A final unit has been added to show the application of spreadsheeting. It can be used to organize, calculate and process data. Tnis unit will establish the foundation for the student's future use of the computer.

The Instructor's Guide contains comprehensive tests. These tests may be used to test basic principles. Used in part or in full, these may be employed as a pretest, a post-test, or as an evaluation of progress during the course of study. The Instructor's Guide includes all answers, helpful hints, and other aids. The tests and other aids may be reproduced for classroom use.

The authors have many years of combined experience in mathematics, science and technology education. Currently both are associated with the McLean County Unit District No. 5 school district in Normal, Illinois.

ACKNOWLEDGMENTS

A text of this nature represents a team effort. Its initial writing can only begin with the authors. Many individuals have contributed to the end product. These include: Elizabeth A. Foeller, Staff Development Coordinator, Brokaw Hospital, Normal, Illinois; Dr. Jacqueline Kinder, Director, School of Nursing, Mennonite Hospital, Bloomington, Illinois; Merle J. Wurth, Director of Laboratory Technology, St. Joseph's Hospital Medical Center, Bloomington, Illinois; Patricia Payne, Nursing Instructor, Loyola and DePaul Universities, Chicago, Illinois; and Corn Belt Biochemical Laboratory, Bloomington, Illinois.

A significant contribution to this text was the critical review given to the problems and general manuscript by Sandra Slingsby, Math Department Chairperson, Chiddix Junior High School, Normal, Illinois.

LEARNER VERIFICATION
McLean County Unit District No. 5
    Chiddix Junior High School — Normal, Illinois
    Parkside Junior High School — Normal, Illinois
    Normal Community High School — Normal, Illinois

PHOTOGRAPHS
William Rainey Harper College — Palatine, Illinois
B. Blair Brooks — Montgomery, Alabama
Pfizer Inc. — New York, New York
City College of Chicago — Chicago, Illinois
Abbott Laboratories
U. S. Army — Washington, D. C.
South Georgia College — Douglas, Georgia

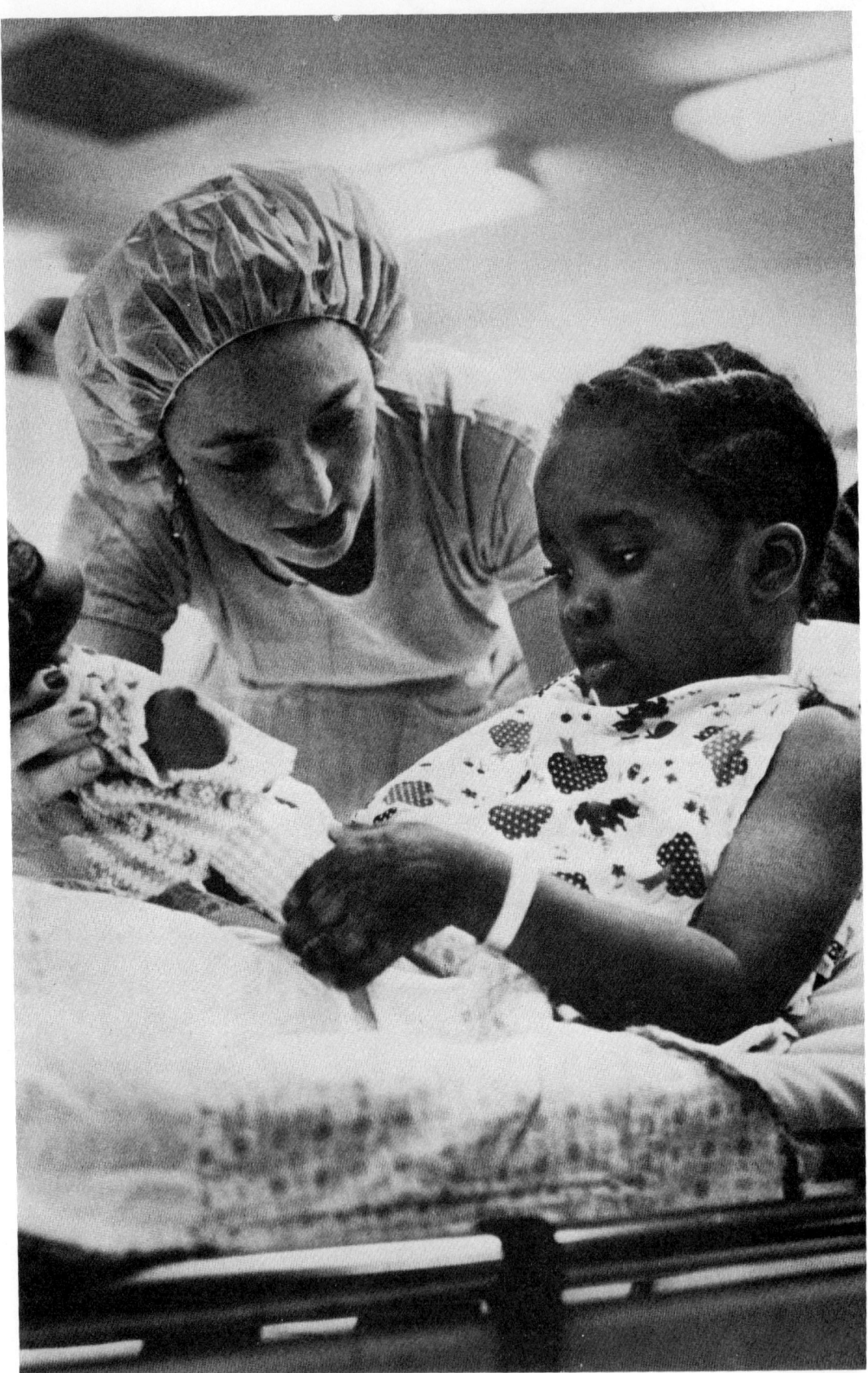

SECTION 1 COMMON FRACTIONS

unit 1 introduction to the mathematical system

Whole numbers are the basis of mathematics. Together with the basic operations of addition, subtraction, multiplication, and division, the mathematical system is developed. Understanding the proper mathematical terminology is essential for using this mathematical system.

DEFINITIONS

- ▼ *Addition* is a fast way of counting. The result is the *sum*.
- ▼ *Subtraction* is the opposite of addition. The result is the *difference*.
- ▼ *Multiplication* is repeated addition. The numbers that are multiplied are the *factors*. The result is the *product*.
- ▼ *Division* is the opposite of multiplication. The result is the *quotient*.

1.1 EXERCISES

Find each result.

1. 3,254
    2,730
    3,149
    + 5,682

2. 531
    − 207

3. 243
    × 17

4. 46) 2,392

5. 79,413
    65,042
    + 73,294

6. 9,028
    − 6,139

7. 256
    × 904

8. 104) 25,584

9. 643
    805
    1,307
    94,315
    + 61

10. 49,271
    − 1,046

11. 4,361
    × 7,831

12. 471) 256,224

Section 1 Common Fractions

Numbers may be considered in many ways. Numbers are compared to find the greater or lesser quantity and to determine primes, multiples, factors, and common numbers.

DIVISIBILITY

Divisible means that there is no remainder in the quotient. Divisibility tests are a quick way of finding out if one number is divisible by another number without exactly dividing.

- **Divisible by 2**: A number is divisible by 2 if the units digit is divisible by 2. The number 39,484 <u>is divisible by 2</u> since 4 is divisible by 2. The number 126,989 <u>is not divisible by 2</u> since 9 is not divisible by 2.

- **Divisible by 5**: A number is divisible by 5 if the last digit is 0 or 5. The number 26,175 <u>is divisible by 5</u> since the last digit is 5. The number 199,990 <u>is divisible by 5</u> since the last digit is 0.

- **Divisible by 10**: A number is divisible by 10 if the last digit is 0. The number 6,780 <u>is divisible by 10</u> since the last digit is 0. The number 11,945 <u>is not divisible by 10</u> since the last digit is not 0.

1.2 EXERCISES

Group these numbers according to divisibility.

1,764	11,130	296,048
3,278	49,000	446,075
65	6,775	786,312
365	82,722	954,560
7,420	24,835	1,526,200

1. Divisible by 2.
2. Divisible by 5.
3. Divisible by 10.

COMPARING WHOLE NUMBERS

Numbers that represent the same quantity are *equal*. The symbol used to show equality is =.

Examples: $3 + 5 = 18 - 10$
$7 \times 3 = 84 \div 4$

Numbers that do not represent the same quantity are *unequal*. The symbol used to show that two numbers are not equal is $\neq$.

Examples: $88 - 13 \neq 75 + 13$
$36 \div 3 \neq 3 \times 3$

Numbers that do not represent the same quantity are *greater than* the quantity or *less than* the quantity. The symbol for greater than is >. The symbol for less than is <.

Examples: $88 - 13 < 75 + 13$ since $75 < 86$.
$36 \div 3 > 3 \times 3$ since $12 > 9$.

DIVISION INVOLVING ZERO

In a division problem involving zero, there are three possibilities:
- Zero is the dividend.
- Zero is the divisor.
- Zero is the dividend and the divisor.

Example: Zero is the dividend.

$$0 \div 5 = ?$$

$0 \div 5 = ?$ means $? \times 5 = 0$

Since any number times zero is zero, $0 \times 5 = 0$ and $0 \div 5 = 0$.

$0 \div 5 = 0 \qquad 0 \times 5 = 0$

- Zero divided by any number equals zero.

Example: Zero is the divisor.

$$4 \div 0 = ?$$

$4 \div 0 = ?$ means $? \times 0 = 4$

Since there is no number times zero that equals 4, $? \times 0 = 4$ is not possible and $4 \div 0 = ?$ is not possible. It is said that $4 \div 0$ is not defined.

$4 \div 0 =$ not defined   no number $\times 0 = 4$

- Any number divided by zero is not defined.

Example: Zero is the dividend and the divisor.

$$0 \div 0 = ?$$

$0 \div 0 = ?$ means $? \times 0 = 0$

Since any number times zero equals zero, it is said that $0 \div 0$ is not defined.

$0 \div 0 =$ not defined   any number $\times 0 = 0$

- Zero divided by zero is not defined.

1.3 EXERCISES

Compare each pair of numbers. Use the symbols $<, >, =$.

1. 5 _?_ 7
2. 13×3 _?_ 3×13

4 Section 1 Common Fractions

3. 7 × 2 × 3 __?__ 7 × 6
4. 36 + 2 __?__ 40 − 8
5. 99 − 9 __?__ 90 ÷ 9
6. 0 × 8 __?__ 0 ÷ 8
7. 16 × 3 __?__ 42 ÷ 6
8. 23 × 5 __?__ 15 + 25 + 75
9. 1,000 − 72 __?__ 459 × 2

FACTORS, MULTIPLES, PRIME NUMBERS

Factors and multiples are a valuable tool in using the mathematical system. Prime numbers help to simplify the process of finding factors and multiples.

DEFINITIONS

- ▼ *Factors* are the numbers being multiplied to find a product.
- ▼ *Common factors* of two or more numbers are the factors that are common to both numbers.
- ▼ *Factorization* is the process of finding the factors of a number.
- ▼ A *multiple* is the product of a given number and another factor.
- ▼ A *common multiple* is a number which is a multiple of each of two or more numbers.
- ▼ A *prime number* is a natural number, other than 1, having only 1 and itself as factors.
- ▼ A *prime factor* is a prime number that is a factor of a number.
- ▼ *Prime factorization* is the process of finding the factors of a number using only prime numbers.

Counting by 3 gives the numbers

  3, 6, 9, 12, 15, 18, 21, 24, 27, 30, . . .

The numbers are multiples of 3.
The number 12 is a multiple of 3.

  12 = 4 × 3

Three is a factor of 12. Four is a factor of 12.

  Counting by 5 gives the numbers

  5, 10, 15, 20, 25, 30, 35, 40, 45, 50, . . .

The numbers are multiples of 5.
The number 35 is a multiple of 5.

  35 = 7 × 5

Five is a factor of 35. Seven is a factor of 35.

The numbers 15 and 30 are multiples of both 3 and 5. The numbers 15 and 30 are common multiples. Any number can be expressed using factors.

Example: Find two factors of 28.

28 = 7 × 4

Four is a factor of 28. Seven is a factor of 28.

Since 7 is also a prime number, it is called a <u>prime factor.</u>

Example: Find the factors of 33.

33 = 11 × 3 *or* 1 × 33

Eleven is a factor of 33. Three is a factor of 33.

Since both 11 and 3 are prime numbers, both numbers are <u>prime factors</u> of 33.

Example: Use prime factorization to find the prime factors of 60. Possible factor trees:

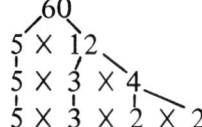

60 = 5 × 2 × 2 × 3

The numbers 5, 2, and 3 are prime factors.

Note: The prime factors are the same. Only the order is different.

1.4 EXERCISES

Find two common multiples of each group of numbers.

1. 2, 5
2. 7, 6, 8
3. 9, 4
4. 5, 9, 2, 7
5. 3, 4, 5

Find the prime factorization of each number.

6. 42
7. 68
8. 99
9. 60
10. 125

APPLICATIONS

Almost four million people work in health-related occupations. Of this number, hospitals employ about one-half of the workers in the health field. Clinics, laboratories, pharmacies, nursing homes, public health agencies, mental health centers, private offices, and patients' homes are places of employment for the other one-half of the workers.

1.5 EXERCISES

1. Using a city directory, determine the number of hospitals, clinics, laboratories, pharmacies, nursing homes and other health care centers that are located in the community.

2. Tour one or more of these health care facilities and list the type of health care positions that are available. Group the health care workers and observe the distribution. Note the differences between smaller and larger facilities.

3. Inquire about one or more of the health care positions. Find out the nature of the job, training and other qualifications, and employment outlook. Compare the finding with smaller and larger facilities.

4. Develop a list of additional sources that may be used to obtain further information about health-related occupations.

5. Consult with a county hospital or clinic supervisor to determine how they estimate the need for health care services in their community.

6. Consult the "Help Wanted" advertisements in at least one major city newspaper to determine the opportunities for health care related employment in that community.

7. Through consultation with your instructor, medical supervisor, or others employed in the health care area, develop a list of courses and degrees you must complete to advance to the level of health care service you want to provide during your career.

unit 2 introduction to common fractions and mixed numbers

OBJECTIVES

After studying this unit the student should be able to:
- Express fractions in lowest terms.
- Express fractions as equivalent fractions.
- Compare fractional values.

FRACTIONAL PARTS

A fraction is a comparison between a part of a whole and the whole.

Example:

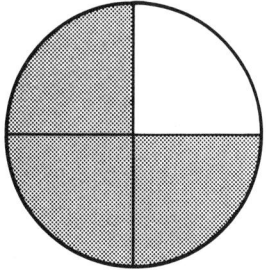

In this figure 3 of the 4 regions are shaded.
The fraction $\frac{3}{4}$ represents this comparison.

A fraction is also a comparison of a part of a group to the whole group.

Example:

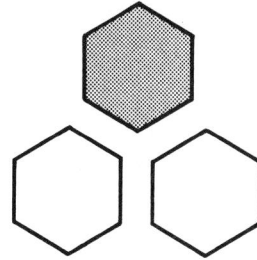

In this figure, 1 hexagon of the 3 hexagons is shaded.
The fraction $\frac{1}{3}$ represents this comparison.

DEFINITIONS OF FRACTIONS

- ▼ The *numerator* is the number of parts being used. It is the number above the fraction bar.
- ▼ The *denominator* is the number of equal parts needed to make a whole object. It is the number below the fraction bar.

$$\frac{3}{4}$$

- ▼ *Equivalent fractions* are two or more fractions which represent the same part of the whole or the same part of a group.
- ▼ The *greatest common factor* (GCF) of two or more numbers is the largest factor common to all numbers.
- ▼ A fraction is in *lowest terms* if the greatest common factor (GCF) of both the numerator and the denominator is 1.
- ▼ The *lowest-term fraction* is the simplest fraction in a group of equivalent fractions.
- ▼ A *mixed number* is a number having a whole number part and a fractional part.

EQUIVALENT FRACTIONS

These fractions name the shaded part of each region.

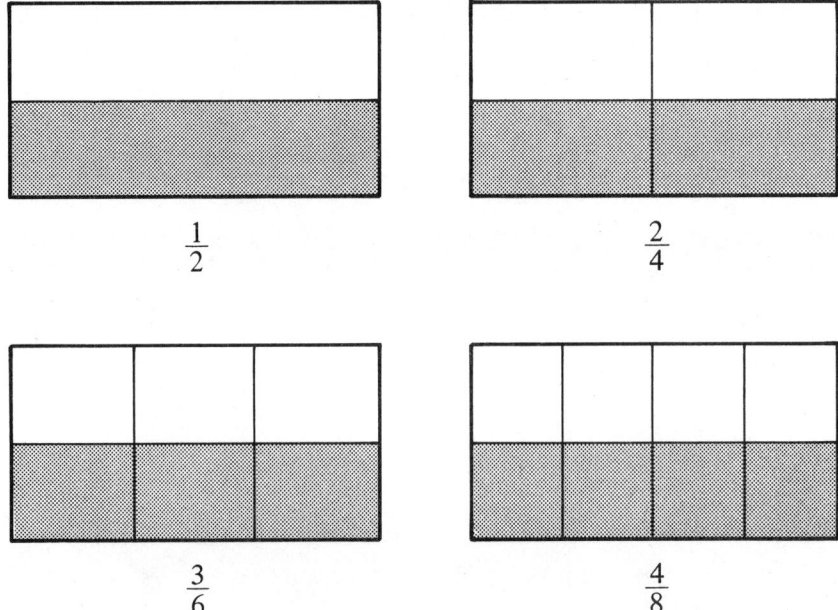

The same part is named by each of these fractions. The fractions $\frac{1}{2}$, $\frac{2}{4}$, $\frac{3}{6}$, and $\frac{4}{8}$ are equivalent fractions.

Multiplication is used to find equivalent fractions. The fraction is multiplied by a fractional form of 1. This means that the numerator and the denominator are multiplied by the same number.

Example: Find four fractions that are equivalent to $\frac{1}{2}$.

FRACTION	EQUIVALENT FRACTIONS			
$\frac{1}{2}$	$\frac{1 \times 2}{2 \times 2} = \frac{2}{4}$	$\frac{1 \times 3}{2 \times 3} = \frac{3}{6}$	$\frac{1 \times 4}{2 \times 4} = \frac{4}{8}$	$\frac{1 \times 5}{2 \times 5} = \frac{5}{10}$

The fractions $\frac{2}{4}$, $\frac{3}{6}$, $\frac{4}{8}$, and $\frac{5}{10}$ are equivalent to $\frac{1}{2}$.

2.1 EXERCISES

Each figure suggests a pair of equivalent fractions. Name the pair of equivalent fractions for each.

1.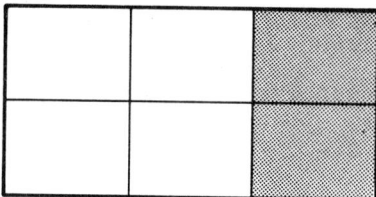

2.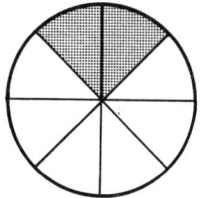

3.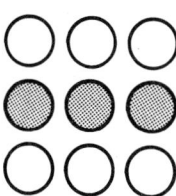

4.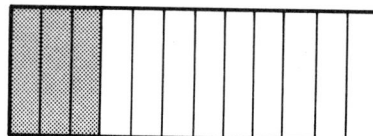

Using multiplication, find the equivalent fractions for each fraction in this chart.

	FRACTION	EQUIVALENT FRACTIONS				
5.	two fifths	$\frac{2}{5}$	$\frac{4}{10}$	$\frac{6}{15}$		
6.	one fourth	$\frac{1}{4}$	$\frac{2}{8}$			
7.	three halves	$\frac{3}{2}$	$\frac{6}{4}$	$\frac{9}{6}$		
8.	one third	$\frac{1}{3}$				
9.	nine tenths	$\frac{9}{10}$				
10.	three fourths					
11.	four fifths					
12.	seven tenths					

Fractions can be shown to be equivalent by using cross products. Cross products are found this way.

$$\frac{2}{5} \searrow \frac{4}{10} \qquad \frac{2}{5} \nearrow \frac{4}{10}$$

$$2 \times 10 = 20 \qquad 4 \times 5 = 20$$

Since 20 = 20, the fractions are equal. This equivalence is written $\frac{2}{5} = \frac{4}{10}$.

Example: Using cross products determine if $\frac{1}{3}$ is equivalent to $\frac{2}{6}$.

$\frac{1}{3} \searrow \frac{2}{6}$ $\frac{1}{3} \nearrow \frac{2}{6}$

$1 \times 6 = 6$ $3 \times 2 = 6$

Since $6 = 6$, the fractions are equivalent. $\frac{1}{3} = \frac{2}{6}$

Example: Is $\frac{3}{5}$ equivalent to $\frac{5}{10}$?

$\frac{3}{5} \searrow \frac{5}{10}$ $\frac{3}{5} \nearrow \frac{5}{10}$

$3 \times 10 = 30$ $5 \times 5 = 25$

Since $30 \neq 25$, the fractions are not equivalent. $\frac{3}{5} \neq \frac{5}{10}$

■ Two fractions are equivalent if the cross products are equal.
Cross products can also be used to find equivalent fractions.

Example: Find the denominator which makes $\frac{3}{4}$ and $\frac{6}{?}$ equivalent fractions.

$\frac{3}{4} = \frac{6}{?}$

$3 \times ? = 6 \times 4$

$3 \times ? = 24$

$3 \times 8 = 24$, so

$\frac{3}{4} = \frac{6}{8}$

Example: Find the numerator which makes $\frac{1}{2}$ and $\frac{?}{12}$ equivalent fractions.

$\frac{1}{2} = \frac{?}{12}$

$2 \times ? = 1 \times 12$

$2 \times ? = 12$

$2 \times 6 = 12$

$\frac{1}{2} = \frac{6}{12}$

2.2 EXERCISES

Using cross products, determine if these fractions are equivalent or nonequivalent. Use the symbol = for equivalent fractions and the symbol ≠ for nonequivalent fractions.

1. $\frac{1}{2}$ ___?___ $\frac{5}{10}$

2. $\frac{1}{3}$ ___?___ $\frac{3}{6}$

3. $\frac{4}{8}$ ___?___ $\frac{8}{16}$

Unit 2 Introduction to Common Fractions and Mixed Numbers 11

4. $\dfrac{4}{6}$ —?— $\dfrac{6}{9}$

5. $\dfrac{10}{12}$ —?— $\dfrac{12}{14}$

6. $\dfrac{1}{3}$ —?— $\dfrac{2}{9}$

7. $\dfrac{80}{100}$ —?— $\dfrac{8}{10}$

8. $\dfrac{3}{6}$ —?— $\dfrac{6}{3}$

9. $\dfrac{0}{3}$ —?— $\dfrac{2}{4}$

10. $\dfrac{3}{1}$ —?— $\dfrac{9}{3}$

11. $\dfrac{2}{4}$ —?— $\dfrac{4}{8}$

12. $\dfrac{2}{2}$ —?— $\dfrac{4}{4}$

Use cross products to find the numerator or denominator that makes each pair of fractions equivalent.

13. $\dfrac{5}{10} = \dfrac{?}{12}$

14. $\dfrac{?}{3} = \dfrac{2}{6}$

15. $\dfrac{10}{?} = \dfrac{15}{30}$

16. $\dfrac{4}{10} = \dfrac{?}{20}$

17. $\dfrac{2}{5} = \dfrac{4}{?}$

18. $\dfrac{?}{7} = \dfrac{6}{14}$

19. $\dfrac{30}{?} = \dfrac{30}{100}$

20. $\dfrac{40}{50} = \dfrac{?}{10}$

21. $\dfrac{25}{100} = \dfrac{50}{?}$

22. $\dfrac{?}{15} = \dfrac{2}{3}$

23. $\dfrac{18}{?} = \dfrac{24}{4}$

12 Section 1 Common Fractions

EXPRESSING FRACTIONS IN LOWEST TERMS

Numbers being multiplied to find a product are called <u>factors.</u>

Examples: $5 \times 2 = 10$ $\qquad$ $21 = 3 \times 7$

$\qquad\qquad$ factors $\quad$ product $\qquad$ product factors

The <u>common factors</u> of two or more numbers are the factors that are common to both numbers.

Example: Find the common factors of 20 and 12.

 $\quad$ The factors of 20 are 1, 2, 4, 5, 10, 20.
 $\quad$ The factors of 12 are 1, 2, 3, 4, 6, 12.
 $\quad$ The common factors are 1, 2, and 4.

The number 4 is the greatest number that is common to both 20 and 12. It is called the <u>greatest common factor.</u>

$\quad$ A fraction is in lowest terms if the greatest common factor (GCF) of both the numerator and the denominator is 1. To find a lowest-term fraction, the numerator and denominator can be divided by the greatest common factor. This means dividing by a fractional form of 1.

Example: Express $\frac{12}{20}$ in lowest terms.

FRACTION	FACTORS	GCF
$\frac{12}{20}$	1, 2, 3, 4, 6, 12 1, 2, 4, 5, 10, 20	4

$\dfrac{\text{Numerator} \div \text{GCF}}{\text{Denominator} \div \text{GCF}}$ $\quad$ Equals $\quad$ Lowest-term Fraction

$\qquad \dfrac{12 \div 4}{20 \div 4} \qquad\quad = \qquad\quad \dfrac{3}{5}$

The fraction $\frac{3}{5}$ is in lowest terms since the greatest common factor of 3 and 5 is 1.
$\quad$ A lowest-term fraction can also be found by <u>prime factorization</u>.

Example: Using prime factorization, find the lowest-term fraction for $\frac{42}{105}$.

 $\quad$ The prime factors of 42 are 3, 7, and 2. $\qquad$ $42 = 3 \times 7 \times 2$
 $\quad$ The prime factors of 105 are 3, 7, and 5. $\quad\;\,$ $\overline{105 = 3 \times 7 \times 5}$
 $\quad$ The greatest common multiple is 3×7, or 21.
 $\quad$ Divide both the numerator and denominator by 21. $\quad \dfrac{42}{105} = \dfrac{2}{5}$

Note: The division can be shown as $\dfrac{42}{105} = \dfrac{\overset{1}{\cancel{3}} \times \overset{1}{\cancel{7}} \times 2}{\underset{1}{\cancel{3}} \times \underset{1}{\cancel{7}} \times 5} = \dfrac{2}{5}$.

2.3 EXERCISES

Name the lowest-term fraction for each fraction or each group of fractions.

1. $\frac{6}{12}$
2. $\frac{4}{10}$
3. $\frac{5}{20}$
4. $\frac{15}{15}$
5. $\frac{25}{50}$
6. $\frac{2}{6}$
7. $\frac{3}{9}$
8. $\frac{2}{14}$
9. $\frac{4}{16}$
10. $\frac{45}{60}$
11. $\frac{2}{6}, \frac{3}{9}, \frac{4}{12}$
12. $\frac{2}{8}, \frac{3}{12}, \frac{4}{16}$
13. $\frac{6}{20}, \frac{9}{30}, \frac{12}{40}$
14. $\frac{4}{10}, \frac{6}{15}, \frac{8}{20}$

Decide which fractions are in lowest terms. For those not in lowest terms, give the lowest-term fraction.

15. $\frac{3}{4}$
16. $\frac{5}{10}$
17. $\frac{8}{12}$
18. $\frac{35}{50}$
19. $\frac{6}{20}$
20. $\frac{4}{15}$
21. $\frac{20}{60}$
22. $\frac{18}{24}$

Use these prime factorizations to find each lowest-term fraction.

23. $\frac{2 \times 3 \times 5}{2 \times 3 \times 7}$
24. $\frac{3 \times 2 \times 5 \times 2}{5 \times 2 \times 2 \times 7}$
25. $\frac{2 \times 2 \times 5 \times 3}{7 \times 5 \times 2}$
26. $\frac{3 \times 3 \times 2 \times 3 \times 2}{2 \times 2 \times 7 \times 3}$
27. $\frac{11 \times 7 \times 5}{13 \times 5 \times 7}$
28. $\frac{7 \times 3 \times 5 \times 1}{31 \times 7 \times 5 \times 3}$
29. $\frac{3 \times 3 \times 11 \times 11}{11 \times 2 \times 2 \times 3 \times 13}$

FRACTIONS AND THE NUMBER LINE

Fractions can be represented on a number line. For each fraction, there corresponds exactly one point on the number line.

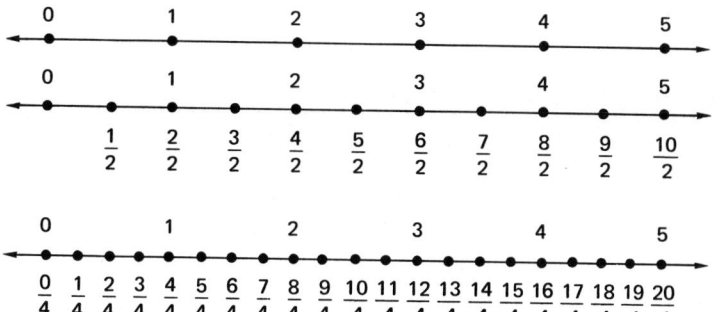

14 Section 1 Common Fractions

Fractions which name the same point on the number line are called *equivalent fractions*. The fractions $\frac{1}{2}$ and $\frac{2}{4}$ are equivalent fractions. The fraction $\frac{1}{2}$ is the lowest-term fraction for the fraction $\frac{2}{4}$.

Example: Using the number line, find fractions which are equivalent to 3.
$\frac{6}{2}$, $\frac{12}{4}$, and 3 name the same point on the number line. The fractions $\frac{6}{2}$ and $\frac{12}{4}$ are equivalent to 3.

Example: Find the whole number equivalent to $\frac{20}{4}$.
The number 5 and $\frac{20}{4}$ name the same point on the number line.
The number 5 is equivalent to $\frac{20}{4}$.

2.4 EXERCISES

Name the fraction that corresponds to the point indicated by each letter.

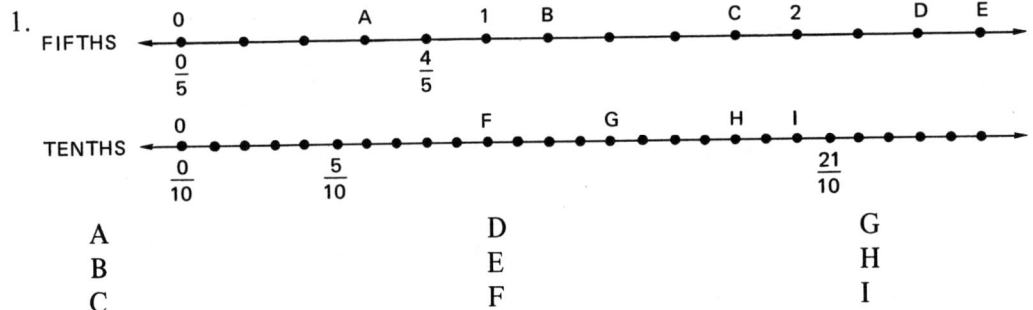

A	D	G
B	E	H
C	F	I

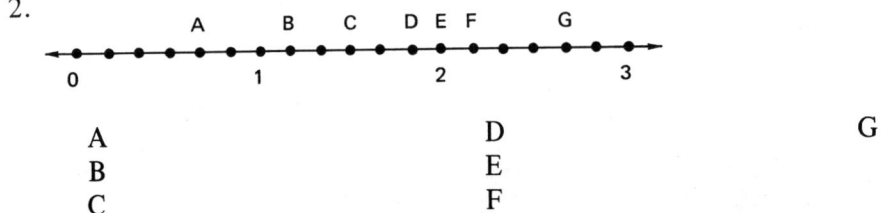

A	D	G
B	E	
C	F	

Draw a number line. Label the points for the whole numbers 0, 1, 2, 3, 4, and 5. On this number line mark equal divisions and locate these points. Use equivalent fractions and lowest-term fractions as an aid.

3. $\frac{2}{3}$ 8. $\frac{11}{4}$ 13. $\frac{16}{4}$

4. $\frac{4}{3}$ 9. $\frac{18}{6}$ 14. $\frac{5}{12}$

5. $\frac{3}{2}$ 10. $\frac{10}{3}$ 15. $\frac{9}{2}$

6. $\frac{7}{4}$ 11. $\frac{7}{2}$ 16. $\frac{19}{4}$

7. $\frac{5}{2}$ 12. $\frac{15}{4}$ 17. $\frac{30}{6}$

COMPARING FRACTIONS

Different methods can be used to compare fractions. One method is by comparing shaded regions.

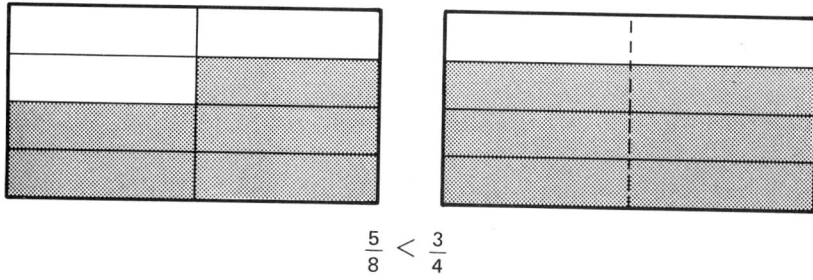

$$\frac{5}{8} < \frac{3}{4}$$

Another method is by using the number line.

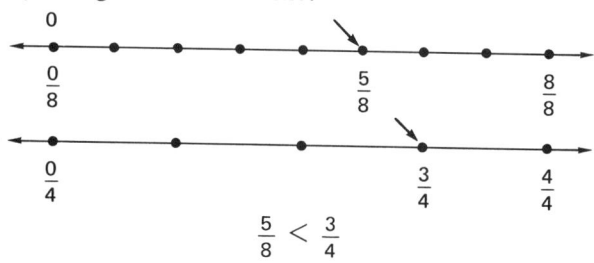

$$\frac{5}{8} < \frac{3}{4}$$

Both methods show that $\frac{5}{8} < \frac{3}{4}$.

Example: Using shaded regions compare $\frac{1}{2}$ and $\frac{3}{4}$.

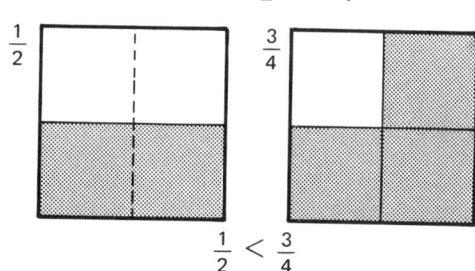

$$\frac{1}{2} < \frac{3}{4}$$

Example: Using the number line, compare $\frac{3}{4}$ and $\frac{4}{3}$.

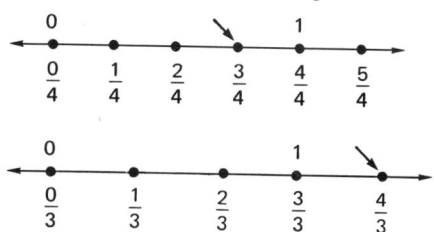

Since $\frac{3}{4}$ is to the left of $\frac{4}{3}$, $\frac{3}{4} < \frac{4}{3}$.

2.5 EXERCISES

Compare each pair of fractions by using shaded regions. Use the symbols $<, >, =$.

1. $\frac{2}{3}$ __?__ $\frac{5}{6}$
2. $\frac{1}{2}$ __?__ $\frac{3}{8}$
3. $\frac{2}{5}$ __?__ $\frac{5}{10}$
4. $\frac{3}{4}$ __?__ $\frac{5}{12}$
5. $\frac{1}{5}$ __?__ $\frac{2}{10}$

Compare each pair of fractions by using the number line. Use the symbols $<, >, =$.

6. $\frac{9}{10}$ __?__ $\frac{9}{11}$
7. $\frac{8}{2}$ __?__ $\frac{16}{4}$
8. $\frac{2}{3}$ __?__ $\frac{3}{4}$
9. $\frac{4}{10}$ __?__ $\frac{2}{5}$
10. $\frac{1}{16}$ __?__ $\frac{1}{32}$
11. $\frac{1}{8}$ __?__ $\frac{1}{7}$
12. 7 __?__ $\frac{7}{1}$

Determine the larger fractions in each pair. To decide which is larger, use either shaded regions or number lines.

13. $\frac{1}{2}, \frac{2}{3}$
14. $\frac{3}{4}, \frac{7}{8}$
15. $\frac{9}{12}, \frac{7}{10}$
16. $\frac{4}{5}, \frac{3}{8}$
17. $\frac{3}{5}, \frac{2}{3}$
18. $\frac{3}{4}, \frac{4}{5}$
19. $\frac{2}{10}, \frac{2}{11}$
20. $\frac{1}{9}, \frac{2}{8}$
21. $\frac{2}{16}, \frac{3}{32}$
22. $\frac{9}{8}, \frac{8}{7}$
23. $\frac{4}{10}, \frac{5}{9}$
24. $\frac{4}{3}, \frac{3}{2}$

MIXED NUMBERS

The numerator of a fraction may be less than, equal to, or greater than the denominator of the fraction. When the numerator is greater than the denominator, the fraction may be written as a <u>mixed number</u>. A *mixed number* is a number having a whole number part and a fractional part. Different methods may be used to express a fraction as a mixed number.

Example: Express $\frac{23}{4}$ as a mixed number.

METHOD 1

STEP 1	STEP 2	STEP 3
$\frac{20}{4}$ is the largest fraction in $\frac{23}{4}$ that equals a whole number.	Rename $\frac{20}{4}$ as 5.	Perform the addition.
$\frac{23}{4} = \frac{20}{4} + \frac{3}{4}$	$\frac{20}{4} + \frac{3}{4} = 5 + \frac{3}{4}$	$5 + \frac{3}{4} = 5\frac{3}{4}$

METHOD 2

STEP 1	STEP 2	STEP 3
Divide the numerator by the denominator.	Use the quotient for the whole number part.	Write the remainder 3 over the divisor 4.
$\frac{23}{4} = 4\overline{)23}\underline{20}3$ (quotient 5)	$4\overline{)23} = 5$ remainder 3	$4\overline{)23} = 5\frac{3}{4}$

At times a mixed number is expressed as a fraction. This is the opposite of expressing a fraction as a mixed number.

Example: Express $5\frac{3}{4}$ as a fraction.

METHOD 1

STEP 1	STEP 2	STEP 3
5 equals $\frac{20}{4}$.	Add the numerators.	Write the sum 23 over the denominator 4.
$5\frac{3}{4} = \frac{20}{4} + \frac{3}{4}$	$20 + 3 = 23$	$\frac{23}{4}$

METHOD 2

STEP 1	STEP 2	STEP 3
Multiply the whole number 5 by the denominator 4.	Add the numerator 3.	Write the sum 23 over the denominator 4.
$5\frac{3}{4}$ $5 \times 4 = 20$	$20 + 3 = 23$	$\frac{23}{4}$

2.6 EXERCISES

Express each fraction as a mixed number. Express the fractional part of the mixed number in lowest terms.

1. $\frac{5}{3}$
2. $\frac{7}{3}$
3. $\frac{9}{4}$
4. $\frac{11}{2}$
5. $\frac{6}{3}$
6. $\frac{11}{7}$
7. $\frac{19}{10}$
8. $\frac{16}{5}$
9. $\frac{13}{3}$
10. $\frac{28}{10}$
11. $\frac{42}{32}$
12. $\frac{48}{8}$
13. $\frac{121}{100}$
14. $\frac{90}{60}$
15. $\frac{3{,}250}{1{,}000}$

Express each mixed number as a fraction.

16. $1\frac{1}{3}$
17. $2\frac{3}{4}$
18. $5\frac{1}{10}$
19. $8\frac{1}{2}$
20. $3\frac{2}{3}$
21. $6\frac{5}{6}$
22. $11\frac{1}{8}$
23. $9\frac{1}{11}$
24. $30\frac{1}{4}$
25. $33\frac{1}{3}$
26. $90\frac{4}{5}$
27. $21\frac{9}{10}$
28. $10\frac{3}{32}$
29. $50\frac{1}{4}$
30. $25\frac{9}{16}$

APPLICATIONS

Medications may be stored in screw cap or plastic-stoppered glass containers. Glass bottles are used because glass does not react chemically with most drugs. Some drugs must be stored in dark bottles to prevent deterioration when exposed to light. Absorbent materials are sometimes placed in the bottles to remove moisture that may cause deterioration.

When a medication is to be divided into equal portions, it may be placed in vials, flasks, medicine glasses, or minim glasses.

▼ A *vial* is a small bottle.
▼ A *flask* is a laboratory vessel usually made of glass and having a constricted neck.
▼ A *medicine glass* is a graduated container. It may be graduated in millilitres, ounces, or drams.
▼ A *minim glass* is another graduated container. It is used to measure smaller portions and is graduated in minims and drams.

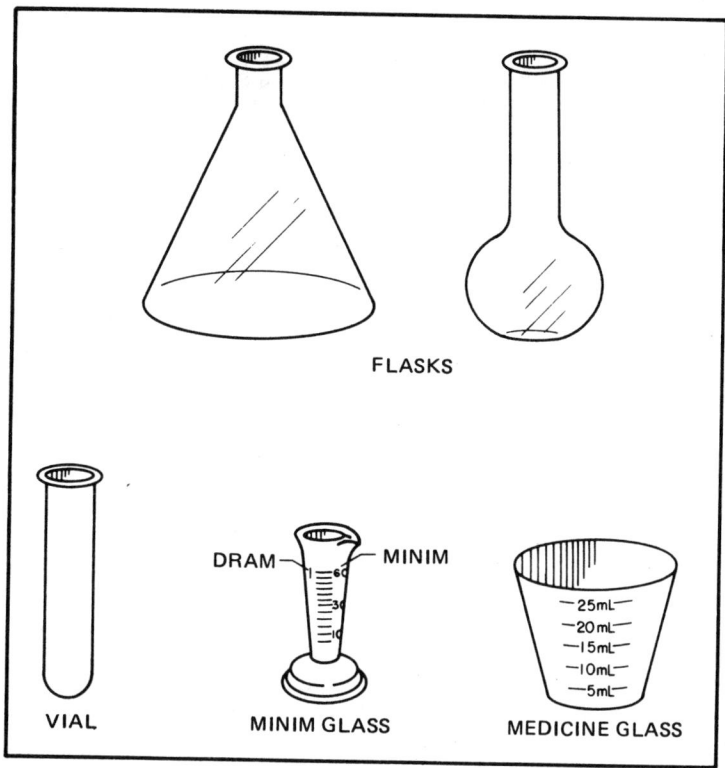

2.7 EXERCISES

1. A screw cap bottle contains a granulated compound. The compound is divided into 9 equal portions and placed in vials. What fractional part of the whole does each portion represent?

2. The contents of a plastic-stoppered glass bottle is divided into 325 equal parts. A flask contains 27 of these equal parts. What fractional part of the whole does the 27 parts represent?

3. One nurse works 1/6 of every day in the operating room. Another nurse works 1/3 of every day in the operating room. Which nurse works more time in the operating room?

4. The increase in the length of two babies is compared. Baby **A** grows 3/8 inch while Baby **B** grows 5/16 inch. Which baby increases the most?

5. A 250 milligram tablet is divided into 4 equal parts. Each part represents what fractional part of the whole?

6. Orderly A spends 1/4 of his 8-hour shift working in the emergency room. Orderly B spends 3/8 of her 8-hour shift working in the emergency room. Which orderly spends less time per day working in the emergency room?

7. In two different doses, a patient receives 3/20 grain and 3/32 grain of morphine sulfate. Which is the larger dose?

unit 3 addition and subtraction of common fractions and mixed numbers

OBJECTIVES
After studying this unit the student should be able to:
- Find least common denominators.
- Express fractions as equivalent fractions with least common denominators.
- Add fractions and mixed numbers.
- Subtract fractions and mixed numbers.

ADDITION AND SUBTRACTION OF FRACTIONS WITH LIKE DENOMINATORS

To add or subtract fractions the denominators must be common denominators. *Common denominator* means that the denominator of each fraction is the same, such as $\frac{3}{4}$ and $\frac{2}{4}$. When the denominators are the same, the numerators are added or subtracted.

Example: $\frac{3}{4} + \frac{2}{4}$

STEP 1	STEP 2	STEP 3
Since the denominators are the same the fractions can be added.	Add the numerators. $3 + 2 = 5$	Express the answer in lowest terms. $\frac{5}{4} = \frac{4}{4} + \frac{1}{4}$ or $1\frac{1}{4}$
$\frac{3}{4}$ → DENOMINATORS $+\frac{2}{4}$	$\frac{3}{4}$ → NUMERATORS $+\frac{2}{4}$ $\overline{}$ $\frac{5}{4}$	$\frac{3}{4}$ $+\frac{2}{4}$ $\overline{}$ $\frac{5}{4} = 1\frac{1}{4}$

Example: $\frac{3}{4} - \frac{2}{4}$

STEP 1	STEP 2
Since the denominators are the same the fractions can be subtracted.	Subtract the numerators $3 - 2 = 1$
$\frac{3}{4}$ → DENOMINATORS $-\frac{2}{4}$	$\frac{3}{4}$ → NUMERATORS $-\frac{2}{4}$ $\overline{}$ $\frac{1}{4}$

3.1 EXERCISES

Find each sum or difference. Express all answers in lowest terms.

Sum

1. $\dfrac{1}{7}$
   $+\dfrac{3}{7}$

2. $\dfrac{1}{3}$
   $+\dfrac{2}{3}$

3. $\dfrac{7}{8}$
   $+\dfrac{4}{8}$

4. $\dfrac{2}{5}$
   $+\dfrac{5}{5}$

5. $\dfrac{4}{3}$
   $+\dfrac{4}{3}$

Difference

6. $\dfrac{9}{8}$
   $-\dfrac{8}{8}$

7. $\dfrac{5}{2}$
   $-\dfrac{3}{2}$

8. $\dfrac{6}{3}$
   $-\dfrac{6}{3}$

9. $\dfrac{12}{8}$
   $-\dfrac{6}{8}$

10. $\dfrac{18}{10}$
    $-\dfrac{3}{10}$

COMMON DENOMINATORS

When fractions have unlike denominators the common denominator must be found. Least common multiples and prime factorization can be used to find the common denominator.

▼ The *least common multiple* (LCM) of two or more numbers is the smallest number that has each of the two numbers as a factor. If two numbers are prime numbers, the product is the least common multiple.

▼ *Prime factorization* is the process of finding the factors of a number using only prime numbers.

Example: Find the least common multiple of 6 and 8.

The multiples of 6 are 0, 6, 12, 18, 24, 30, 42, 48, ...

The multiples of 8 are 0, 8, 16, 24, 32, 40, 48, ...

The common multiples of 6 and 8 are 24 and 48.

The number 24 is the smallest number that is common to both 6 and 8. It is the <u>least common multiple</u> of 6 and 8.

Example: Use prime factorization to find the least common multiple of 16 and 24.

The prime factorization of 16 is $\quad 2 \times 2 \times 2 \times 2$.

The prime factorization of 24 is $\quad 2 \times 2 \times 2 \quad\quad \times 3$.

The prime factors common to 16 and 64 are $2 \times 2 \times 2 \times 2 \times 3$.

The least common multiple is the product of the prime factors, or 48.

▼ The product of the prime numbers common to two or more fractions is the *least common denominator*. The <u>least common denominator</u> (LCD) of two or more fractions is found by factoring the denominator into the product of prime numbers.

Example: Find the least common denominator of $\frac{2}{16}$ and $\frac{3}{24}$.

The product of the prime factors common to 16 and 24 is 48.

The <u>least common denominator</u> of $\frac{2}{16}$ and $\frac{3}{24}$ is 48.

Example: Find the least common denominator of $\frac{1}{10}$ and $\frac{3}{16}$.

The prime factorization of 10 is $\quad 5 \times 2$.

The prime factorization of 16 is $\quad\quad\quad 2 \times 2 \times 2 \times 2$.

The LCM of 10 and 16 is $\quad\quad\quad 5 \times 2 \times 2 \times 2 \times 2$.

The LCD of 10 and 16 is 80.

3.2 EXERCISES

Find the least common denominator (LCD) for each pair of fractions.

1. $\frac{1}{6}, \frac{1}{8}$

2. $\frac{1}{3}, \frac{1}{2}$

3. $\frac{1}{3}, \frac{3}{5}$

4. $\frac{2}{10}, \frac{4}{5}$

5. $\frac{2}{9}, \frac{3}{12}$

6. $\frac{3}{4}, \frac{1}{16}$

7. $\frac{3}{8}, \frac{4}{32}$

8. $\frac{1}{10}, \frac{3}{100}$

9. $\frac{2}{6}, \frac{4}{16}$

10. $\frac{9}{16}, \frac{3}{32}$

Unit 3 Addition and Subtraction of Common Fractions and Mixed Numbers

ADDING AND SUBTRACTING FRACTIONS WITH UNLIKE DENOMINATORS

In adding fractions with unlike denominators the fractions are expressed as equivalent fractions using the least common denominator. Then, the numerators are added.

Example: $\frac{1}{4} + \frac{5}{6}$

STEP 1	STEP 2	STEP 3
Since the denominators are different, common denominators must be found. $\frac{1}{4}$ $+\frac{5}{6}$	The least common denominator is 12. It is the smallest number that is divisible by 4 and 6. $\frac{1}{4} = \frac{?}{12}$ $+\frac{5}{6} = \frac{?}{12}$	Express the fractions as equivalent fractions using the least common denominator. $4\overline{)12} \rightarrow 3 \times 1 = 3$ $6\overline{)12} \rightarrow 2 \times 5 = 10$ $\frac{1}{4} = \frac{3}{12}$ $+\frac{5}{6} = \frac{10}{12}$

STEP 4	STEP 5
Add the numerators. $3 + 10 = 13$ $\frac{1}{4} = \frac{3}{12}$ $+\frac{5}{6} = \frac{10}{12}$ $\frac{13}{12}$	Express the answer in lowest terms. $\frac{13}{12} = \frac{12}{12} + \frac{1}{12}$ $\frac{13}{12} = 1 + \frac{1}{12} = 1\frac{1}{12}$ $\frac{3}{12}$ $+\frac{10}{12}$ $\frac{13}{12} = 1\frac{1}{12}$

Subtracting fractions with unlike denominators is similar to adding fractions with unlike denominators. In subtraction the numerators are subtracted rather than added.

3.3 EXERCISES

Find each sum or difference. Express all answers in lowest terms.

1. $\frac{1}{2}$
   $+\frac{1}{8}$

2. $\frac{1}{10}$
   $+\frac{3}{20}$

3. $\dfrac{2}{8}$
   $+ \dfrac{3}{16}$

4. $\dfrac{3}{4}$
   $+ \dfrac{3}{8}$

5. $\dfrac{4}{3}$
   $+ \dfrac{5}{6}$

6. $\dfrac{4}{4}$
   $+ \dfrac{10}{8}$

7. $\dfrac{3}{8}$
   $- \dfrac{1}{4}$

8. $\dfrac{1}{2}$
   $- \dfrac{3}{7}$

9. $\dfrac{2}{5}$
   $- \dfrac{3}{10}$

10. $\dfrac{3}{3}$
    $- \dfrac{1}{6}$

11. $\dfrac{8}{5}$
    $- \dfrac{1}{10}$

12. $\dfrac{5}{3}$
    $- \dfrac{10}{6}$

13. $\dfrac{4}{5}$
    $- \dfrac{1}{20}$

14. $\dfrac{11}{6}$
    $- \dfrac{2}{3}$

15. $\dfrac{18}{8}$
    $- \dfrac{6}{4}$

3.4 EXERCISES

Rename two of the three fractions so all three fractions have the same denominator. Find the sum and express all answers as mixed numbers in lowest terms.

1. $\dfrac{1}{2}, \dfrac{1}{3}, \dfrac{1}{6}$

2. $\dfrac{3}{8}, \dfrac{2}{16}, \dfrac{1}{32}$

3. $\dfrac{2}{5}, \dfrac{4}{10}, \dfrac{5}{20}$

4. $\dfrac{1}{4}, \dfrac{2}{50}, \dfrac{3}{100}$

5. $\dfrac{1}{2}, \dfrac{2}{4}, \dfrac{3}{8}$

6. $\dfrac{1}{8}, \dfrac{4}{8}, \dfrac{5}{16}$

7. $\dfrac{5}{2}, \dfrac{4}{5}, \dfrac{3}{10}$

8. $\dfrac{1}{4}, \dfrac{2}{8}, \dfrac{3}{16}$

9. $\dfrac{2}{3}, \dfrac{3}{2}, \dfrac{4}{6}$

10. $\dfrac{4}{2}, \dfrac{3}{8}, \dfrac{4}{16}$

ADDITION AND SUBTRACTION OF MIXED NUMBERS

Addition of mixed numbers is exactly the same as addition of fractions except that the whole numbers must also be added.

Example: $4\frac{1}{4} + 2\frac{5}{6}$

STEP 1	STEP 2	STEP 3
Find a common denominator for the fractions.	The least common denominator is 12. It is the smallest number that is divisible by 4 and 6.	Express the fractions as equivalent fractions using the least common denominator. $4\overline{)12}^{\;3} \rightarrow 3 \times 1 = 3$ $6\overline{)12}^{\;2} \rightarrow 2 \times 5 = 10$
$4\frac{1}{4}$ $+\,2\frac{5}{6}$	$4\frac{1}{4} = 4\frac{?}{12}$ $+\,2\frac{5}{6} = 2\frac{?}{12}$	$4\frac{1}{4} = 4\frac{3}{12}$ $2\frac{5}{6} = 2\frac{10}{12}$

STEP 4	STEP 5	STEP 6
Add the fractions. $\frac{3}{12} + \frac{10}{12} = \frac{13}{12}$	Add the whole numbers. $4 + 2 = 6$	Express the answer in lowest terms. $6\frac{13}{12} = 6 + \frac{12}{12} + \frac{1}{12}$ $6 + 1\frac{1}{12} = 7\frac{1}{12}$
$4\frac{1}{4} = 4\frac{3}{12}$ $+\,2\frac{5}{6} = 2\frac{10}{12}$ $\phantom{+\,2\frac{5}{6} =\;} \frac{13}{12}$	$4\frac{1}{4} = 4\frac{3}{12}$ $+\,2\frac{5}{6} = 2\frac{10}{12}$ $\phantom{+\,2\frac{5}{6} =\;} 6\frac{13}{12}$	$4\frac{1}{4} + 2\frac{5}{6} = 7\frac{1}{12}$

Subtraction of mixed numbers involves the same process as addition. In order to subtract the fractional part, it is sometimes necessary to express the whole number part as a mixed number.

Example: $4\frac{1}{4} - 2\frac{5}{6}$

26 Section 1 Common Fractions

STEP 1	STEP 2	STEP 3
Find a common denominator for the fractions.	The least common denominator for 4 and 6 is 12.	Express as equivalent fractions. $4\overline{)12}^{\,3} \rightarrow 3 \times 1 = 3$ $6\overline{)12}^{\,2} \rightarrow 2 \times 5 = 10$
$4\frac{1}{4}$ $-2\frac{5}{6}$	$4\frac{1}{4} = 4\frac{?}{12}$ $-2\frac{5}{6} = 2\frac{?}{12}$	$4\frac{1}{4} = 4\frac{3}{12}$ $-2\frac{5}{6} = 2\frac{10}{12}$

STEP 4	STEP 5	STEP 6
Express the whole number 4 as the mixed number $3\frac{12}{12}$ $4\frac{3}{12} = 3 + \frac{12}{12} + \frac{3}{12} = 3\frac{15}{12}$	Subtract the numerators. $15 - 10 = 5$	Subtract the whole numbers. $3 - 2 = 1$
$4\frac{3}{12} = 3\frac{15}{12}$ $-2\frac{10}{12} = 2\frac{10}{12}$	$3\frac{15}{12}$ $-2\frac{10}{12}$ $\frac{5}{12}$	$3\frac{15}{12}$ $-2\frac{10}{12}$ $1\frac{5}{12}$

3.5 EXERCISE

Find the sum or difference. Express all answers in lowest terms.

1. $8\frac{1}{5}$
   $+ 6\frac{2}{5}$

2. $3\frac{1}{3}$
   $+ 5\frac{3}{4}$

3. $2\frac{3}{4}$
   $+ 4\frac{8}{16}$

4. $9\frac{3}{6}$
   $+ 11\frac{4}{12}$

5. $30\frac{7}{8}$
   $+ 1\frac{3}{4}$

6. $4\frac{3}{5}$
   $+ 24\frac{9}{10}$

7. $8\frac{1}{12}$
   $+ 3\frac{5}{36}$

8. $2\frac{1}{16}$
   $+ 5\frac{3}{32}$

9. $5\frac{1}{2}$
   $+ 9\frac{7}{10}$

10. $4\frac{4}{5}$
    $+ 13\frac{1}{3}$

11. $3\frac{11}{12}$
    $- 2\frac{2}{10}$

12. $10\frac{3}{4}$
    $- 4\frac{1}{8}$

13. $16\frac{4}{5}$
    $- 9\frac{3}{10}$

14. $18\frac{37}{100}$
    $- 3\frac{1}{10}$

15. 5
    $- 2\frac{1}{4}$

16. $37\frac{2}{3}$
    $- 14\frac{3}{4}$

17. $11\frac{4}{32}$
    $- 2\frac{3}{8}$

18. $53\frac{13}{100}$
    $- 12\frac{3}{25}$

19. $16\frac{2}{3}$
    $- 5$

20. $18\frac{1}{2}$
    $- 9\frac{7}{10}$

COMPARING FRACTIONS USING COMMON DENOMINATORS

To compare two fractions that have a common denominator compare the numerators. The larger fraction has the greater numerator.

Example: Compare $\frac{1}{2}$ and $\frac{3}{5}$.

The common denominator is 10.

Express each fraction as an equivalent fraction.

$\frac{1}{2} = \frac{?}{10}$ $2\overline{)10}^{\,5} \longrightarrow 5 \times 1 = 5$ $\frac{1}{2} = \frac{5}{10}$

$\frac{3}{5} = \frac{?}{10}$ $5\overline{)10}^{\,2} \longrightarrow 2 \times 3 = 6$ $\frac{3}{5} = \frac{6}{10}$

Since $5 < 6$, $\frac{5}{10} < \frac{6}{10}$ or $\frac{1}{2} < \frac{3}{5}$

3.6 EXERCISES

Express each fraction as an equivalent fraction using the given denominator. Compare the two fractions. Use the symbols, <, >, =, to show the relationship.

1. $\frac{1}{2} = \frac{?}{4}$; $\frac{3}{4} = \frac{?}{4}$

   $\frac{1}{2}$ __?__ $\frac{3}{4}$

2. $\frac{2}{3} = \frac{?}{6}$; $\frac{5}{6} = \frac{?}{6}$

   $\frac{2}{3}$ __?__ $\frac{5}{6}$

3. $\frac{1}{3} = \frac{?}{12}$; $\frac{1}{4} = \frac{?}{12}$

   $\frac{1}{3}$ __?__ $\frac{1}{4}$

4. $\frac{2}{5} = \frac{?}{30}$; $\frac{3}{6} = \frac{?}{30}$

   $\frac{2}{5}$ __?__ $\frac{3}{6}$

5. $\frac{3}{4} = \frac{?}{20}$; $\frac{2}{5} = \frac{?}{20}$

   $\frac{3}{4}$ __?__ $\frac{2}{5}$

6. $\frac{1}{10} = \frac{?}{100}$; $\frac{10}{100} = \frac{?}{100}$

   $\frac{1}{10}$ __?__ $\frac{10}{100}$

Rename each pair of fractions using a common denominator. Compare the numerators of each pair. The larger fraction has the greater numerator. Name the larger fraction for each pair of fractions.

7. $\frac{4}{5}$, $\frac{2}{3}$

8. $\frac{5}{12}$, $\frac{4}{6}$

9. $\frac{2}{3}$, $\frac{3}{2}$

10. $\frac{9}{3}$, $\frac{9}{4}$

11. $\frac{1}{2}$, $\frac{3}{4}$

12. $\frac{13}{20}$, $\frac{4}{5}$

13. $3\frac{1}{2}$, $3\frac{1}{4}$

14. $\frac{10}{5}$, $\frac{3}{2}$

15. $\frac{1}{6}$, $\frac{2}{5}$

16. $\frac{2}{3}$, $\frac{2}{4}$

17. $\frac{5}{3}$, $2\frac{1}{2}$

18. $5\frac{1}{5}$, $\frac{26}{4}$

19. $\frac{3}{8}$, $\frac{3}{4}$

20. $\frac{11}{2}$, 5

21. $6\frac{1}{3}$, $5\frac{2}{3}$

22. $\frac{11}{2}$, $\frac{11}{3}$

APPLICATIONS

Medication may be in the form of a liquid or a solid (crystals, powders, or tablets). Liquid medication may be measured in ounces, millilitres, or pints. Crystals, powders, and tablets are weighed in grains, grams, or milligrams.

Medication is administered by a trained health care person. The portion of the drug that is to be administered at one time is the *dose*. The *dosage* is the total quantity that is to be administered.

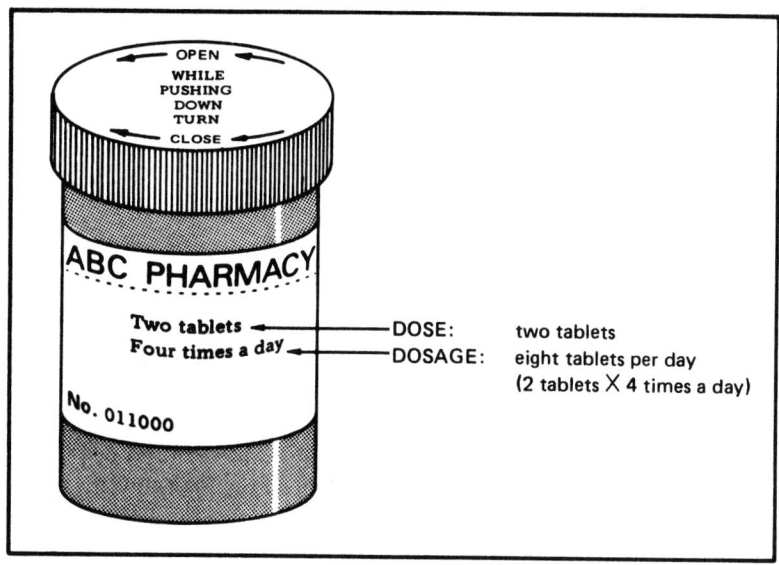

3.7 EXERCISES

1. David drinks 1/3 ounce of medication and 2 hours later he drinks 4/5 ounce. How much medication does David consume during this period?

2. A patient is given 2 1/2 grains of medication followed by 1 2/3 grains. What is the total dosage the patient receives?

3. A *medical assistant* is responsible for maintaining a record of laboratory supplies. When purchased, a bottle contains 7 1/2 ounces of liquid. When the medical assistant conducts an inventory, only 3 3/4 ounces of liquid remain. How much liquid has been removed?

4. An *operating room technician* assists surgeons before, during, and after an operation. One of the technician's responsibilities is to set up the operating room with instruments, equipment, and fluids that may be needed. The surgeon requests that the operating room technician supply 10 pints of dextrose solution. After the operation, the operating room technician finds that 6 2/3 pints of dextrose solution remain. How many pints of solution were used for the operation?

5. In two doses, a patient receives 1/20 grain and 3/32 grain of morphine sulfate, respectively. What is the total dosage that the patient receives?

6. A new baby grew 3/8 inch in January. In February the baby grew 7/16 inch. How many total inches did the baby grow during January and February?

7. A prescription calls for a first dose of 2 1/4 grains followed three hours later by a dose of 1 1/2 grains. The second dose is how many grains less than the first dose?

unit 4 multiplication and division of common fractions and mixed numbers

OBJECTIVES

After studying this unit the student should be able to:
- Multiply fractions and mixed numbers.
- Divide fractions and mixed numbers.

MULTIPLICATION OF FRACTIONS

Multiplication of fractions can be illustrated by using the concept that fractions are part of a whole.

Example: What part of a whole is $\frac{1}{2}$ of $\frac{1}{3}$?

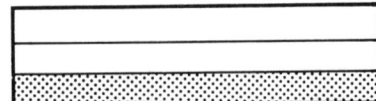

$\frac{1}{3}$ of the total region is dotted.

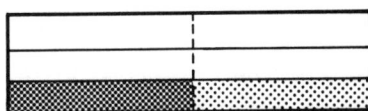

Darken $\frac{1}{2}$ of the $\frac{1}{3}$ region.

$\frac{1}{6}$ of the total region is darkened.

The mathematical notation is: $\frac{1}{2}$ of $\frac{1}{3} = \frac{1}{2} \times \frac{1}{3} = \frac{1}{6}$

Example: What part of the total region is $\frac{1}{2}$ of $\frac{2}{3}$?

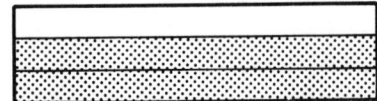

$\frac{2}{3}$ of the total region is dotted.

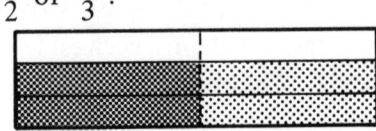

Darken $\frac{1}{2}$ of the $\frac{2}{3}$ region.

$\frac{2}{6}$ or $\frac{1}{3}$ of the total region is darkened.

The mathematical notation is: $\frac{1}{2}$ of $\frac{2}{3} = \frac{1}{2} \times \frac{2}{3} = \frac{2}{6}$ or $\frac{1}{3}$

Example: What part of the whole is $\frac{1}{2}$ of $\frac{3}{3}$?

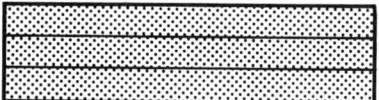 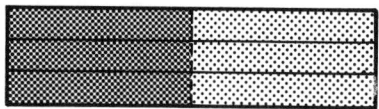

$\frac{3}{3}$ of the total region is dotted.   Darken $\frac{1}{2}$ of the $\frac{3}{3}$ region.

$\frac{3}{6}$ or $\frac{1}{2}$ of the total region is darkened.

The mathematical notation is: $\frac{1}{2}$ of $\frac{3}{3} = \frac{1}{2} \times \frac{3}{3} = \frac{3}{6}$ or $\frac{1}{2}$

- To multiply two fractions find the product of the numerators, then find the product of the denominators. This may be written:

$$\frac{a}{b} \times \frac{c}{d} = \frac{a \times c}{b \times d} = \frac{ac}{bd}$$

Example: $\frac{2}{5} \times \frac{1}{3}$

Multiplication of fractions involves multiplying numerators then multiplying denominators.

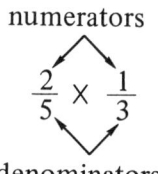

STEP 1	STEP 2	STEP 3
Multiply the numerators. $2 \times 1 = 2$	Multiply the denominators. $5 \times 3 = 15$	Express the answer, or product, as a fraction. $\frac{2}{15}$
$\frac{2}{5} \times \frac{1}{3} = \frac{2 \times 1}{?} = \frac{2}{?}$	$\frac{2}{5} \times \frac{1}{3} = \frac{2 \times 1}{5 \times 3} = \frac{2}{15}$	$\frac{2}{5} \times \frac{1}{3} = \frac{2}{15}$

The product of fractions is usually expressed in lowest terms. The product may be expressed in lowest terms after the multiplication is performed.

Example: $\frac{2}{5} \times \frac{3}{4}$

STEP 1	STEP 2
Multiply the numerators. $2 \times 3 = 6$ Multiply the denominators. $5 \times 4 = 20$	Express the answer in lowest terms. $\frac{6}{20} = \frac{(6 \div 2)}{(20 \div 2)} = \frac{3}{10}$ $\frac{6}{20} = \frac{3}{10}$
$\frac{2}{5} \times \frac{3}{4} = \frac{2 \times 3}{5 \times 4} = \frac{6}{20}$	$\frac{2}{5} \times \frac{3}{4} = \frac{6}{20}$ or $\frac{3}{10}$

Fractions may also be expressed in lowest terms before multiplying. This process involves dividing a numerator and denominator by the same number. Dividing a numerator and a denominator by the same number is commonly called *cancellation*.

Example: $\frac{2}{5}$ of $\frac{5}{6}$

$\frac{2}{5}$ of $\frac{5}{6}$ means $\frac{2}{5} \times \frac{5}{6}$.

STEP 1	STEP 2	STEP 3
Divide a numerator and denominator by the same number, 5. In the numerator, $5 \div 5 = 1$. In the denominator, $5 \div 5 = 1$.	Divide a numerator and a denominator by the same number, 2. In the numerator, $2 \div 2 = 1$. In the denominator, $6 \div 2 = 3$.	Multiply the numerators and the denominators. $\frac{1}{1} \times \frac{1}{3} = \frac{1 \times 1}{1 \times 3} = \frac{1}{3}$
$\frac{2}{5} \times \frac{5}{6} = \frac{2}{(5 \div 5)} \times \frac{(5 \div 5)}{6}$ $= \frac{2}{1} \times \frac{1}{6}$	$\frac{2}{1} \times \frac{1}{6} = \frac{(2 \div 2)}{1} \times \frac{1}{(6 \div 2)}$ $= \frac{1}{1} \times \frac{1}{3}$	$\frac{2}{5} \times \frac{5}{6} = \frac{1}{3}$

Note: Since the fractions have already been expressed in lowest terms, no simplification is necessary.

4.1 EXERCISES

Find the product of each pair of fractions. When possible express the fractions in lowest terms before multiplying. Express all answers in lowest terms. (Remember that *of* indicates multiplication.)

1. $\frac{1}{2}$ of 50
2. $\frac{1}{3}$ of 45
3. $\frac{1}{10}$ of 100
4. $\frac{1}{2}$ of $\frac{1}{3}$
5. $\frac{1}{3}$ of $\frac{1}{2}$
6. $\frac{1}{2}$ of $\frac{3}{5}$
7. $\frac{1}{4}$ of $\frac{3}{7}$
8. $\frac{1}{5}$ of $\frac{2}{3}$
9. $\frac{2}{3}$ of $\frac{3}{3}$
10. $\frac{1}{2}$ of $\frac{2}{4}$
11. $\frac{3}{4} \times \frac{2}{5}$
12. $\frac{1}{8} \times \frac{2}{3}$
13. $\frac{1}{16} \times \frac{2}{5}$
14. $\frac{4}{3} \times \frac{3}{4}$
15. $\frac{1}{2} \times \frac{8}{5}$
16. $\frac{7}{12} \times \frac{6}{7}$
17. $\frac{3}{8} \times \frac{1}{2}$
18. $\frac{14}{5} \times \frac{10}{7}$
19. $\frac{1}{3} \times \frac{2}{2}$
20. $\frac{2}{9} \times \frac{4}{7}$
21. $\frac{5}{6} \times \frac{2}{3}$
22. $\frac{24}{5} \times \frac{5}{10}$
23. $\frac{5}{10} \times \frac{10}{5}$
24. $\frac{2}{3} \times \frac{3}{5}$
25. $\frac{7}{8} \times \frac{4}{5}$
26. $\frac{1}{4} \times 0$
27. $\frac{2}{5} \times \frac{1}{4}$
28. $\frac{1}{8} \times \frac{3}{4}$
29. $\frac{3}{4} \times \frac{2}{9}$
30. $\frac{7}{10} \times \frac{2}{3}$

MULTIPLICATION OF MIXED NUMBERS

When mixed numbers are multiplied, the mixed numbers are first expressed as fractions. Whole numbers are also expressed as fractions. The same process as in multiplication of fractions can then be performed.

Example: $2 \times 3\frac{1}{4}$

STEP 1	STEP 2	STEP 3
Express the first number as a fraction. $2 = \frac{2}{1}$ Express the second number as a fraction. $3\frac{1}{4} = \frac{(3 \times 4)+1}{4} = \frac{13}{4}$	Multiply the numerators. $2 \times 13 = 26$ Multiply the denominators. $1 \times 4 = 4$	Express the answer as a mixed number. $\frac{26}{4} = \frac{(26 \div 2)}{(4 \div 2)} = \frac{13}{2}$ $13 \div 2 = 2\overline{)13}$ $= 6\frac{1}{2}$
$2 \times 3\frac{1}{4} = \frac{2}{1} \times \frac{13}{4}$	$\frac{2}{1} \times \frac{13}{4} = \frac{2 \times 13}{1 \times 4} = \frac{26}{4}$	$2 \times 3\frac{1}{4} = 6\frac{1}{2}$

34 Section 1 Common Fractions

Example: $3\frac{3}{4} \times 6\frac{1}{3}$

STEP 1	STEP 2	STEP 3	STEP 4
Express the first number as a fraction. $3\frac{3}{4} = \frac{(3 \times 4) + 3}{4} = \frac{15}{4}$ Express the second number as a fraction. $6\frac{1}{3} = \frac{(6 \times 3) + 1}{3} = \frac{19}{3}$	Simplify. Divide 3 and 15 by 3.	Multiply the numerators. $5 \times 19 = 95$ Multiply the denominators. $4 \times 1 = 4$	Express the answer as a mixed number. $95 \div 4 = 23\frac{3}{4}$
$3\frac{3}{4} \times 6\frac{1}{3} = \frac{15}{4} \times \frac{19}{3}$	$\frac{15}{4} \times \frac{19}{3} = \frac{\overset{5}{\cancel{15}} \times 19}{4 \times \cancel{3}}$ 1	$\frac{5 \times 19}{4 \times 1} = \frac{95}{4}$	$3\frac{3}{4} \times 6\frac{1}{3} = \frac{95}{4} = 23\frac{3}{4}$

Example: $2\frac{2}{5} \times 6\frac{1}{4}$

STEP 1	STEP 2	STEP 3	STEP 4
Express the numbers as fractions. $2\frac{2}{5} = \frac{(2 \times 5) + 2}{5} = \frac{12}{5}$ $6\frac{1}{4} = \frac{(6 \times 4) + 1}{4} = \frac{25}{4}$	Simplify. Divide 5 and 25 by 5. Divide 4 and 12 by 4.	Multiply the numerators and the denominators.	Express the answer in lowest terms. $\frac{15}{1} = 15$
$2\frac{2}{5} \times 6\frac{1}{4} = \frac{12}{5} \times \frac{25}{4}$	$\frac{12}{5} \times \frac{25}{4} = \frac{\overset{3}{\cancel{12}} \times \overset{5}{\cancel{25}}}{\cancel{5} \times \cancel{4}}$ $1 1$	$\frac{3 \times 5}{1 \times 1} = \frac{15}{1}$	$2\frac{2}{5} \times 6\frac{1}{4} = \frac{15}{1} = 15$

4.2 EXERCISES

Find each product. When possible, express the fractions in lowest terms before multiplying.

1. $1\frac{1}{3} \times \frac{2}{5}$
2. $3\frac{1}{4} \times \frac{1}{6}$
3. $4\frac{2}{8} \times \frac{2}{3}$

4. $4\frac{1}{2} \times \frac{1}{4}$
5. $1\frac{1}{3} \times 2\frac{3}{4}$
6. $3\frac{1}{2} \times 4\frac{2}{3}$

7. $4\frac{1}{3} \times 5\frac{1}{2}$
8. $3\frac{1}{2} \times 4\frac{3}{8}$
9. $3\frac{1}{5} \times 5\frac{1}{3}$

10. $3\frac{1}{5} \times 2\frac{3}{4}$ 14. $2\frac{5}{6} \times 4\frac{1}{3}$ 18. $2\frac{4}{10} \times \frac{20}{6}$

11. $1\frac{5}{6} \times 2\frac{1}{4}$ 15. $2\frac{2}{5} \times 0$ 19. $20\frac{5}{8} \times 2\frac{4}{5}$

12. $2\frac{7}{8} \times 2\frac{1}{4}$ 16. $1\frac{1}{10} \times 3\frac{2}{5}$ 20. $0 \times 8\frac{1}{3}$

13. $3\frac{1}{3} \times 10$ 17. $4\frac{1}{4} \times \frac{4}{17}$

DIVISION OF FRACTIONS

Division of fractions can also be illustrated by using the concept that fractions are part of a whole.

Example: How many halves are there in 4?

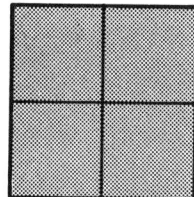   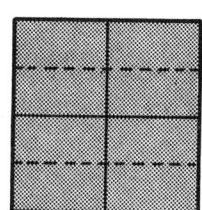

4 regions   Each of the 4 regions is divided in half.
                         8 regions are formed.

The mathematical notation is: 4 divided by $\frac{1}{2}$ = $4 \div \frac{1}{2}$ = 8

Example: How many fourths are there in 3?

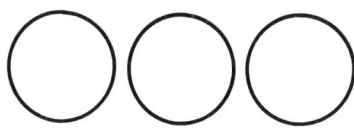   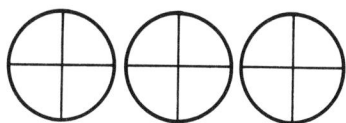

3 regions   Each of the 3 regions is divided in fourths.
                         12 regions are formed.

The mathematical notation is: 3 divided by $\frac{1}{4}$ = $3 \div \frac{1}{4}$ = 12

4.3 EXERCISES

Find each answer. Use diagrams if necessary.

1. How many thirds are there in 2?

   $2 \div \frac{1}{3} = ?$

2. How many fifths are there in 4?

   $4 \div \frac{1}{5} = ?$

3. How many fourths are there in 4?

   $4 \div \frac{1}{4} = ?$

4. How many tenths are there in 2?

   $2 \div \frac{1}{10} = ?$

5. How many eighths are there in 3?

   $3 \div \frac{1}{8} = ?$

6. How many sixths are there in 1?

   $1 \div \frac{1}{6} = ?$

7.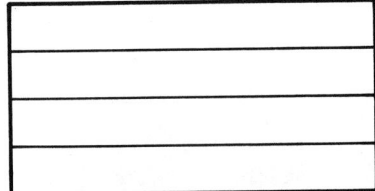

   a. How many $\frac{1}{4}$s are there in 1?

   b. How many $\frac{2}{4}$s are there in 1?

8.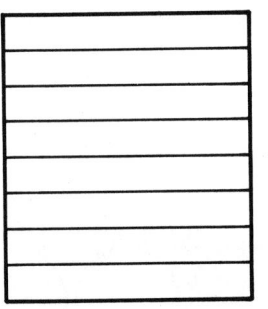

   a. How many $\frac{1}{8}$s are there in 1?

   b. How many $\frac{2}{8}$s are there in 1?

   c. How many $\frac{4}{8}$s are there in 1?

9.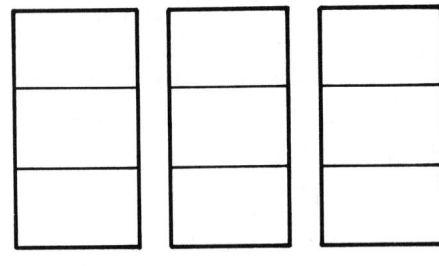

   a. How many $\frac{1}{3}$s are there in 3?

   b. How many $\frac{2}{3}$s are there in 3?

   c. How many $\frac{3}{3}$s are there in 3?

10.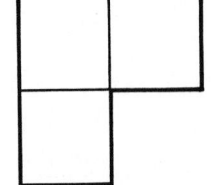

    a. How many $\frac{1}{4}$s are there in $\frac{3}{4}$?

    b. How many $\frac{2}{4}$s are there in $\frac{3}{4}$?

    c. How many $\frac{3}{4}$s are there in $\frac{3}{4}$?

Unit 4 Multiplication and Division of Common Fractions and Mixed Numbers

The division process can be generalized by using reciprocals or multiplicative inverses.

▼ Two numbers whose products are 1 are reciprocals or multiplicative inverses of each other.

Examples: The numbers $\frac{9}{1}$ and $\frac{1}{9}$ are reciprocals since $\frac{9}{1} \times \frac{1}{9} = 1$.

The expressions $\frac{a}{b}$ and $\frac{b}{a}$ are reciprocals since $\frac{a}{b} \times \frac{b}{a} = 1$.

4.4 EXERCISES

Find each reciprocal.

1. 7
2. $\frac{1}{3}$
3. 22
4. $\frac{5}{9}$
5. 1
6. $\frac{c}{d}$
7. $6\frac{1}{4}$
8. $\frac{76}{44}$
9. $8\frac{4}{7}$
10. 0

Using reciprocals, the division process can be generalized this way.

■ Dividing by a fraction is the same as multiplying by its reciprocal. This may be written:

If $\frac{a}{b}$ and $\frac{c}{d}$ are fractions, and $\frac{c}{d} \neq 0$, then

$$\frac{a}{b} \div \frac{c}{d} = \frac{a}{b} \times \frac{d}{c} = \frac{ad}{bc}.$$

Example: $\frac{1}{3} \div \frac{5}{8}$

Division of fractions involves finding the reciprocal and then multiplying.

	Fraction	Reciprocal
	$\frac{5}{8}$	$\frac{8}{5}$

STEP 1	STEP 2	STEP 3
The reciprocal of $\frac{5}{8}$ is $\frac{8}{5}$.	Multiply the numerators. $1 \times 8 = 8$ Multiply the denominators. $3 \times 5 = 15$	Express the answer in lowest terms. $\frac{8}{15}$ is in lowest terms.
$\frac{1}{3} \div \frac{5}{8} = \frac{1}{3} \times \frac{8}{5}$	$\frac{1}{3} \times \frac{8}{5} = \frac{1 \times 8}{3 \times 5} = \frac{8}{15}$	$\frac{1}{3} \div \frac{5}{8} = \frac{8}{15}$

As in multiplication, the fractions can be expressed in lowest terms before performing the operation. Expressing the fraction in lowest terms is done <u>after</u> the reciprocal is found.

Example: $\frac{5}{12} \div \frac{4}{3}$

STEP 1	STEP 2	STEP 3
The reciprocal of $\frac{4}{3}$ is $\frac{3}{4}$.	Simplify. Divide 12 and 3 by 3.	Multiply the numerators and the denominators. $\frac{5 \times 1}{4 \times 4} = \frac{5}{16}$
$\frac{5}{12} \div \frac{4}{3} = \frac{5}{12} \times \frac{3}{4}$	$\frac{5}{12} \times \frac{3}{4} = \frac{5 \times \cancel{3}^{1}}{\cancel{12}_{4} \times 4}$	$\frac{5}{12} \div \frac{4}{3} = \frac{5}{16}$

Note: Since the fractions have already been expressed in lowest terms, no simplification is necessary.

4.5 EXERCISES

Find each quotient. Express answers as mixed numbers in lowest terms.

1. $\frac{1}{6} \div \frac{2}{5}$
2. $\frac{4}{9} \div \frac{1}{3}$
3. $\frac{1}{2} \div \frac{3}{4}$
4. $\frac{10}{1} \div \frac{2}{5}$
5. $\frac{3}{4} \div \frac{10}{7}$
6. $\frac{6}{7} \div \frac{1}{8}$
7. $\frac{3}{5} \div \frac{3}{4}$
8. $\frac{2}{5} \div \frac{4}{10}$
9. $\frac{1}{2} \div \frac{1}{4}$
10. $22 \div \frac{11}{2}$
11. $\frac{6}{7} \div \frac{2}{14}$
12. $\frac{3}{6} \div \frac{2}{3}$
13. $2 \div \frac{4}{3}$
14. $\frac{18}{3} \div 5$
15. $0 \div \frac{2}{3}$

DIVISION OF MIXED NUMBERS

When mixed numbers are used in division, the mixed numbers are first expressed as fractions. Expressing whole numbers as fractions also simplifies the process. The same procedure as in division of fractions can then be performed.

Unit 4 Multiplication and Division of Common Fractions and Mixed Numbers

Example: $2\frac{1}{6} \div 3\frac{1}{3}$

STEP 1	STEP 2
Express the first number as a fraction. $$2\frac{1}{6} = \frac{(2 \times 6) + 1}{6} = \frac{13}{6}$$ Express the second number as a fraction. $$3\frac{1}{3} = \frac{(3 \times 3) + 1}{3} = \frac{10}{3}$$ $$2\frac{1}{6} \div 3\frac{1}{3} = \frac{13}{6} \div \frac{10}{3}$$	The reciprocal of $\frac{10}{3}$ is $\frac{3}{10}$. $$\frac{13}{6} \div \frac{10}{3} = \frac{13}{6} \times \frac{3}{10}$$

STEP 3	STEP 4
Simplify. Divide 3 and 6 by 3. $$\frac{13}{6} \times \frac{3}{10} = \frac{13 \times \cancel{3}^{1}}{\cancel{6}_{2} \times 10}$$	Multiply the numerators and the denominators. $$\frac{13 \times 1}{2 \times 10} = \frac{13}{20}$$ $$2\frac{1}{6} \div 3\frac{1}{3} = \frac{13}{20}$$

Example: $5\frac{1}{5} \div 1\frac{3}{10}$

STEP 1	STEP 2
Express the numbers as fractions. $$5\frac{1}{5} = \frac{(5 \times 5) + 1}{5} = \frac{26}{5}$$ $$1\frac{3}{10} = \frac{(1 \times 10) + 3}{10} = \frac{13}{10}$$	The reciprocal of $\frac{13}{10}$ is $\frac{10}{13}$
$5\frac{1}{5} \div 1\frac{3}{10} = \frac{26}{5} \div \frac{13}{10}$	$\frac{26}{5} \div \frac{13}{10} = \frac{26}{5} \times \frac{10}{13}$

STEP 3	STEP 4
Simplify.	Multiply the numerators and the denominators. $$\frac{2 \times 2}{1 \times 1} = \frac{4}{1} = 4$$
$\frac{26}{5} \times \frac{10}{13} = \frac{\overset{2}{\cancel{26}} \times \overset{2}{\cancel{10}}}{\underset{1}{\cancel{5}} \times \underset{1}{\cancel{13}}}$	$5\frac{1}{5} \div 1\frac{3}{10} = 4$

4.6 EXERCISES

Find each quotient. Express answers as mixed numbers in lowest terms.

1. $1\frac{1}{2} \div 2\frac{1}{4}$
2. $3\frac{1}{3} \div 4\frac{2}{9}$
3. $6\frac{3}{5} \div 2\frac{1}{2}$
4. $4\frac{7}{8} \div 2\frac{1}{6}$
5. $2\frac{2}{3} \div 1\frac{1}{2}$
6. $2\frac{3}{4} \div 1\frac{2}{3}$
7. $16\frac{2}{3} \div 3\frac{1}{3}$
8. $100 \div 3\frac{1}{3}$
9. $4\frac{3}{8} \div 2\frac{5}{6}$
10. $\frac{1}{28} \div 7\frac{1}{2}$
11. $18\frac{1}{2} \div 1$
12. $15 \div 2\frac{1}{2}$
13. $4\frac{1}{3} \div 3$
14. $1 \div 8\frac{1}{3}$
15. $0 \div 3\frac{1}{4}$

APPLICATIONS

Health care assistants are a vital part of the medical field. *Health care assistants* maintain the control of medications, drugs, and medical records by keeping an accurate inventory. The assistant occupations enable the health care field to run smoothly.

Medical records clerks are one type of assistant. The medical records clerk is responsible for assembling, in sequence, information for medical records. They may also gather statistical data for reports.

Medical assistants help physicians examine and treat patients. The medical assistant may be responsible for arranging instruments and equipment and for checking office and laboratory supplies.

A *medical laboratory assistant* aids the medical technologist in the laboratory. The medical laboratory assistant is responsible for cleaning and sterilizing laboratory equipment, glassware, and instruments. The medical laboratory assistant may prepare solutions following standard laboratory formulas.

4.7 EXERCISES

1. A medical records clerk gathers data about patients with broken bones. It is found that 1/3 of the medical records are for individuals with broken bones. A total of 14,391 records are in the files. How many records are for individuals with broken bones?
2. How many 1/2-gram doses can be obtained from a 5-gram vial of medication?
3. A medical laboratory assistant prepares a solution using a standard laboratory formula. The solution in the flask weighs 6 1/3 ounces. What is the weight of 3/5 of the solution?
4. How many fourths can be produced from one scored medication tablet?
5. A medical assistant fills a storage cabinet with 14 bottles of dextrose. Each bottle is filled with 16 2/3 ounces of the solution. How many ounces of this solution are in the cabinet?

unit 5 section one applications to health work

OBJECTIVES

After studying this unit the student should be able to:

- Use the basic operations of fractions to solve health work problems.

A *drug* is a substance or a mixture of substances which have been found to have a definite value in the detection, prevention, or treatment of diseases. Drugs may be used to cure diseases, assist the body in overcoming diseases, or help to prevent diseases. Drugs may also be used to help diagnose a disease.

In administering medication, accuracy is of the utmost importance. Errors in the amount of medication may have fatal results. Medications that are a mixture of two or more substances must be accurately prepared; liquid medication must be accurately measured.

The ways in which drugs are administered are: oral, injection, intramuscular, and topical.

▼ Administering a drug *orally* means that the drug is taken via the mouth. If the drug is to be given orally, it is usually in the form of a liquid, tablet, or powder.

▼ Administering a drug by *injection* means that the drug enters the body through the blood system. For injection purposes, the medication must be in a liquid form. The medication is administered by using a syringe.

▼ An *intramuscular* administration of a drug means that the drug is placed directly into the muscle. A syringe is used for this purpose and the preparation must be in a liquid form.

▼ A *topical* application of a drug means that the medication is placed on the external body. Topical drugs cannot be administered internally. Topical drugs are usually in a liquid, powder, or semisolid form.

The portion of a drug to be administered at one time is the *dose*. The total quantity that is to be administered is the *dosage*. Drug dosage depends on:

- The weight, sex, and age of the patient.
- The disease being treated.
- How the drug is to be administered.
- The patient's tolerance of the drug.

In calculating doses and dosages, these terms are used.

▼ An *average dose* is the amount of medication which has been proven most effective with minimal toxic effects.

▼ An *initial dose* is the first dose.

▼ A *maximum dose* is the largest amount of medication which can be safely administered at one time.

▼ A *lethal* dose is the amount that could cause death to a patient.

In administering doses of medication, more than one tablet may be used or a scored tablet may have to be divided. Liquid preparations may have to be divided into equal portions or additional portions may have to be made. Care must always be taken when preparing the medications and administering the drugs.

5.1 EXERCISES

1. A physician prescribes a 90-milligram dosage of thyroid tablets. Each tablet contains 30 milligrams, or 1/2 grain, of medication.
   a. What fractional part of the prescribed dosage does one tablet represent?
   b. How many 30-milligram tablets would be needed to administer the prescribed dosage to the patient?
   c. How many total grains are present in the total dosage?

2. A patient is allergic to natural thyroid preparations. The physician prescribes a synthetic thyroid preparation which is available in 25-microgram tablets. The prescribed dose is 37 1/2 micrograms. How many tablets are needed?

3. An unlocked medical cabinet contains 67 different compounds. A total of 23 are used for skin conditions and are applied topically. A total of 15 are used for intestinal disorders and are administered orally. A registered nurse removes the chemical compounds used for intestinal disorders. What fractional part of the remaining chemicals are used for skin disorders?

4. In a community hospital, a medical records technician is responsible for preparing statistical reports. The medical records clerk assists the technician in the gathering of data that is needed. The clerk finds that the hospital is composed of 60 people. There are 3 maintenance personnel, 2 secretaries, and 1 billing clerk. Find the fractional part represented by each group.
   a. maintenance personnel
   b. medical secretaries
   c. billing clerks
   d. others

5. A health service administrator determines that a medical staff of 127 people must be decreased by approximately 1/12. How many staff positions must be eliminated?

6. Each day, a doctor administers 2 1/2 milligrams of medication to a patient. There are 25 milligrams of medication left in the bottle. How many more 2 1/2-milligram doses can the doctor administer from the bottle?

7. One poison is known to cause death in amounts as small as 1/250 ounce. A solution of 4/5 ounce poison in 1 gallon of distilled water will produce the lethal results. If this solution is divided into equal amounts, how many lethal doses can be prepared? Note: 1 gallon = 128 ounces

8. Death may be caused by 1/20 ounce of arsenic. How many lethal doses are represented in 8/9 ounce?

9. A pharmacist prepares a mixture containing six grams of compound *A* and three grams of compound *B*.

   a. What part of the mixture is compound *A*?
   b. What part of the mixture is compound *B*?

10. A powder to be used topically is prepared by mixing 5 grams of compound *C* and 7 grams of compound *D*.

    a. How many grams does the mixture contain?
    b. What fractional part of the mixture is compound *C*?
    c. What fractional part of the mixture is compound *D*?

11. A medical laboratory assistant prepares containers of a saline solution. Each container has 4 3/8 ounces of solution in it. How many ounces of solution are present in

    a. 3 1/2 containers?
    b. 1 3/5 containers?
    c. 2/3 container?
    d. 17 1/3 containers?

12. A certain medical assistant is allowed to administer injections. The assistant has a vial of medication containing 2 ounces of medication. The average dose is 3/5 ounce. How many full 3/5-ounce doses can be obtained from the vial?

13. An average dose of medicine is 3/4 ounce. One patient is given an initial dose of 2/5 of the 3/4-ounce dose. A second patient is given an initial dose of 2 1/2 times the 3/4-ounce dose.

    a. How many ounces of medicine does the first patient receive?
    b. How many ounces of medicine does the second patient receive?

14. A *health services administrator* makes management decisions about personnel, space requirements, and budgets. The administrator determines that for the coming year, the proposed budget must be decreased by $237,000. The decrease is 1/15 of the proposed budget. How much is the proposed budget?

15. Two file cabinets for medical records are the same size. One cabinet is 4/5 full and the other is 1/4 full. A medical records clerk wants to combine the cabinets. Can the contents of these two cabinets be combined? Explain.

16. Ann receives a gradually decreasing dose of medication. She drinks 3/4 ounce of medication at 1 P.M.; 1/2 ounce at 3 P.M.; and 1/4 ounce at 6 P.M. What is the total amount of medication that Ann consumes during this time period?

17. A registered nurse removes two scored medication tablets from the same container. One patient is given 1/2 tablet and another is given 1/4 tablet. Which patient is given the larger dose?

18. A dietitian knows that a box containing 566 grams of cereal is composed of 100 grams protein, 400 grams carbohydrates, and 20 grams fat. Find the amounts present in 1/9 of the box.

   a. protein
   b. carbohydrates
   c. fat
   d. other substances

19. A pharmacist in a hospital weighs a capsule of medication. The capsule weighs 4/90 ounce.

   a. What is the weight of three capsules?
   b. What is the weight of a capsule containing 1/2 the amount of this same medication?

20. Margaret has a condition requiring the administration of colchicine. The maximum dose of colchicine is 1/50 grain; each tablet contains 1/100 grain of medication.

   a. How many tablets are in the maximum dose?
   b. How many maximum doses could be obtained from a bottle containing 100 tablets of colchicine?

21. Two vials of liquid, one 2/3 full and a second 3/8 full, are to be combined in a third vial of the same size. Will the third vial hold the combined contents?

22. A nurse has a vial containing 8 ounces of medication. The average dose is 1/2 ounce. After 5 doses how many ounces of medication are left in the vial?

23. A powder is to be prepared by mixing 7 grams of substance A and 3 grams of substance B.

   a. Substance A is what fractional part of the mixture?
   b. Substance B is what fractional part of the mixture?

24. Flasks, each containing 6 2/5 ounces of an iodine solution, are prepared in a lab. How many ounces of solution are present in:
   a. 1/4 flask?
   b. 2 1/2 flasks?

25. The $125,000 supply budget for maintenance in a nursing home must be reduced by 1/10. How much money will remain in the budget for supplies?

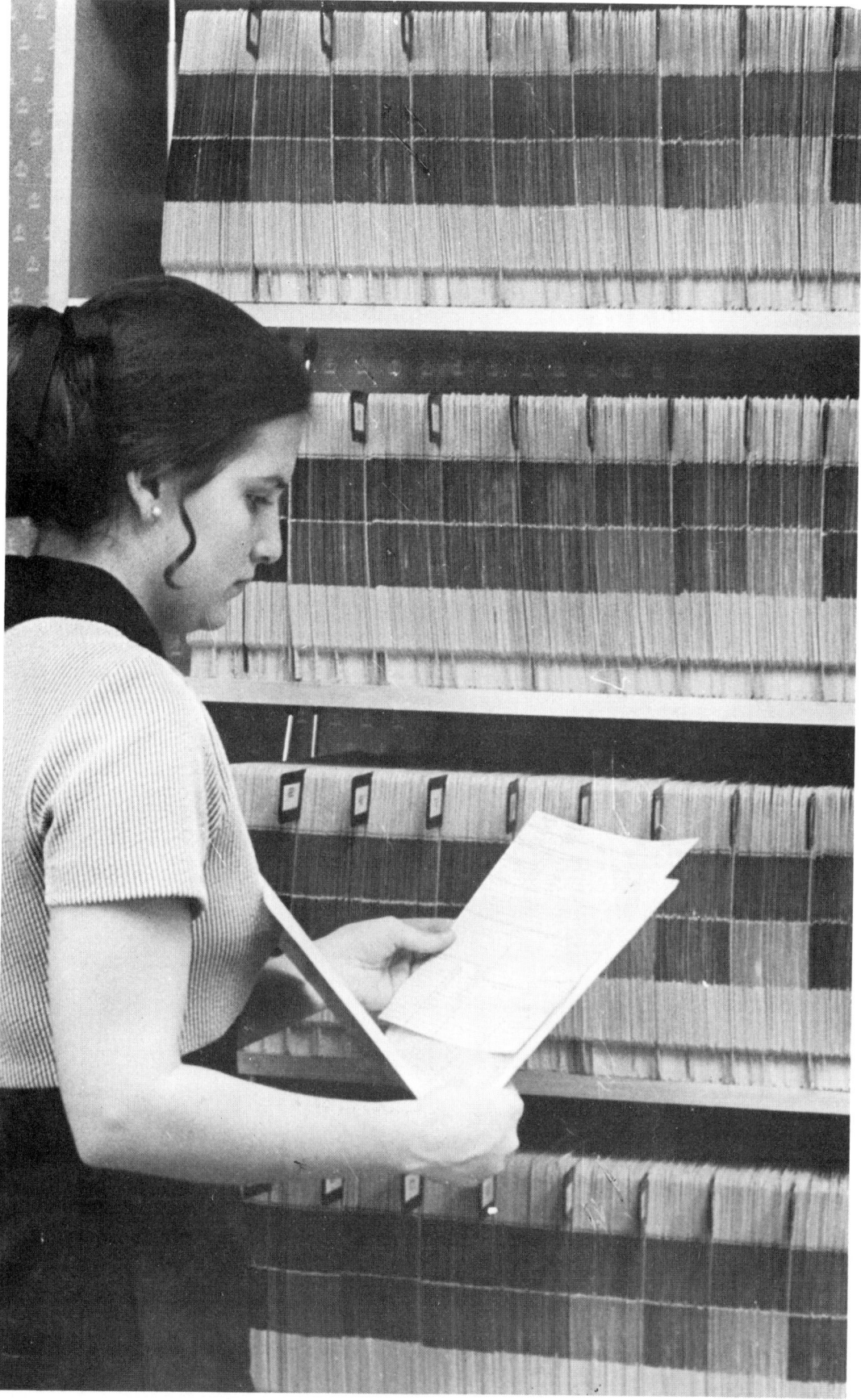

SECTION 2 DECIMAL FRACTIONS

unit 6 introduction to decimal fractions

OBJECTIVES

After studying this unit the student should be able to:
- Express a common fraction with a denominator which is a power of ten as a decimal fraction.
- Express a decimal fraction as a mixed number with a denominator which is a power of ten.
- Compare decimal fractions.

DECIMAL FRACTIONS

A decimal fraction is used to express a common fraction whose denominators are powers of 10, such as 10; 100; 1,000; 10,000; 100,000; and 1,000,000.

Example: The fraction $\frac{2}{5}$ is equivalent to $\frac{4}{10}$, $\frac{40}{100}$ and $\frac{400}{1,000}$. These denominators are powers of 10.

$\frac{4}{10} = 0.4$ This is read "4 tenths."

$\frac{40}{100} = 0.40$ This is read "40 hundredths."

$\frac{400}{1,000} = 0.400$ This is read "400 thousandths."

Similarly, any decimal fraction can be expressed as a common fraction with a denominator as a power of ten.

Example:

five tenths	0.5	$\frac{5}{10}$
seven hundredths	0.07	$\frac{7}{100}$
eleven thousandths	0.011	$\frac{11}{1,000}$
two hundred nineteen ten-thousandths	0.0219	$\frac{219}{10,000}$
forty-three hundred-thousandths	0.00043	$\frac{43}{100,000}$
eight hundred seventeen millionths	0.000817	$\frac{817}{1,000,000}$

DECIMAL FRACTIONS IN THE PLACE-VALUE SYSTEM

The base ten place-value system is a decimal system. The place-value system is extended to give meaning to decimals. The decimal point separates the whole numbers from the decimal fractions.

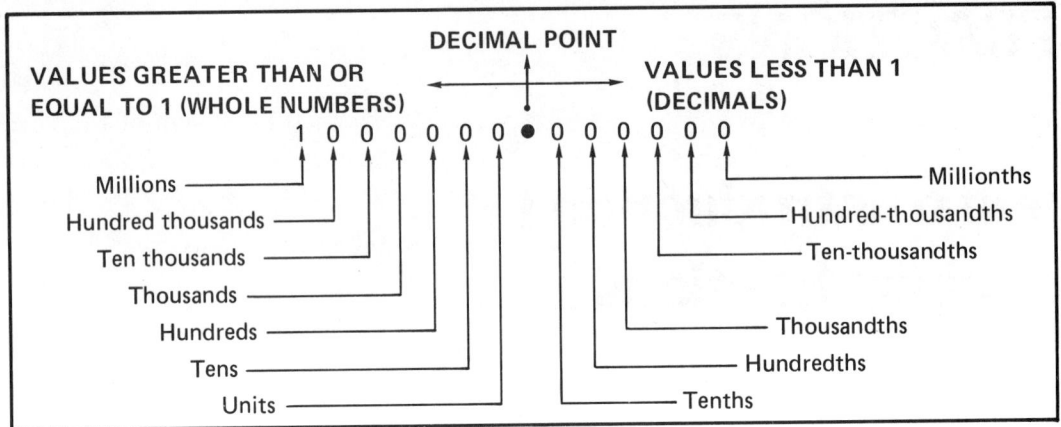

Example: The sum $86 + \frac{3}{10} + \frac{7}{100} + \frac{4}{1,000}$ can be written as a decimal using the place-value system.

$86 + \frac{3}{10} + \frac{7}{100} + \frac{4}{1,000}$ is written

TENS	UNITS	•	TENTHS		HUNDREDTHS		THOUSANDTHS
8	6	•	3		7		4

Example: Express 4.517 as a mixed number. Use the sum of fractions whose denominators are powers of ten.

$4.517 = 4 + \frac{5}{10} + \frac{1}{100} + \frac{7}{1,000} = 4 + \frac{500}{1,000} + \frac{10}{1,000} + \frac{7}{1,000} = 4\frac{517}{1,000}$

6.1 EXERCISES

Express each quantity as a decimal.

1. $\frac{3}{10}$
2. $\frac{21}{100}$
3. $\frac{137}{1,000}$
4. $\frac{1,571}{10,000}$
5. $\frac{9}{1,000}$
6. $\frac{7}{100}$
7. $\frac{31}{10,000}$
8. $\frac{1}{1,000}$
9. $\frac{7}{10,000}$
10. $\frac{80}{1,000}$
11. $4 + \frac{2}{10}$
12. $5 + \frac{13}{100}$

13. $6 + \frac{21}{100}$ 16. $11 + \frac{17}{1,000}$ 19. $15 + \frac{3}{10,000}$

14. $23 + \frac{137}{1,000}$ 17. $10 + \frac{1}{100}$

15. $42 + \frac{8,131}{10,000}$ 18. $0 + \frac{107}{10,000}$

Express each decimal as a fraction or mixed number. Use the sum of fractions whose denominators are powers of ten.

20. 3.462   22. 17.803
21. 0.981   23. 9.012

Express each decimal as a mixed number. Do not express in lowest terms.

24. 5.9   28. 42.657   32. 17.00570
25. 7.31   29. 14.057   33. 111.00072
26. 8.90   30. 92.705   34. 9.7005
27. 2.5   31. 1.0057   35. 15.82090

COMPARING DECIMAL FRACTIONS

Comparing decimals is similar to comparing whole numbers. Starting from the place value to the far left, each number is compared. This process continues until unequal values are found in corresponding place values.

Example: Which number is smaller: 3.1478 or 3.1468?

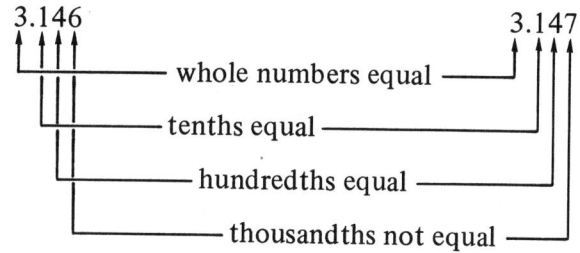

Since, in the thousandths place, $6 < 7$, $3.1468 < 3.1478$.

Example: Which number is larger: 0.279 or 0.27?

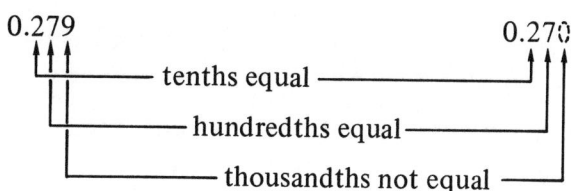

Since $9 > 0$, $0.279 > 0.27$.

6.2 EXERCISES

Compare each pair of decimals. Use the symbols, <, >, =.

1. 0.56 __?__ 0.59
2. 0.68 __?__ 0.680
3. 0.325 __?__ 0.327
4. 2.398 __?__ 2.389
5. 3.765 __?__ 2.765
6. 4.001 __?__ 3.999
7. 0.3 __?__ 0.99
8. 0.005 __?__ 0.012
9. 0.19 __?__ 0.989
10. 7.304 __?__ 7.3
11. 0.009 __?__ 0.010
12. 4.7690 __?__ 4.769
13. 0.0099 __?__ 0.100
14. 4.342 __?__ 4.0342
15. 0.32 __?__ 0.32001

APPLICATIONS

A patient in a hospital is given 0.4 grams of medication instead of 0.04 gram. The patient dies. The cause of death might read: MISPLACED DECIMAL. This tragic example of carelessness — or perhaps lack of knowledge — with decimals can occur.

Decimals are a vital part of the health care field. Each health care worker should understand and use decimals carefully. Preparing medications, comparing and administering doses, and compiling statistical reports are only a few examples of instances where decimals are used.

6.3 EXERCISES

1. Two patients receive the same medication. The first patient receives 0.125 gram and the second receives 0.325 gram. Which patient receives the larger dose?

2. *Occupational therapists* design and direct vocational, educational and recreational activities for handicapped people. There are about 9,600 occupational therapists in the United States of which 4/10 work with the emotionally handicapped and 6/10 work with the physically handicapped. Express these fractional parts as decimals.

3. During an operation, a patient receives 2 8/10 pints of blood. Express the amount of blood as a decimal.

4. *Chiropractic* is based on the principle that a person's health is determined mainly by the nervous system. *Chiropractors* treat their patients by manipulating parts of the body to correct interferences in the nervous system. More than 4/10 of the total chiropractors are located in California, Michigan, Missouri, New York, Pennsylvania, and Texas. Express this fraction as a decimal.

5. A medical record technician calculates that 0.323 of all optometrists are women and that 0.332 of all veterinarians are women. Which health career has more women?

6. Megan grew 1.34 centimetres since her last checkup. Jamie grew 1.43 centimetres in the same time period. Which one grew the most?

unit 7 rounding decimal numbers and finding equivalents

OBJECTIVES

After studying this unit the student should be able to:
- Round decimal numbers to any required number of places.
- Express common fractions as decimal fractions.
- Express decimal fractions as common fractions.

After solving a problem using decimal numbers the answer may have more decimal places than are needed. In these cases, the numbers may be rounded. Rounding is an expression used when referring to an approximation for a number.

ROUNDING DECIMAL NUMBERS

- To round a decimal number:
  - Determine the number of decimal places required.
  - If the digit directly to the right of the last decimal place required is less than 5, the last required digit is not altered.
  - If the digit directly to the right of the last decimal place required is 5 or larger, the last required digit is increased by one.

The symbol $\approx$ is used in rounding numbers. It means *is approximately equal to*.

Example: The place-value names for the number 5,250.849 are:

Thousands	Hundreds	Tens	Units	Tenths	Hundredths	Thousandths
5	2	5	0	8	4	9

This number is rounded to various places.

Round to the nearer hundredth.

5,250.84̲9̸ Check the digit to the right of the hundredths place. Since $9 > 5$, the preceding digit is increased by 1.

$$5,250.849 \approx 5,250.85 \text{ (hundedths)}$$

54 Section 2 Decimal Fractions

Round to the nearer tenth.

5,250.8̲4́9 Check the digit to the right of the tenths place. Since $4 < 5$, the preceding digit is not altered.
$$5{,}250.849 \approx 5{,}250.8 \text{ (tenths)}$$

Round to the nearer whole number.

5,250̲.8́49 Check the digit to the right of the units place. Since $8 > 5$, the preceding digit is increased by 1.
$$5{,}250.849 \approx 5{,}251 \text{ (units)}$$

Round to the nearer ten.

5,25̲0́.849 Check the digit to the right of the tens place. Since $0 < 5$, the preceding digit is not altered.
$$5{,}250.849 \approx 5{,}250 \text{ (tens)}$$

Round to the nearer hundred.

5,2̲5́0.849 Check the digit to the right of the hundreds place. Since $5 = 5$, the preceding digit is increased by 1.
$$5{,}250.849 \approx 5{,}300 \text{ (hundreds)}$$

Round to the nearer thousand.

5̲,2́50.849 Check the digit to the right of the thousandths place. Since $2 < 5$, the preceding digit is not altered.
$$5{,}250.849 \approx 5{,}000 \text{ (thousands)}$$

7.1 EXERCISES

Round each number to the indicated place.

Thousandth

1. 2.8925
2. 74.51930
3. 0.43276
4. 0.01875
5. 100.0264
6. 35.0552
7. 0.2509
8. 1.2170
9. 73.6050
10. 432.9215

Hundredth

11. 16.321
12. 0.895
13. 4.7166
14. 0.0875
15. 0.0074
16. 3.1416
17. 74.2785
18. 0.3704
19. 17.00347
20. 322.751

Tenth

21. 5.74
22. 289.86
23. 0.68
24. 3.512
25. 706.475
26. 23.07
27. 0.21794
28. 29.059
29. 0.00243
30. 1,323.019

Whole Number

31. 3.719
32. 0.1
33. 29.61
34. 44.099
35. 317.268
36. 9.09
37. 40.17
38. 410.71
39. 0.692
40. 0.50

Ten

41. 273
42. 145.9
43. 308.29
44. 1,872.65
45. 29.31
46. 1,607.48
47. 470.91
48. 502.67
49. 2,106.39
50. 14,007.46

Hundred

51. 6,234.9
52. 1,760.81
53. 3,909
54. 1,200.675
55. 15,650.125
56. 3,100.875
57. 6,849
58. 9,025.6
59. 1,989.1
60. 23,992

EXPRESSING COMMON FRACTIONS AS DECIMAL FRACTIONS

Expressing a decimal as a fraction is not difficult since the denominator is a power of ten, for example $0.13 = \frac{13}{100}$. However, the method is more difficult when expressing a common fraction as a decimal.

Example: Express $\frac{1}{2}$ as a decimal.

$$\frac{1}{2} = \frac{5}{10}$$

$$\frac{5}{10} = 0.5$$

$$\frac{1}{2} = 0.5$$

This method uses multiplication to find an equivalent fraction with a denominator that is a power of ten.

56 Section 2 Decimal Fractions

Example: Using multiplication to find an equivalent fraction, express $\frac{5}{8}$ as a decimal.

$$\frac{5}{8} \times \frac{?}{?} = \frac{?}{1{,}000}$$

$$\frac{5}{8} \times \frac{125}{125} = \frac{625}{1{,}000}$$

$$\frac{625}{1{,}000} = 0.625$$

$$\frac{5}{8} = 0.625$$

Finding the number to be used as a factor in forming equivalent fractions can become increasingly difficult. For this reason division is usually used to express fractions as decimals.

Example: Using division, express $\frac{5}{8}$ as a decimal.

$\frac{5}{8}$ means $5 \div 8$.

$$\begin{array}{r} 0.625 \\ 8\overline{)5.000} \\ \underline{4\;8} \\ 20 \\ \underline{16} \\ 40 \\ \underline{40} \\ 0 \end{array}$$

$$\frac{5}{8} = 0.625$$

Note: Although either method will produce correct results, the problem with the multiplication method is in finding the number to be used as a factor so that the new divisor is a power of ten. Consequently, in actual practice the division method is used most often.

7.2 EXERCISES

Using the indicated method, express each fraction as a decimal.

Use Multiplication to Find Equivalent Fractions

1. $\frac{4}{5} = \frac{?}{10} = ?$

2. $\frac{13}{50} = \frac{?}{100} = ?$

3. $\frac{3}{4} = \frac{?}{100} = ?$

4. $\frac{17}{25} = \frac{?}{100} = ?$

5. $\frac{1}{20} = \frac{?}{100} = ?$

6. $\frac{3}{8} = \frac{?}{1{,}000} = ?$

7. $\frac{17}{20} = \frac{?}{100} = ?$

8. $\frac{0}{50} = \frac{?}{100} = ?$

9. $\frac{9}{16} = \frac{?}{10,000} = ?$

10. $\frac{5}{32} = \frac{?}{100,000} = ?$

Use Division

11. $\frac{3}{5} \longrightarrow 5\overline{)3}$

12. $\frac{7}{8} \longrightarrow 8\overline{)7}$

13. $\frac{3}{200} \longrightarrow 200\overline{)3}$

14. $\frac{5}{2} \longrightarrow 2\overline{)5}$

15. $\frac{171}{500} \longrightarrow 500\overline{)171}$

16. $\frac{9}{20} \longrightarrow 20\overline{)9}$

17. $\frac{32}{25} \longrightarrow 25\overline{)32}$

18. $\frac{7}{16} \longrightarrow 16\overline{)7}$

19. $\frac{25}{2} \longrightarrow 2\overline{)25}$

20. $\frac{3}{16} \longrightarrow 16\overline{)3}$

Use Either Method

21. $\frac{1}{2}$

22. $\frac{5}{8}$

23. $\frac{9}{10}$

24. $\frac{13}{25}$

25. $2\frac{3}{4}$

26. $\frac{11}{25}$

27. $\frac{7}{2}$

28. $\frac{21}{80}$

29. $\frac{11}{5}$

30. $\frac{23}{50}$

31. $\frac{11}{16}$

32. $\frac{9}{40}$

33. $\frac{13}{8}$

34. $\frac{121}{100}$

35. $\frac{17}{20}$

36. $\frac{3}{75}$

37. $\frac{115}{250}$

38. $\frac{3}{32}$

39. $\frac{0}{100}$

40. $\frac{1}{64}$

REPEATING DECIMAL FRACTIONS

When expressing a fraction as a decimal only one of two things can happen.

- The decimal *terminates*. This means that the last remainder is 0.

- The decimal *repeats*. This means that the remainders repeat again and again.

Example: When expressing $\frac{1}{4}$ as a decimal, the last remainder is 0.

$$\frac{1}{4} = 4 \overline{)\begin{array}{l} 0.25 \\ 1.00 \\ \underline{8} \\ 20 \\ \underline{20} \\ 0 \end{array}}$$

The decimal equivalent, 0.25, is a <u>terminating decimal.</u>

Example: When expressing $\frac{2}{3}$ as a decimal, the remainders repeat again and again.

$$\frac{2}{3} = 3 \overline{)\begin{array}{l} 0.666\ldots \\ 2.000 \\ \underline{1\,8} \\ 20 \\ \underline{18} \\ 20 \\ \underline{18} \\ 2 \end{array}}$$

The remainder, 2, repeats again and again. The decimal equivalent 0.666 . . . is a <u>repeating decimal.</u>

In a repeating decimal the three dots, . . . , show that the indicated pattern continues indefinitely. Another way to represent a repeating decimal is to place a bar over the digit or group of digits that repeats. For example, 0.666 . . . can be written $0.\overline{6}$. This shows that the digit 6 repeats indefinitely. It is read "point 6 repetend."

The *period* of a repeating decimal is the number of digits in the repeating block. The period of the repeating decimal 0.185185 . . . is 3. The period of $0.\overline{16}$ is 2.

7.3 EXERCISES

Using division find the repeating decimal for each fraction. Use proper notation to indicate that the decimal repeats.

1. $\frac{7}{3}$
2. $\frac{7}{12}$
3. $\frac{1}{6}$
4. $\frac{2}{11}$
5. $\frac{5}{3}$
6. $\frac{1}{7}$
7. $\frac{5}{9}$
8. $\frac{4}{3}$
9. $\frac{11}{13}$
10. $\frac{19}{12}$

Use the bar notation to represent those repeating decimals which have been expressed with three dots.

Use the three dot notation to represent those repeating decimals which have been expressed with the bar.

Find the period for each repeating decimal.

11. $0.\bar{5}$
12. $5.7\bar{4}$
13. $0.\overline{02}$
14. $0.\overline{004}$
15. $0.\overline{037}$
16. $9.72317231\ldots$
17. $32.608608\ldots$
18. $1.243243\ldots$
19. $0.55\ldots$
20. $0.5833\ldots$
21. $0.\overline{18}$
22. $41.28\bar{9}$
23. $4.\overline{27}$
24. $1.\overline{142857}$
25. $15.\bar{0}$
26. $0.166\ldots$
27. $0.4545\ldots$
28. $0.428571428571\ldots$
29. $0.076923076923\ldots$
30. $27.6262\ldots$

APPLICATIONS

When calculating the amount of medication to be administered, values that are too small may be meaningless for the kinds of measurements that are to be used. A calculation which results in 3.003 tablets to be administered is meaningless since it would be almost impossible to find out what 0.003 tablet is. A tablet can not be divided into such a small portion. Conversely, a calculation which results in 0.003 grams of medication to be placed into a solution would not be meaningless.

When confronted with a "rounding situation," use common sense. Always follow the directions of the doctor or the supervisor in the laboratory or pharmacy. If in doubt, consult a pharmacist or a technician in that particular field.

7.4 EXERCISES

1. Through calculations it is determined that 4.689 320 0 grams of glucose are required in the preparation of a solution. The available balance can weigh to thousandths of a gram. Find the number of grams of glucose used in preparing the solution.

2. The lengths of four babies are compared. These birth lengths are recorded: 43.5 centimetres; 44.125 centimetres; 42.025 centimetres; 46.65 centimetres. Round each measurement to the number of decimal places in the least accurate measurement.

3. A standard adult dose for a specific medication is 0.025 litre. The central supply has 5.692 litres on hand. Using this information, the number of human doses is found to be 227.68. Can 227.68 doses be rounded to 228 doses?

4. The instructions are to prepare 1 700 millilitres of an alcohol solution containing one-third ethyl alcohol and two-thirds distilled water.

   a. Find the number of millilitres of ethyl alcohol required to prepare the solution.
   b. Find the number of millilitres of distilled water in the preparation.
   c. The graduated measuring device measures to 0.01 millilitre. Find the number of millilitres of ethyl alcohol used.

5. Five individuals were weighed with the following results: 14.65 kilograms, 21.15 kilograms, 13.09 kilograms, 15.16 kilograms, and 17.26 kilograms.

   a. What is the total weight of all five individuals?
   b. What is the average weight of these five individuals?
      (1) To the nearest one hundredth of a kilogram?
      (2) To the nearest tenth of a kilogram?

6. The death rate in the community is found to be one person per 1,500 annually. If the current population is 152,375, how many people can be anticipated to die in the next 12 months?

7. It has been determined that an average of 35 cotton swabs are used per patient in one week. These swabs are purchased in packages of 100 each. If the patient load is determined to average 62 patients per week, how many packages of swabs must be ordered to provide a twenty-six week supply?

unit 8 basic operations with decimal fractions

OBJECTIVES

After studying this unit the student should be able to:

- Add decimal fractions.
- Subtract decimal fractions.
- Multiply decimal fractions.
- Divide decimal fractions.

Remember that different symbols express the same decimal. For example 0.5 can be written 0.50, 0.500, 0.5000 etc. The number 1 can be written as 1, 1.0, 1.00 etc. Keep this fact in mind when adding and subtracting decimals.

ADDITION OF DECIMAL FRACTIONS

In adding decimals, using zeros as placeholders reduces the possibility of errors. Zeros are used so that all the values have the same number of places to the right of the decimal point. This does not affect the value of the numbers.

Example: 36.014 + 7.28 + 14.9

STEP 1	STEP 2	STEP 3
Align the decimal points.	Use zeros as placeholders so that each value has the same number of decimal places.	Add as in whole numbers. The decimal point in the answer is aligned with the decimal points in the values that are added.
36.014 7.28 + 14.9	36.014 7.280 + 14.900	36.014 7.280 + 14.900 58.194

SUBTRACTION OF DECIMAL FRACTIONS

In subtraction as in addition, decimal points are aligned and zeros are used as placeholders.

Example: 62.7 − 29.38

STEP 1	STEP 2	STEP 3
Align the decimal points.	Use zeros as placeholders so that each value has the same number of decimal places.	Subtract as in whole numbers. The decimal point in the answer is aligned with the decimal points in the values that are subtracted.
62.7 − 29.38	62.70 − 29.38	62.70 − 29.38 33.32

8.1 EXERCISES

Find each sum or difference. Use zeros as placeholders as needed.

1. 0.12
 0.45
 + 0.14

2. 16.7
 0.23
 + 0.08

3. 25.37
 6.05
 + 7.2

4. 3.478
 2.32
 + 17.9

5. 4.216
 0.35
 + 1.2

6. 45
 0.78
 + 13.2

7. 32.6
 16.73
 + 0.003

8. 1.003
 0.0379
 + 16.4

9. 3.8
 − 2.9

10. 7.0
 − 5.28

11. 92.37
 − 57.56

12. 18.97
 − 9.248

13. 13.403
 − 9.7

14. 4.702
 − 3.278

15. 15.2
 − 0.003

16. 1.0
 − 0.789

17. 2.6
 1.5
 + 0.48

18. 0.45
 2.6
 + 0.7

19. 4.56
 21.7
 + 0.08

20. 6
 4.25
 + 0.008

21. 18.7
 0.124
 + 7.0

22. 6.654
 0.398
 + 14.822

23. 132.1
 17.813
 + 0.999

24. 37.41
 13.3
 + 7.345

25. 28.2
 − 8.28

26. 0.8
 − 0.77

27. 123.6
 − 15.74

28. 5.87
 − 3.242

29. 2.01
 − 0.998

30. 0.01
 − 0.001

31. 189.01
 − 0.987

32. 10
 − 0.0012

MULTIPLICATION OF DECIMAL FRACTIONS

Decimals are an expression for fractions whose denominators are powers of ten. Multiplication of decimals can be illustrated by using these fractions whose denominators are powers of ten.

Examples:

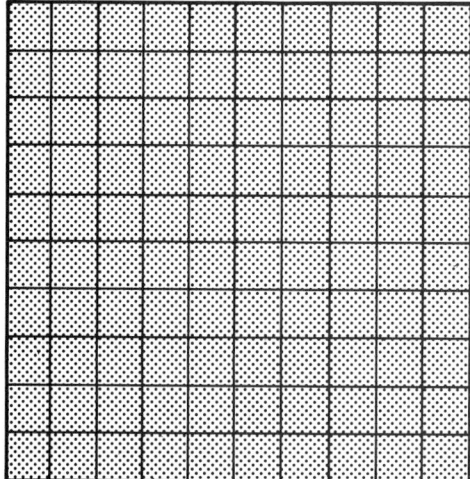
Shade the total region.

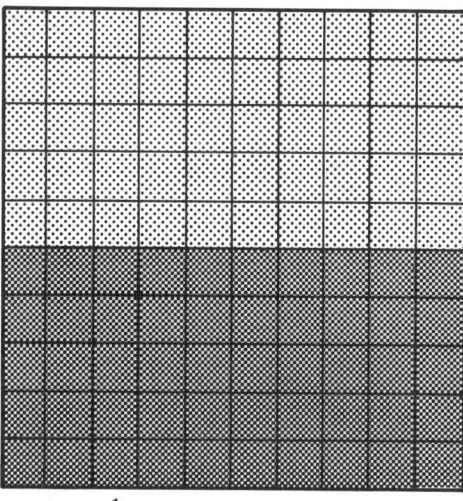
Darken $\frac{1}{2}$ or 0.5 of the total region.
50 regions in 100 are darkened.

The mathematical notation is:
$$\frac{1}{2} \times 1 = \frac{1}{2} \text{ or } \frac{50}{100}$$
$$\frac{5}{10} \times 1 = \frac{5}{10} \text{ or } \frac{50}{100}$$
$$0.5 \times 1 = 0.5 \text{ or } \frac{50}{100}$$

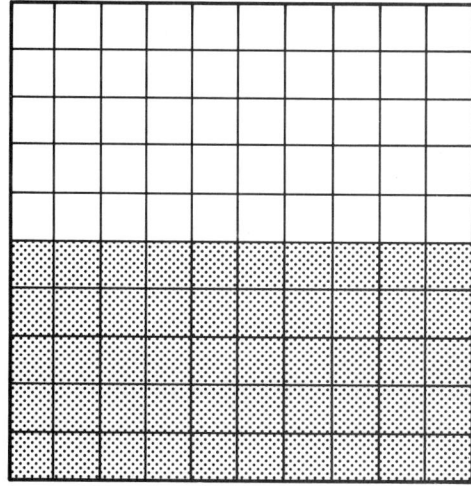
Shade $\frac{1}{2}$ or 0.5 of the total region.

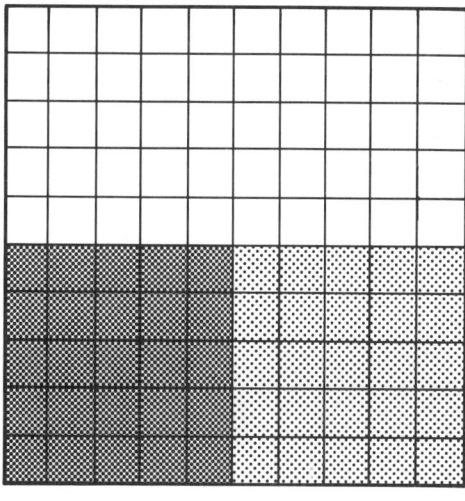
Darken $\frac{1}{2}$ or 0.5 of the $\frac{1}{2}$ (0.5) region.
25 regions in 100 are darkened.

The mathematical notation is: $\frac{1}{2} \times \frac{1}{2} = \frac{1}{4}$ or $\frac{25}{100}$

$$\frac{5}{10} \times \frac{5}{10} = \frac{25}{100}$$

$$0.5 \times 0.5 = 0.25 \text{ or } \frac{25}{100}$$

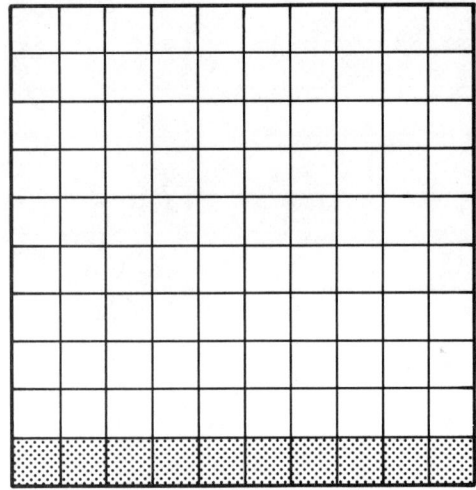

Shade $\frac{1}{10}$ or 0.1 of the total region.

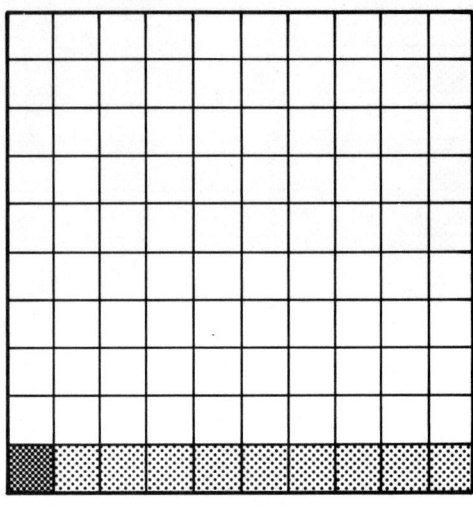

Darken $\frac{1}{10}$ or 0.1 of the $\frac{1}{10}$ (0.1) region.
1 region in 100 is darkened.

The mathematical notation is: $\frac{1}{10} \times \frac{1}{10} = \frac{1}{100}$

$$0.1 \times 0.1 = 0.01 \text{ or } \frac{1}{100}$$

The notation for multiplication of decimals can be generalized this way.

COMMON FRACTIONS	DECIMAL FRACTIONS
$\frac{1}{10} \times \frac{1}{10} = \frac{1}{100}$	$0.1 \times 0.1 = 0.01$ (tenths X tenths = hundredths)
$\frac{1}{10} \times \frac{1}{100} = \frac{1}{1,000}$	$0.1 \times 0.01 = 0.001$ (tenths X hundredths = thousandths)
$\frac{1}{10} \times \frac{1}{1,000} = \frac{1}{10,000}$	$0.1 \times 0.001 = 0.0001$ (tenths X thousandths = ten-thousandths)

Note that the number of decimal places in the product depends on the number of decimal places in each factor. The number of decimal places in the product is the sum of the decimal places in the factors.

Example: 2.3 × 45.

STEP 1	STEP 2	STEP 3
Multiply as in whole numbers.	Count the number of decimal places in each factor.	The number of decimal places in the product is the sum of the decimal places in the factors. Locate the decimal point to indicate that number.
2.3 × 45 115 92 1035	2.3 1 × 45 + 0 1035 1	2.3 × 45 103.5 ↳ 1 decimal place

Example: 2.3 × 4.5

STEP 1	STEP 2	STEP 3
Multiply as in whole numbers.	Count the number of decimal places in each factor.	The number of decimal places in the product is the sum of the decimal places in the factors. Locate the decimal point to indicate that number.
2.3 × 4.5 115 92 1035	2.3 1 × 4.5 + 1 1035 2	2.3 × 4.5 10.35 ↳ 2 decimal places

8.2 EXERCISES

Find each product.

1. 4.8 × 3
2. 0.48 × 3
3. 0.048 × 3
4. 5.2 × 31
5. 5.2 × 3.1
6. 0.52 × 3.1
7. 5.2 × 0.031
8. 0.13 × 72
9. 34.95 × 0.96
10. 0.007 × 0.008
11. 251.3 × 0.15
12. 15.34 × 31.3
13. 0.371 × 4.24
14. 0.063 × 0.0006
15. 0.75 × 83.60
16. 421.25 × 416.40

66 Section 2 Decimal Fractions

DIVISION OF DECIMAL FRACTIONS

Division of decimals can also be illustrated using fractions whose denominators are powers of ten.

Example:

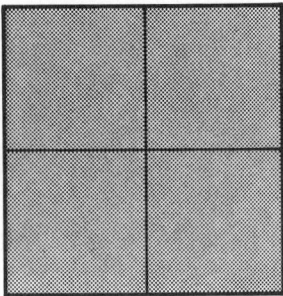

4 regions

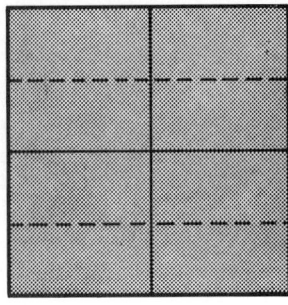

Each of the 4 regions is divided in half *or* 0.5.

8 regions are formed.

The mathematical notation is: $4 \div \frac{1}{2} = 4 \times \frac{2}{1}$ or 8

$$4 \div 0.5 = 8$$

Division of decimals can be performed by first finding equivalent fractions which have whole numbers as numerators and denominators. Then, the division of whole numbers is performed.

Example: $75.50 \div 2.5$

$75.50 \div 2.5$ means $\frac{75.50}{2.5}$.

$$\frac{75.50}{2.5} \times \frac{10}{10} = \frac{755}{25}$$

```
        30.2
    25 ) 755.0
         75
         ‾‾
         05
          0
         ‾‾
         5 0
         5 0
         ‾‾‾
           0
```

Example: 2.3 × 45.

STEP 1	STEP 2	STEP 3
Multiply as in whole numbers.	Count the number of decimal places in each factor.	The number of decimal places in the product is the sum of the decimal places in the factors. Locate the decimal point to indicate that number.
2.3 × 45 ――― 115 92 ――― 1035	2.3 1 × 45 + 0 ――― ――― 1035 1	2.3 × 45 ――― 103.5 └― 1 decimal place

Example: 2.3 × 4.5

STEP 1	STEP 2	STEP 3
Multiply as in whole numbers.	Count the number of decimal places in each factor.	The number of decimal places in the product is the sum of the decimal places in the factors. Locate the decimal point to indicate that number.
2.3 × 4.5 ――― 115 92 ――― 1035	2.3 1 × 4.5 + 1 ――― ――― 1035 2	2.3 × 4.5 ――― 10.35 └― 2 decimal places

8.2 EXERCISES

Find each product.

1.   4.8
   ×   3

2.   0.48
   ×   3

3. 0.048
   ×   3

4.   5.2
   × 31

5.   5.2
   × 3.1

6.   0.52
   × 3.1

7.   5.2
   × 0.031

8.   0.13
   × 72

9. 34.95
   × 0.96

10. 0.007
    × 0.008

11. 251.3
    × 0.15

12. 15.34
    × 31.3

13. 0.371
    × 4.24

14. 0.063
    × 0.0006

15. 0.75
    × 83.60

16. 421.25
    × 416.40

DIVISION OF DECIMAL FRACTIONS

Division of decimals can also be illustrated using fractions whose denominators are powers of ten.

Example:

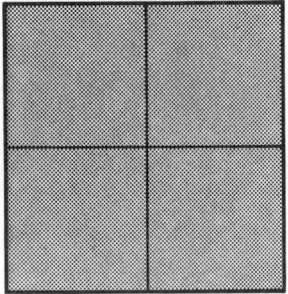

4 regions

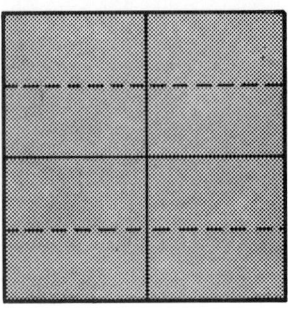

Each of the 4 regions is divided in half *or* 0.5.

8 regions are formed.

The mathematical notation is: $4 \div \frac{1}{2} = 4 \times \frac{2}{1}$ or 8

$$4 \div 0.5 = 8$$

Division of decimals can be performed by first finding equivalent fractions which have whole numbers as numerators and denominators. Then, the division of whole numbers is performed.

Example: $75.50 \div 2.5$

$75.50 \div 2.5$ means $\frac{75.50}{2.5}$.

$$\frac{75.50}{2.5} \times \frac{10}{10} = \frac{755}{25}$$

```
          30.2
   25 ) 755.0
        75
        ‾‾
         05
          0
         ‾‾
          50
          50
          ‾‾
           0
```

Example: 75.50 ÷ 0.25

75.50 ÷ 0.25 means $\frac{75.50}{0.25}$.

$\frac{75.50}{0.25} \times \frac{100}{100} = \frac{7,550}{25}$

```
        302
    ┌───────
 25 ) 7,550
      7 5
      ───
        05
         0
        ──
        50
        50
        ──
         0
```

Example: 75.50 ÷ 0.025

75.50 ÷ 0.025 means $\frac{75.50}{0.025}$.

$\frac{75.50}{0.025} \times \frac{1,000}{1,000} = \frac{75,500}{25}$

```
         3,020
    ┌────────
 25 ) 75,500
       75
       ──
        05
        00
        ──
        50
        50
        ──
        00
        00
        ──
         0
```

Note: All solutions should be checked. The solution may be checked by multiplying the quotient by the divisor. The result of this calculation should be the dividend.

Notice that in finding the equivalent fractions, the form of 1 is a power of ten. Each time a number is multiplied by a power of ten, the place value of the number increases by the same power. Zeros serve as placeholders in the multiplication of powers of ten and the division process.

Example: 1.178 ÷ 0.69
Round the answer to the nearer hundredth.

STEP 1	STEP 2	STEP 3
Multiply both numbers by 100 and locate the decimal point in the answer.	Divide to the thousandths place.	Since 7 > 5, the preceding digit is increased by 1.

0₍69.⟌1₍17.80
 	
69⟌117.8
	1.707
	69⟌117.800
	   69
	   48 8
	   48 3
	      500
	      483
	       17
		1.707
		69⟌117.800
		
		1.178 ÷ 0.69 = 1.71
		(rounded)

Example: 14 ÷ 1.5
Round the answer to the nearer tenth.

STEP 1	STEP 2	STEP 3
Multiply both numbers by 10 and locate the decimal point in the answer.	Divide to the hundredths place.	Since 3 < 5, the preceding digit is not altered.

1₍5.⟌14₍0. 15⟌140.	9.33
	15⟌140.00
	   135
	      5 0
	      4 5
	         4 50
	           45
	            5
		9.33
		15⟌140.00
		
		1.5 ÷ 14 = 9.3
		(rounded)

8.3 EXERCISES

Find each quotient. Round when indicated.

1. 3)21.9
2. 5)4.25
3. 7)0.714
4. 12)24.36
5. 15)4.575
6. 28)0.5684
7. 123)246.123
8. 248)7.44
9. 514)15.42
10. 628)2.512
11. 0.2)31
12. 0.3)132.3
13. 0.004)0.8204
14. 2.1)4.221
15. 0.34)6.8
16. 0.51)306
17. 0.006)03618
18. 0.032)649.6
19. 813)0.3252
20. 1.48)7,919.924
21. 39.2)19,603.92
22. 21.2)1,696.424
23. 0.040)1.2060
24. 0.612)42,840
25. 0.0035)756.0

Round to the nearer hundredth.

26. 1.7)21.3
27. 0.08)1.573
28. 0.12)2.15
29. 6.1)0.178
30. 17.2)2.59732
31. 0.135)0.2946732

Round to the nearer thousandth.

32. 0.003)172.0
33. 2.02)57.74
34. 0.09)14.78234

APPLICATIONS

When administering medications certain basic procedures are followed. These procedures ensure that the correct amount of medication is administered to the correct patient at the correct time.

When administering any type of medication, there are certain general considerations.

- Avoid handling the medications with the fingers. Use the cap of the container and a medicine glass when administering pills or capsules.
- Never try to divide a tablet that is not scored.
- When administering a part of a scored tablet, always throw away the unused part.
- While pouring a medication, take care not to contaminate the bottle.
- Never pour unused liquids back into the stock bottle or container.
- Always replace bottle caps after pouring the medicine.
- Check to see if the correct dose is being given. If the dose is not the same as what is ordered, calculate the correct dose.

8.4 EXERCISES

1. A patient receives this series of doses of medication: 1.25 millilitres; 0.5 millilitre; 2.125 millilitres; and 1 millilitre. What is the total dosage?

2. A total of 4.5 millilitres of medication is in a vial. An injection of 1.125 millilitres is withdrawn into a syringe. How much remains in the vial?

3. A container holds 12.5 millilitres of streptomycin sulfate. How many 1.25-millilitre doses can be administered from the container?

4. Fifteen people are each to receive 1.25-millilitre doses of streptomycin sulfate. How many millilitres of streptomycin sulfate are needed?

5. Small vials are purchased at a cost of $0.1062 each. Assuming no discount is given, how much does the clinic pay for 15 dozen vials of this size?

6. The hospital places a request for individual servings of meat. The supplier provides this meat at a cost of $0.4289 per serving. The cost of preparing and serving this meat to the patient is an additional $0.1364 per serving. What is the cost to the hospital for 250 servings of meat?

7. The mass of a patient is recorded over a thirty-day period at ten-day intervals.

    | Start | 88.904 kilograms |
    | 10th day | 87.772 kilograms |
    | 20th day | 86.592 kilograms |
    | 30th day | 84.036 kilograms |

    a. Find the mass loss over the 30-day period.
    b. If the loss occurs uniformly for each day, find the loss in mass for one 24-hour period. Round the answer to the nearer thousandth kilogram.
    c. Find the average mass for the four recorded masses. Average = total mass divided by number of recorded masses.

8. If 1.5 millilitres of an experimental drug is administered daily to each of 12 patients, how many millilitres of the drug will be used in 30 days?

9. You are to prepare 1,500 millilitres of an alcohol solution containing 0.3 ethyl alcohol and 0.7 distilled water.
    a. How many millilitres of distilled water will be used?
    b. How many millilitres of ethyl alcohol are used?

10. For a $5.00 fee, a person can receive a flu shot at a local clinic. It costs the clinic $0.50 per shot for the vaccine. Yesterday the clinic gave 178 people flu shots. What was the clinic's gross profit for the day?

unit 9 exponents and scientific notation

OBJECTIVES

After studying this unit the student should be able to:
- Multiply and divide powers of ten.
- Express numbers using scientific notation.
- Perform multiplication using scientific notation.

EXPONENTS

Numbers that are multiplied to find a product are <u>factors.</u>

Examples: $4 \times 5 = 20$
$4 \cdot 5 = 20$
$(4)\ (5) = 20$

Notice that three different symbols can be used to denote multiplication. These symbols will be used interchangeably to denote multiplication.

Examples: $(10)\ (10) = 100$
$10 \times 10 \times 10 = 1{,}000$
$10 \cdot 10 \cdot 10 \cdot 10 = 10{,}000$

Notice that in each case the factors are the same. The number 10 is used as a factor 2, 3, and 4 times respectively. Each product is a power of ten.

- ▼ A *power* is the product of two or more equal factors.
- ▼ A *base* is the number used as a factor.
- ▼ An *exponent* is the number of times the base is used as a factor.
- ▼ The mathematical notation for expressing exponential numbers is:

$$b^n = P$$

where b means the base; n means the exponent; and P means the product.

Example: 10^4

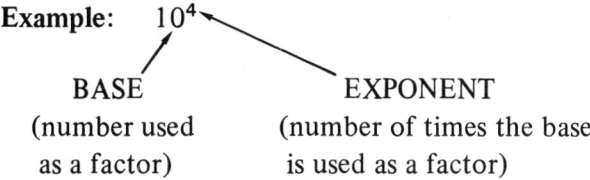

BASE
(number used as a factor)

EXPONENT
(number of times the base is used as a factor)

10^4 means $10 \cdot 10 \cdot 10 \cdot 10$ or $10,000$.
It is read "ten to the fourth power" or "the fourth power of ten."

Example: 6^3

BASE   EXPONENT
(number used as   (number of times the
a factor)   base is used as a factor)

6^3 means $6 \times 6 \times 6$ or 216.
It is read "six to the third power" or "the third power of six."
In the base ten place-value system, each place can be represented as a power of 10.

Example: The thousands place can be represented by 10^3. This means $10 \cdot 10 \cdot 10$ or $1,000$.

Example: The hundredths place can be represented by $\frac{1}{10^2}$. This means $\frac{1}{10} \times \frac{1}{10}$ or $\frac{1}{100}$.

The number $\frac{1}{10^2}$ can also be represented by 10^{-2}. This is read "ten to the negative second power." The negative number indicates that the product is a fraction.

▼ Any *negative exponent* may be expressed as:
$b^{-n} = \frac{1}{b^n}$, where n is any whole number and $b \neq 0$

Example: The units place can be represented by 10^0 or 1. It is read "ten to the zero power."

▼ Any number raised to the *zero power* is <u>one</u>.
This is expressed as:
$b^0 = 1$, where $b \neq 0$. The symbol 0^0 is undefined.

This chart illustrates the usage of powers of ten in the place-value system.

Place-Value Name	TEN THOUSANDS	THOUSANDS	HUNDREDS	TENS	UNITS	TENTHS	HUNDREDTHS	THOUSANDTHS	TEN-THOUSANDTHS
Powers Of Ten	10^4	10^3	10^2	10^1	10^0	10^{-1}	10^{-2}	10^{-3}	10^{-4}
Number The Power Represents	$10 \cdot 10 \cdot 10 \cdot 10$ = 10,000	$10 \cdot 10 \cdot 10$ = 1,000	$10 \cdot 10$ = 100	10	1	$\frac{1}{10}$ = $\frac{1}{10}$	$\frac{1}{10 \cdot 10}$ = $\frac{1}{100}$	$\frac{1}{10 \cdot 10 \cdot 10}$ = $\frac{1}{1,000}$	$\frac{1}{10 \cdot 10 \cdot 10 \cdot 10}$ = $\frac{1}{10,000}$

9.1 EXERCISES

Express each set of factors using exponents.

1. $4 \cdot 4$
2. $2 \cdot 2 \cdot 2 \cdot 2 \cdot 2$
3. $10 \cdot 10 \cdot 10 \cdot 10$
4. $9 \cdot 9 \cdot 9 \cdot 9$
5. $7 \cdot 7 \cdot 7$

Indicate each exponent.

6. 10^5
7. 2^3
8. 5^1
9. 10^9
10. 10^{100}

Determine the number or symbol ($<, >, =$) which makes each sentence true.

11. $16 = 2^n$
12. $b^4 = 256$
13. 1^5 __?__ 5^1
14. 0^4 __?__ 4^0
15. $5^n = 625$
16. $P = 8^2$
17. 8^0 __?__ 1
18. $27 = b^3$
19. $100^n = 1$
20. 2^4 __?__ 4^2

Use positive exponents to rewrite those expressions having negative exponents.
Use negative exponents to rewrite those expressions having positive exponents.

21. 10^{-3}
22. 7^{-1}
23. 4^{-5}
24. 10^{-4}
25. 8^{-2}
26. 5^{-3}
27. 9^{-6}
28. 10^{-10}
29. $\dfrac{1}{3^5}$
30. $\dfrac{1}{10^1}$
31. $\dfrac{1}{2^4}$
32. $\dfrac{1}{3^2}$
33. $\dfrac{1}{10^5}$
34. $\dfrac{1}{9^3}$
35. $\dfrac{1}{1{,}000^4}$
36. $\dfrac{1}{3^1}$

USING EXPONENTS IN MULTIPLICATION AND DIVISION

Multiplication and division of exponents use the same method as multiplication and division of whole numbers and powers of ten. The numbers being multiplied or divided must have the same base. The exponent form of the numbers is written using the base as the factors. Then, the multiplication or division is performed.

Example: $10^2 \cdot 10^3$

$10^2 \cdot 10^3 = (10 \cdot 10)(10 \cdot 10 \cdot 10)$

$(10 \cdot 10)(10 \cdot 10 \cdot 10) = 100{,}000$

$100{,}000 = 10^5$

Note: $10^2 \cdot 10^3 = 10^5$; the sum of the exponents, $2 + 3$ or 5, is the exponent in the answer. The numbers 10^2, 10^3, and 10^5 have the same base, 10.

Example: $10^3 \div 10^1$

$$10^3 \div 10^1 = \frac{10^3}{10^1}$$

$$\frac{10^3}{10} = \frac{10 \cdot 10 \cdot 10}{10}$$

$$\frac{\cancel{10}^1 \cdot 10 \cdot 10}{\cancel{10}_1} = 100$$

$$100 = 10^2$$

Note: $10^3 \div 10^1 = 10^2$; the difference of the exponents, 3 − 1 or 2, is the exponent in the answer. The numbers 10^3, 10^1, and 10^2 have the same base, 10.

Multiplication and division of numbers having exponents can be simplified by using the idea of adding and subtracting exponents.

▼ Multiplication of numbers having exponents can be expressed as:

$$b^x \cdot b^y = b^{x+y}$$

This means that in multiplication, when the bases are the same, the exponents are added. The exponent of the product is the sum of the exponents of the factors.

▼ Division of numbers having exponents can be expressed as:

$$b^x \div b^y = b^{x-y} \qquad \text{if } x > y$$

$$b^x \div b^y = \frac{1}{b^{y-x}} \qquad \text{if } y > x$$

$$b^x \div b^y = 1 \qquad \text{if } x = y$$

This means that in division, when the bases are the same, the exponents are subtracted. The exponent of the quotient is the difference of the exponents.

At times a number containing an exponent is raised to another power, such as $(10^3)^2$. This is read "ten to the third power raised to the second power." This means that the number 10^3 is raised to the second power. The value of this expression can be found by using the definition of exponents.

Example: $(10^3)^2$

$(10^3)^2 = (10 \cdot 10 \cdot 10)^2$

$(10 \cdot 10 \cdot 10)^2 = (10 \cdot 10 \cdot 10)(10 \cdot 10 \cdot 10)$

$(10 \cdot 10 \cdot 10)(10 \cdot 10 \cdot 10) = 1,000,000$

$1,000,000 = 10^6$

Note: $(10^3)^2 = 10^6$; the product of the exponents, 3 × 2 or 6, is the exponent in the answer.

▼ Raising a number containing an exponent to a power can be expressed as:
$$(b^x)^y = b^{x \cdot y}$$

This means that in raising a number containing an exponent to a power, multiplication is used. The exponent of the result is the product of the exponents.

9.2 EXERCISES

Find each product or quotient. Write each answer using exponents.

1. $10^1 \cdot 10^2$
2. $4^3 \cdot 4^3$
3. $6^{-4} \cdot 6^2$
4. $2^5 \cdot 2^{-5}$
5. $4^0 \cdot 4^3$
6. $10^{-2} \cdot 10^1$
7. $0.5^2 \cdot 0.5^1$
8. $(\frac{1}{2})^3 \cdot (\frac{1}{2})^2$
9. $0.3^{-2} \cdot 0.3^2$
10. $0.1^{-4} \cdot 0.1^1$
11. $3^4 \div 3^2$
12. $10^5 \div 10^5$
13. $2^4 \div 2^3$
14. $5^0 \div 5^2$
15. $0.7^3 \div 0.7^2$
16. $8^0 \div 8^0$
17. $10^3 \div 10^0$
18. $2^3 \div 2^4$
19. $10^3 \div 10^1$
20. $0.6^2 \div 0.6^2$
21. $(10^2)^2$
22. $(10^3)^1$
23. $(4^4)^2$
24. $(2^5)^2$
25. $(0.7^1)^0$

SCIENTIFIC NOTATION

Very large or very small numbers may be written as a product of a number from 1 to 10 (not including 10) and a power of ten. This number is then said to be expressed in scientific notation. The number is written with the decimal point after the first nonzero digit. The place value of the number is indicated by the power of ten.

Example: In scientific notation, the number 8.5 acquires different values depending on the power of ten.

NUMBER		SCIENTIFIC NOTATION
8,500.	$8.5 \times 1,000$	8.5×10^3
850.0	8.5×100	8.5×10^2
85.00	8.5×10	8.5×10^1
8.5	8.5×1	8.5×10^0
0.85	8.5×0.1	8.5×10^{-1}
0.085	8.5×0.01	8.5×10^{-2}
0.0085	8.5×0.001	8.5×10^{-3}

Section 2 Decimal Fractions

- To express a number in decimal form as a number in scientific notation:
  - Place the decimal point after the first nonzero number.
  - Determine the power of ten that is needed.

Example: Express 238,400 and 0.000597 in scientific notation.

$$238,400 = 2.384 \times 100,000 = 2.384 \times 10^5$$
$$0.000597 = 5.97 \times \frac{1}{10,000} = 5.97 \times 10^{-4}$$

- To express a number in scientific notation as a number in decimal form:
  - Determine the number that the power of ten represents.
  - Multiply the number that the power of ten represents by the number from 1 to 10.

Example: Express 6.203×10^4 and 7.13×10^{-5} in decimal form.

$$6.203 \times 10^4 = 6.203 \times 10,000 = 62,030$$
$$7.13 \times 10^{-5} = 7.13 \times \frac{1}{100,000} = 0.0000713$$

9.3 EXERCISES

Express in decimal form each number that is in scientific notation.
Express in scientific notation each number that is not in scientific notation.

1. 2.7×10^0
2. 3.8×10^{-1}
3. 1.45×10^2
4. 1.000×10^3
5. 3.7×10^1
6. 6.3×10^{-4}
7. 1.1×10^5
8. 342
9. 0.072
10. 20,000,000
11. 0.35×10^1
12. 0.062×10^2
13. 0.735×10^0
14. 3.7×10^0
15. 5.314×10^6
16. 6.17×10^{-2}
17. 41.8
18. 1,000
19. 0.173000
20. 54.2×10^2
21. 385×10^{-2}
22. 0.0579×10^2
23. 8.92×10^3
24. 6.15×10^{-3}
25. 2.73
26. 528,000
27. 4.08×10^5
28. 4.00×10^{-4}
29. 0.45
30. 0.00342

Using scientific notation facilitates multiplication. The place value, and the placement of decimal point is regulated by the powers of ten. Thus, the multiplication of the numbers and powers of ten can be done separately. All results are expressed using scientific notation. Multiplying the results indicates the place value of the answer.

Example: 500 × 5,000 or $(5 \times 10^2) \times (5 \times 10^3)$

$(5 \times 10^2) \times (5 \times 10^3)$

$(5 \times 5) \times (10^2 \times 10^3)$

25   × 10^5

$(2.5 \times 10^1) \times 10^5$

2.5×10^6 =   2,500,000

Note: The process of multiplication using exponents is shown here. The multiplication is $10^2 \times 10^3 = 10^{2+3}$ or 10^5. The number 25 is expressed in scientific notation. This leads to the final answer of 2,500,000.

Example: 0.003 × 600,000 or $(3 \times 10^{-3}) \times (6 \times 10^5)$

$(3 \times 10^{-3}) \times (6 \times 10^5)$

$(3 \times 6) \times (10^{-3} \times 10^5)$

$18 \times \dfrac{10^5}{10^3}$

18×10^2

$(1.8 \times 10^1) \times 10^2$

1.8   × 10^3 =   1,800

Note: The process of division using exponents is shown here. The power of ten, 10^{-3}, is expressed as $\dfrac{1}{10^3}$. Then $\dfrac{10^5}{10^3}$ is divided. The division is $\dfrac{10^5}{10^3} = 10^{5-3}$ or 10^2. The number 18 is expressed in scientific notation. This leads to the final answer of 1,800.

Example: 400×0.00007 or $(4 \times 10^2) \times (7 \times 10^{-5})$

$(4 \times 10^2) \times (7 \times 10^{-5})$

$(4 \times 7) \times (10^2 \times 10^{-5})$

$28 \times \dfrac{10^2}{10^5}$

$(2.8 \times 10^1) \times \dfrac{1}{10^3}$

$2.8 \times \dfrac{10}{10^3}$

$2.8 \times \dfrac{1}{10^2}$

$2.8 \times 10^{-2} \qquad = \qquad 0.028$

Example: 0.03×0.07 or $3 \times 10^{-2} \times 7 \times 10^{-2}$

$(3 \times 10^{-2}) \times (7 \times 10^{-2})$

$(3 \times 7) \times (10^{-2} \times 10^{-2})$

$21 \times \dfrac{1}{10^2 \cdot 10^2}$

$(2.1 \times 10^1) \times \dfrac{1}{10^4}$

$2.1 \times \dfrac{10^1}{10^4}$

$2.1 \times \dfrac{1}{10^3}$

$2.1 \times 10^{-3} \qquad = \qquad 0.0021$

9.4 EXERCISES

Find each product. Express the answer using scientific notation and place-value notation.

1. $4 \times 10^2 \times 5 \times 10^3$
2. $8 \times 10^2 \times 7 \times 10^0$
3. 900×0.07
4. $4 \times 10^0 \times 6 \times 10^2$
5. $3 \times 10^{-1} \times 2 \times 10^{-2}$
6. 0.08×0.003
7. $9 \times 10^{-3} \times 8 \times 10^5$
8. $60,000 \times 0.000008$

APPLICATIONS

The prevention and the control of disease are a major function of every health care person. Diseases are caused by microorganisms. The study of microorganisms is microbiology. The microbiologist studies the cause and effect of microorganisms and disease and applies this knowledge to medicine.

By definition, *microbiology* means the study of simple forms of living matter which cannot be seen by the naked eye. This "smallness" has brought about new units of measure. These units are expressed by using powers of ten and exponents.

metre	1×10^0 metre
centimetre	1×10^{-2} metre
millimetre	1×10^{-3} metre
micrometre	1×10^{-6} metre
nanometre	1×10^{-9} metre
picometre	1×10^{-12} metre

Microorganisms are usually measured in micrometres. For example, a bacteria may be 0.002 micrometre long. Using scientific notation, this measure would be 2×10^{-3} micrometre or 2×10^{-9} metre ($2 \times 10^{-3} \cdot 1 \times 10^{-6}$).

9.5 EXERCISES

1. *Protozoa* are the cause of various types of malaria. Other species are responsible for amoebic dysentery. Protozoa range from 3 to 1 000 micrometres.
    a. Express this range in scientific notation using micrometres as the unit of measure.
    b. Express this range in scientific notation using metres as the unit of measure.

2. *Viruses* — the smallest infectious agents — invade the cell, increase in number, and then break through the cell wall and discharge more virus particles into the bloodstream. Smallpox, chickenpox, infectious hepatitis and German measles are among the diseases caused by viruses. Viruses range from $\frac{1}{2\,500}$ micrometre to $\frac{1}{50\,000}$ micrometre.
    a. Express this range in decimals using micrometres as the unit of measure.
    b. Express this range in scientific notation using micrometres as the unit of measure.

3. *Yeast* is a spherical-shaped or oval-shaped plant cell. Yeast is a rich source of vitamin B and is used in making bread and beer. By fermentation, it is also responsible for the spoilage of fruits, syrups, and jellies. The average dimensions of a yeast are 3 to 5 micrometres wide and 5 to 10 micrometres long.
    a. Express these dimensions in scientific notation using micrometres as the unit of measure.
    b. Express these dimensions in decimals using metres as the unit of measure.

4. *Bacteria* are the smallest living things that can be called "living." Nonpathogenic bacteria are helpful and useful bacteria. The curing of tobacco, tea, coffee, cocoa, and leather as well as the making of sauerkraut, vinegar, and cheese are among the accomplishments of bacteria. Pathogenic bacteria, commonly called *germs,* invade plant and animal tissue and are the cause of a multitude of diseases. The average length of a bacteria is $\frac{1}{1\,000}$ micrometre.

   a. Express this length in scientific notation using micrometres as the unit of measure.

   b. Using division, determine how many times larger a bacteria is than the smallest virus. Viruses range from $\frac{1}{2\,500}$ micrometre to $\frac{1}{50\,000}$ micrometre.

5. Bacterial growth is the greatest cause of infectious disease. The greatest defense against bacteria is aseptic procedures, sterilization, disinfection, and isolation techniques. One bacteria cell can become 256 000 cells within 8 generations. Express this new number of cells using scientific notation.

6. Several microorganisms have been measured. Express each of the following values in scientific notations.

   a. 0.0000136
   b. 0.0002893
   c. 0.004682
   d. 0.000000368
   e. 0.0003010
   f. 0.009000

7. Give the decimal value of the following scientific notations.

   a. 1.963×10^{-8}
   b. 4.6×10^{5}
   c. 9.3×10^{1}
   d. 9.3×10^{-1}

unit 10 estimation and significant digits

OBJECTIVES

After studying this unit the student should be able to:

- Estimate products and quotients.
- Round numbers to the indicated significant digit.
- Perform operations with numbers using the process of retention of significant digits.

ESTIMATION

Estimating products and quotients is an important skill in today's calculator world. Estimation involves rounding the numbers to a defined place.

Example: Rounding several numbers to various places is shown in these charts.

NUMBER	ROUNDED TO THE NEARER WHOLE NUMBER	ROUNDED TO THE NEARER TENTH
2.371	2	2.4
6.94	7	6.9
38.5	39	38.5
0.82	1	0.8
0.097	0	0.1

NUMBER	ROUNDED TO THE NEARER HUNDREDTH	ROUNDED TO THE NEARER THOUSANDTH
3.7218	3.72	3.722
0.9706	0.97	0.971
51.0519	51.05	51.052
7.5254	7.53	7.525
19.6108	19.61	19.612

82 Section 2 Decimal Fractions

The rounded numbers are used in performing multiplication or division. The resulting product or quotient is an approximation.

Example: 3.12 × 4.78
3.12 (rounded to nearer whole number) ≈ 3
4.78 (rounded to nearer whole number) ≈ × 5
Therefore, 3.12 × 4.78 ≈ 15

Example: 0.0672 × 6.73
0.0672 (rounded to nearer hundredth) ≈ 0.07
6.73 (rounded to nearer whole number) ≈ × 7
Therefore, 0.0672 × 6.73 ≈ 0.49

Example: 937.82 ÷ 6.39
937.82 (rounded to nearer hundred) ≈ 900/6 = 150
6.39 (rounded to nearer whole number) ≈ 6
Therefore, 937.82 ÷ 6.39 ≈ 150

Example: 3.12 ÷ 4.3
3.12 (rounded to nearer hundredth) ≈ 3.12/4 = 0.78
4.3 (rounded to nearer whole number) ≈ 4
Therefore, 3.12 ÷ 4.3 ≈ 0.78

10.1 EXERCISES

Round each factor as indicated. Using the rounded numbers, estimate each product.

Round the First Factor to the Nearer Whole Number.
Round the Second Factor to the Nearer Whole Number.

1. 7.3 × 9.6
2. 5 × 19.7
3. 0.82 × 3.613
4. 24.67 × 39.78
5. 379.7 × 19.81
6. 100.3 × 0.82
7. 0.98 × 12.302
8. 65 × 10.78
9. 249.75 × 30.2
10. 0.75 × 36.2

Round the First Factor to the Nearer Tenth.
Round the Second Factor to the Nearer Whole Number.

11. 3.17 × 14.5
12. 0.23 × 40.32
13. 0.067 × 319.76
14. 0.3152 × 17.3
15. 2.19 × 3.782

Round The First Factor to the Nearer Hundredth.
Round the Second Factor to the Nearer Whole Number.

16. 42.789 × 3.14
17. 19.207 × 9.93
18. 713.035 × 99.9
19. 47.0765 × 4.61
20. 0.6132 × 59.75

Round the dividend and divisor as indicated. Using the rounded numbers, estimate each quotient.

Round the Divisor to the Nearer Whole Number.
Round the Dividend to the Nearer Whole Number.

21. 32.1 ÷ 15.8
22. 191.7 ÷ 64.1
23. 15.3 ÷ 4.8
24. 80.93 ÷ 9.1
25. 453.12 ÷ 0.87
26. 399.73 ÷ 19.6
27. 53.67 ÷ 3.1
28. 43.5 ÷ 10.6
29. 1,023.71 ÷ 3.92
30. 87.6 ÷ 1.95

Round the Divisor to the Nearer Tenth.
Round the Dividend to the Nearer Whole Number.

31. 31.04 ÷ 6.24
32. 51.68 ÷ 2.62
33. 65.75 ÷ 2.19
34. 76.61 ÷ 1.134
35. 499.782 ÷ 2.54

Round the Divisor to the Nearer Hundredth.
Round the Dividend to the Nearer Whole Number.

36. 176.7318 ÷ 10.004
37. 146.9067 ÷ 0.074
38. 6.18102 ÷ 3.00157
39. 15.3126 ÷ 0.047
40. 2,174.8962 ÷ 0.0479

SIGNIFICANT DIGITS

Often, results of measurements are estimated and rounded to different degrees of accuracy. In measuring, there are some distances which are certain and some that are estimated.

Example: What is the indicated distance between the arrows?

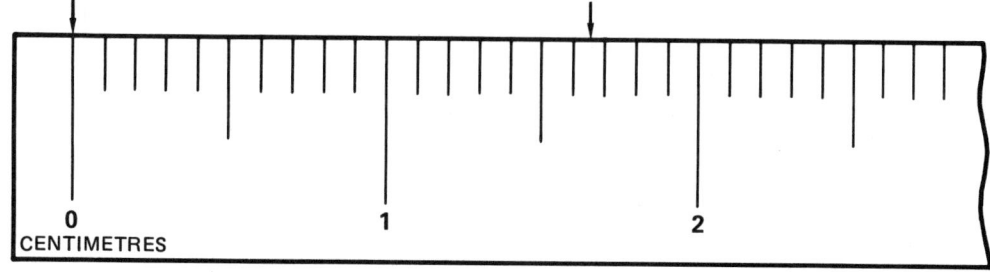

It is certain that the distance is between 1 and 2 centimetres.
It is certain that the distance is between 1.6 and 1.7 centimetres.
It is uncertain what the next reading is. It may be 1.65 centimetres, 1.66 centimetres, or even 1.67 centimetres. In this measurement two digits are certain and one is uncertain. The three digits are called significant digits. *Significant digits* are digits which indicate the number of units that are reasonably sure of having been counted in making a measurement.

- When taking a measurement, the significant digits include:
  - all the digits which are sure, plus
  - one digit which is estimated.

Significant digits are important for finding the product or quotient of approximations. Certain rules are followed when determining how many significant digits a number contains.

- All non-zero digits are significant.
  These numbers have 4, 4, 2, and 5 significant digits, respectively.
  9,763   97.63   4.5   5.4889

- All zeros between significant digits are significant.
  Each of these numbers has 5 significant digits.
  59,002   350.7   99.009   3.0007

- All final zeros to the right of the decimal point are significant.
  These numbers have 4, 4, 5, and 7 significant digits, respectively.
  523.0   28.00   5.5000   11.80000

- If a numeral names a whole number greater than 1 and a decimal point follows the final zero, all zeros are significant.
  These numbers have 2, 3, 4, and 5 significant digits, respectively.
  30.   560.   6,000.   82,000.

- If a numeral names a whole number greater than 1 and no decimal point follows the final zero, the final zeros are not significant.
  Each of these numbers has 2 significant digits. The significant digits are underlined.
  760   9800   88,000   120,000

- If a numeral names a number between 0 and 1, the initial zeros are not significant.
  These numbers have 1, 2, 3, and 1 significant digits, respectively. The significant digits are underlined.
  0.08   0.0081   0.00760   0.00004

- If a number is written in proper scientific notation, all digits are significant except those in the power.
  These numbers have 3, 2, and 4 significant digits, respectively. The significant digits are underlined.
  1.64×10^{-19} 9.7×10^3 6.495×10^7

Note: Zeros representing nonsignificant digits are placeholders stating how large or small the number is.

10.2 EXERCISES

Indicate the number of significant digits for each number.

1. 634
2. 50.037
3. 730
4. 3.14
5. 0.2001
6. 207
7. 0.0278
8. 61.359
9. 0.0319
10. 50.0

Round to the indicated number of significant digits.

Three Significant Digits

11. 5,293
12. 3.7800
13. 7,969
14. 13.489
15. 16.8
16. 14.55
17. 31.708
18. 2.0007
19. 309.09
20. 1.4365

One Significant Digit

21. 217.8
22. 0.07681
23. 37,562
24. 93.82
25. 0.3709
26. 0.00051
27. 2.50
28. 0.000432
29. 4,500,781
30. 0.667

RETENTION OF SIGNIFICANT DIGITS

- Retain as many significant digits in data and results as will give only one uncertain digit.

Example: On reading a burette, the number 15.34 is recorded.

All figures are significant since 15.3 represents actual scale divisions and the 4 represents an estimation between two scale divisions and is the only digit which is uncertain. Another analyst may read this same setting as 15.33 or 15.35.

- To have all of its digits significant, every digit of a number except the last must be correct.

Example: The number 62.73 has four significant digits. The 6, 2, and 7 are correct and the 3 states that the number is closer to 3 hundredths. If the numbers 62.725 or 62.734 are rounded to four significant digits, the result would be 62.73.

- In retaining significant digits, all numbers are rounded to the number which has the least number of significant digits.

Example: The numbers 2.78, 6,282, and 0.5096 are rounded to 3 significant digits.

NUMBER	ROUNDED TO 3 SIGNIFICANT DIGITS
2.78	2.78
6,282	6,280
0.5096	0.510

Example: The numbers 2,457, 0.057, and 378 are rounded to 1 significant digit.

NUMBER	ROUNDED TO 1 SIGNIFICANT DIGIT
2,457	2,000
0.057	0.06
378	400

RETENTION OF SIGNIFICANT DIGITS IN ADDITION AND SUBTRACTION

- In adding or subtracting numbers, the accuracy of the answer is in the column where the uncertain digit has the greatest place value.

Example: 0.0457 + 37.82 + 9.36942

```
  0.0457        The uncertain digits are underlined.
 37.82          The uncertain digit 2 in the number
+ 9.369642      37.82 has the greatest place value of
                the uncertain digits.
```

```
  0.05          The digit 2 in 37.82 has a place value
 37.82          of hundredths.
+ 9.37          Round the numbers to the nearer hundredth.
 -----
 47.24          Add the numbers.
```

The result, 47.24, is accurate to the nearer hundredth.

Example: 96 − 35.8

```
  96            The uncertain digits are underlined.
− 35.8          The uncertain digit 6 in the number 96 has the
                greater place value.
```

```
  96            The digit 6 in 96 has a place value of units.
− 36            Round the numbers to the nearer unit.
 ----
  60.           Subtract the numbers.
```

Placing a decimal point in the answer 60 shows that there are two significant digits in the result.

RETENTION OF SIGNIFICANT DIGITS IN MULTIPLICATION AND DIVISION

- For practical purposes, in multiplying and dividing numbers with differing numbers of digits, retain as many significant figures as are found in the number having the least number of significant digits.

Example: 35.19 × 0.0451 × 4.0787

    35.19   ×   0.0451   ×   4.0787

     4   3   5   SIGNIFICANT DIGITS

Since 0.0451 has the least number of significant digits, round all numbers to 3 significant digits.

35.2 × 0.0451 × 4.08 = 6.4770816; rounds to 6.48

The product, 6.48, is also rounded to 3 significant digits.

Note: When computing with a calculator, retain all digits and round only the final result. In manual computation, retain as many digits as are plausible, then round the final result. This procedure will ensure the proper accuracy.

10.3 EXERCISES

Perform the indicated operations using the process of retaining significant digits.

1.   3.073
       4.28
   + 9.7654

2.   1.8972
   + 0.913

3.   89.7
     14.000
   + 9.302

4.   325.7
     141.72
   +   0.983

5.   29.573
   − 13.84

6.   42.5
   − 27

7.   18.203
   − 7.6

8.   1.7392
   − 0.706

9.   30 × 0.049

10.   71.32
   × 4.814

11. 0.712 × 0.014

12. 15.0 × 7.53

13. 0.4200 ÷ 179

14. 0.1492 ÷ 3,000

15. 1.542 ÷ 71.9

16. 0.0004 ÷ 0.0018

APPLICATIONS

Estimation should never be used when calculating the amount of medication to be administered, the amount of a drug to be added to a liquid, or the amount of liquid to be used with a drug. Estimation does aid the health care worker in judging how much drug, solution, or other substances will be needed. It will prevent unneeded preparations of solutions and incomplete procedures due to a lack of a needed ingredient.

Estimation is a "foresight." It also serves as a check on the calculations that may be necessary to prepare a solution.

The amount of accuracy needed is dependent upon the purpose of the procedure and the measuring instruments that are to be used. For this reason, numbers cannot simply be "dropped." Even a small quantity such as 0.000 08 gram may be meaningful. Expressing measurements using scientific notation aids in determining significant digits and accuracy. This practice may save a life or help to avoid a death.

10.4 EXERCISES

1. A group of researchers each conducted independent studies on determining the size of a pathogenic bacterium. The average length from each researcher is:

    Researcher A   0.001 63 micrometre
    Researcher B   0.001 542 1 micrometre
    Researcher C   0.001 491 micrometre
    Researcher D   0.001 5 micrometre

    Since Researcher **D** provided a measurement only accurate to the nearer ten-thousandth, this becomes the level of significance for all the measurements.

    a. Round the measurements to the nearer ten-thousandth micrometre.
    b. Find the average measurement by adding the four measurements and dividing by four. Round the answer to the nearer ten-thousandth micrometre.

2. A 2.2-litre flask of thiamine assay medium contains 40 grams of dextrose; 0.000 000 8 gram of biotin; 0.02 gram of manganese sulfate; plus other substances. To find the number of grams of each substance present in 1.5 litres of the medium perform the indicated operations. Round each answer to three significant digits.

    a. dextrose: $\frac{1.5}{2.2} \times 40$

    b. biotin: $\frac{1.5}{2.2} \times 0.000\ 000\ 8$

    c. manganese sulfate: $\frac{1.5}{2.2} \times 0.02$

3. A laboratory technician is asked to weigh a specimen provided from the surgical team. The mass is determined to be 12.342 6 grams. A second technician finds the mass to be 12.342 4 grams. A third technician weighs the specimen and records the mass as 12.342 9 grams. Find the average of the recorded masses by adding the three masses and dividing by three. Round the answer to the nearer ten-thousandth gram.

4. The acceptable adult dose of a specific medication is determined to be 0.4 millilitre. A technician is requested to divide a 25-millilitre volume into equal adult doses. Estimate the number of adult doses available.

unit 11 section two applications to health work

OBJECTIVES

After studying this unit the student should be able to:

- Use the basic principles of decimal numbers to solve health work problems.

Every person who is involved in the health care field is dedicated to a common goal — the patient. Moreover, the patient is the whole reason and the very fact for having health care workers. Technicians, technologists, physicians, nurses, and assistants are involved with the "well-being" of the patient.

Laboratory technicians and technologists, in particular, have a significant responsibility to the prevention, diagnosis, and treatment of diseases and illness. The medical laboratory data constitute the bulk of quantitative and objective information about the patient. Errors in computation or in measurement may be fatal. Remember the cause of death could be: MISPLACED DECIMAL. For this reason, it is essential for all health care workers to concentrate on quality control.

- *Quality control* means applying all possible means to guarantee that laboratory findings, administration of medications, and all other health care procedures are reliable and valid. The elements of quality control in the health care field include:

  - *Having a positive and helpful attitude.* Health care workers should not assume that they "know it all." Rather, checking results and seeking advice or assistance when in doubt is the route to follow.

  - *Having a thorough knowledge of health care work principles.* Health care workers should have sound judgment about the proficiency in their particular area.

  - *Checking the equipment for accuracy.* Health care workers should realize that equipment does not maintain its standardization or calibration forever. The time taken to check the equipment may save a life.

  - *Setting standards.* Health care workers should concentrate on labeling solutions, medications, and other items and tools. They should also concentrate on not destroying these standards by being unconcerned or careless. A mislabeled bottle may have grave results.

  - *Calculating with care.* Careless arithmetical errors are one of the most common sources of error. These errors are needless and the carelessness may be fatal.

11.1 EXERCISES

1. A laboratory assistant is asked to prepare dextrose agar. The substances will be dissolved in distilled water to make 500 millilitres of solution. The substances are: beef extract, 1.5 grams; dextrose, 5 grams; tryptose, 5 grams; sodium chloride, 2.5 grams; agar, 7.5 grams. What is the total mass of the ingredients that are to be dissolved?

2. A laboratory assistant prepares a 0.25-preparation of Czapek solution agar. A 1.0-preparation contains: saccharose, 30 grams; sodium nitrate, 2 grams; dipotassium phosphate, 1 gram; magnesium sulfate, 0.5 gram; potassium chloride, 0.5 gram; ferrous sulfate, 0.01 gram; agar, 15 grams. This is dissolved in distilled water to make a 1 000-millilitre solution. Find the mass of each substance in a 0.25-preparation.

   a. saccharose
   b. sodium nitrate
   c. dipotassium phosphate
   d. magnesium sulfate
   e. potassium chloride
   f. ferrous sulfate
   g. agar

3. A 5-gram container of potassium chloride is purchased for bacteriological work. Each culture medium requires 0.25 gram of potassium chloride. How many culture media will the 5-gram container supply?

4. The liquid output for an individual is 2.679 litres on Monday and 3.168 litres on Tuesday. Round each answer to the nearer thousandth.

   a. What is the total output for the two days?
   b. What was the average output for the two days?

   Note: average = $\frac{\text{total output}}{\text{two days}}$

   c. How many times greater is the output on Tuesday than on Monday?

5. A patient is prescribed 2.5 grams of medication. One gram is equal to 15.432 4 grains. How many grains of medication does the patient receive?

6. For each meal, a patient eats 85.05 grams of meat. How many grams of meat are eaten in six meals?

7. To determine the average length of microorganisms, several microorganisms are measured. The measurements are:

0.018 millimicron	0.193 millimicron
0.020 millimicron	0.191 millimicron
0.017 millimicron	0.179 millimicron
0.018 millimicron	0.183 millimicron
0.018 millimicron	0.188 millimicron

   Using the formula: average = total ÷ number of measurements, find the average length. Round the answer to the nearer thousandth.

8. A *manometer* is used to determine the rate at which oxygen is used by a bacteria culture. This rate is measured at 30-minute intervals and recorded in chart form.

INTERVAL	AMOUNT OF OXYGEN USED	INCREASE OR DECREASE OF OXYGEN
First 30-minute interval	1.275 625 millilitres	---
Second 30-minute interval	1.373 75 millilitres	?
Third 30-minute interval	1.413 millilitres	?
Fourth 30-minute interval	1.334 5 millilitres	?
Fifth 30-minute interval	1.775 millilitres	?

a. What is the total oxygen used during all the intervals?
b. Which interval shows the greatest increase in the use of oxygen?
c. What is the greatest increase in the use of oxygen?
d. Which interval shows the least change in the use of oxygen?
e. What is the smallest increase in the use of oxygen?
f. In which interval was there a decrease in the amount of oxygen used?
g. What is the amount of decrease?

9. A storage container holds 9.750 litres of ethyl alcohol.

a. If 150 millilitres, 200 millilitres, 100 millilitres, 1 000 millilitres, and 2 500 millilitres are removed from the container, how many litres of alcohol remain?
Note: 1 litre = 1 000 millilitres
b. In the morning, the 9.750-litre container has 4.250 litres in it. If an additional 3.125 litres are poured in, what is the total?
c. How much alcohol could be stored in 7 of these storage containers?
d. How much alcohol can be stored in a container that is 0.65 the size of the 9.750-litre container?

10. At a certain hospital, eight babies are born during a one-month period. Their masses are: 4.348 kilograms; 4.892 kilograms; 4.621 kilograms; 4.485 kilograms; 4.213 kilograms; 4.077 kilograms; 3.397 kilograms; and 3.533 kilograms.

a. What is the mass of the largest baby born during this month?
b. What is the mass of the smallest baby born during this month?
c. What is the average mass of the babies born during the one-month period? Round the answer to the nearer thousandth.
Note: average = total mass ÷ number of babies

11. It takes 79 millilitres of wax to cover 1 square metre of floor tile. How many millilitres of wax are needed to wax a room 18.183 metres long and 12.89 metres wide?
Note: area = length X width; round the answer to the nearer thousandth square metre.

12. When operating at full capacity, a heating unit consumes 25.693 litres of fuel per hour.

   a. If operated at this level, how many litres will be burned in a 24-hour period?

   b. Assuming that the heating unit must continue to operate at full capacity, what size storage tank must be used to ensure a 10-day supply?

13. The excreted urine is monitored for a patient over a 12-hour period. During the same period of time, liquid intake is also measured. Following is the results of this monitoring process.

	LIQUID INTAKE	URINE EXCRETED
0 hours	250 millilitres	0 millilitres
2 hours	100 millilitres	100 millilitres
4 hours	50 millilitres	75 millilitres
6 hours	125 millilitres	50 millilitres
8 hours	75 millilitres	50 millilitres
10 hours	75 millilitres	25 millilitres
12 hours	0 millilitres	25 millilitres

   a. Find, in millilitres, the total liquid intake.

   b. Find, in millilitres, the total urine excreted.

   c. What can be concluded about the patient?

14. A weight-loss clinic has several patients on a weight-loss program. In one week the following losses are recorded for four patients:

   PATIENT 1 (2.938 kilograms), PATIENT 2 (3.891 kilograms), PATIENT 3 (1.216 kilograms), and PATIENT 4 (0.112 kilograms).

   a. What is the average loss for these four patients?

   b. What is the total mass lost by the four patients?

SI METRICS STYLE GUIDE

SI metrics is derived from the French name Le Systeme International d'Unités. The metric unit names are already in accepted practice. SI metrics attempts to standardize the names and usages so that students of metrics will have a universal knowledge of the application of terms, symbols, and units.

The English system of mathematics (used in the United States) has always had many units in its weights and measures tables which were not applied to everyday use. For example, the pole, perch, furlong, peck, and scruple are not used often. The measurements, however, are used to form other measurements and it has been necessary to include the measurements in the tables. Including these measurements aids in the understanding of the orderly sequence of measurements greater or smaller than the less frequently used units.

The metric system also has units that are not used in everyday application. Only by learning the lesser-used units is it possible to understand the order of the metric system. SI metrics, however, places an emphasis on the most frequently used units.

In using the metric system and writing its symbols, certain guidelines are followed. For the student's reference, some of the guidelines are listed.

1. In using the symbols for metric units, the first letter is capitalized only if it is derived from the name of a person.

SAMPLE:

UNIT	SYMBOL	UNIT	SYMBOL
metre	m	newton	N (named after Sir Isaac Newton)
gram	g	degree Celsius	°C (named after Anders Celsius)

EXCEPTION: The symbol for litre is L. This is used to distinguish it from the number one (1).

2. Prefixes are written with lowercase letters.

SAMPLE:

PREFIX	UNIT	SYMBOL
centi	metre	cm
milli	gram	mg

EXCEPTIONS:

PREFIX	UNIT	SYMBOL
tera	metre	Tm (used to distinguish it from the metric tonne, t)
giga	metre	Gm (used to distinguish it from gram, g)
mega	gram	Mg (used to distinguish it from milli, m)

3. Periods are not used in the symbols. Symbols for units are the same in the singular and the plural (no "s" is added to indicate a plural).

SAMPLE: 1 mm *not* 1 mm. 3 mm *not* 3 mms

4. When referring to a unit of measurement, symbols are not used. The symbol is used only when a number is associated with it.

SAMPLE: The length of the room is expressed in metres. *not* The length of the room is expressed in m. (*The length of the room is 25 m* is correct.)

5. When writing measurements that are less than one, a zero is written before the decimal point.

SAMPLE: 0.25 m *not* .25 m

6. Separate the digits in groups of three, counting from the decimal point to the left and to the right. A space is left between the groups of digits.

SAMPLE: 5 179 232 mm *not* 5,179,232 mm   0.566 23 mg *not* 0.56623 mg   1 346.098 7 L *not* 1,346.0987 L

A space is also left between the digits and the unit of measure.

SAMPLE: 5 179 232 mm *not* 5 179 232 mm

7. Symbols for area measure and volume measure are written with exponents.

SAMPLE: 3 cm^2 *not* 3 sq. cm   4 km^3 *not* 4 cu. km

8. Metric words with prefixes are accented on the first syllable. In particular, kilometre is pronounced "kill'-o-metre." This avoids confusion with words for measuring devices which are generally accented on the second syllable, such as thermometer (ther-mom'-e-ter).

SECTION 3 METRIC MEASURE

unit 12 introduction to metric measure

OBJECTIVES

After studying this unit the student should be able to:

- Identify the base units of measure for length and mass.
- Identify the derived unit of measure for volume.
- Identify metric measures in terms of magnitude.
- Express equivalences for metric measure.

THE MEASURING PROCESS

To measure an object, compare it to a predetermined unit of measure and assign a number in relationship to this standard unit.

- The process of measuring an object consists of:
  - Selecting a unit.
  - Dividing the object into units.
  - Counting the number of units in the object.
  - The number of units is the measure of the object.

Example: Two health career students measure a piece of gauze. Chit measures the width of the gauze and finds the width to be 6 index fingers.

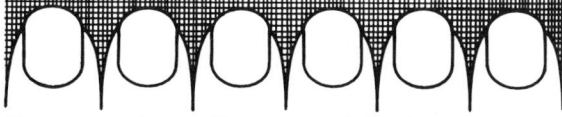

Sara measures the same piece of gauze and finds the width to be 9 index fingers.

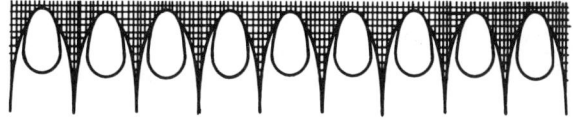

Since very few index fingers are exactly the same width, using the index finger as a unit of measure is unsatisfactory. To have a useful system, there must be uniform or standard units of measure. Among the many systems of measure is the International System of Units — the metric system.

METRIC MEASURE AND THE PLACE-VALUE SYSTEM.

The metric system is a system of measure which uses the base 10, or the decimal system of numeration. The decimal system uses grouping by tens. Since there are only ten digits in the decimal system, 0; 1; 2; 3; 4; 5; 6; 7; 8; 9, two or more digits are used when expressing a number that is larger than nine.

Each digit in a number has place value associated with it. The place values are powers of ten.

Place-value	Thousands	Hundreds	Tens	Units	Tenths	Hundredths	Thousandths
Meaning	1 000	100	10	1	0.1	0.01	0.001
Power of 10	10^3	10^2	10^1	10^0	10^{-1}	10^{-2}	10^{-3}

Example: Illustrate each place value for 5 237.806.

THOUSANDS	HUNDREDS	TENS	UNITS	.	TENTHS	HUNDREDTHS	THOUSANDTHS
5	2	3	7	.	8	0	6

Since the metric system is based upon powers of ten, it is important to be able to mentally multiply by a power of ten.

Example: Mentally multiply 23.57 × 100.

Count the number of zeros in the power of ten.

100

2 zeros

Move the decimal point of the number to the right this same number of zeros.

23.57.

23.57 × 100 = 2 357

Note: The number 100 = 10^2. The exponent, 2, determines the number of places to the right that the decimal point is moved.

Example: Mentally multiply 23.57 × 0.01.

Count the number of places to the right of the decimal point in the power of ten.

0.01

2 decimal places

Move the decimal point of the number to the left this same number of decimal places.

.23̮57

23.57 × 0.01 = 0.235 7

Note: The decimal $0.01 = 10^{-2}$. The exponent, $^-2$, determines the number of places to the left that the decimal point is moved.

12.1 EXERCISES

Mentally, multiply the numbers by the powers of ten.

	1 000	100	10	Number	0.1	0.01	0.001
1.				6.28			
2.				0.913			
3.				57.194			
4.				0.07			
5.				371.721 5			

	10^{-3}	10^{-2}	10^{-1}	Number	10^1	10^2	10^3
6.				37.594			
7.				0.816 3			
8.				407.38			
9.				0.003 57			

UNITS OF MEASURE AND PREFIXES

In the metric system, the three kinds of units are:

- base units
- supplementary units
- derived units

Two of the base units are the quantity of length measure and the quantity of mass measure. The base unit for length measure is the metre (m). The base unit for mass measure is the kilogram (kg). A kilogram is equal to 1 000 grams. For purposes of comparison, the gram (g) will be used.

One of the derived units is the quantity of volume measure. The derived unit for volume measure for fluids is the litre (L) and for solids it is the cubic centimetre (cm^3).

Other units of measure are multiples and sub-multiples of the base or derived units. Every metric measure is a power of ten of the base or derived units. Thus, the metric system is sometimes defined as the decimal system of weights and measures.

Different Greek and Latin prefixes are used as names for the powers of ten. This expansion of the place-value chart shows these prefixes and the meanings.

Place-value	Thousands	Hundreds	Tens	Units	Tenths	Hundredths	Thousandths
Meaning	1 000	100	10	1	0.1	0.01	0.001
Power of 10	10^3	10^2	10^1	10^0	10^{-1}	10^{-2}	10^{-3}
Metric Prefix	kilo	hecto	deka	unit of measurement	deci	centi	milli

To write a measure in the metric system, a prefix and a basic metric unit are combined.

Example: Using the metre and the appropriate prefixes, equivalences can be formed.

1 000 metres	=	1 kilometre
100 metres	=	1 hectometre
10 metres	=	1 dekametre
0.1 metre	=	1 decimetre
0.01 metre	=	1 centimetre
0.001 metre	=	1 millimetre

12.2 EXERCISES

Find each equivalence.

1. 1 thousand = __?__ hundreds
2. 1 hundred = __?__ tens
3. 1 ten = __?__ units
4. 1 unit = __?__ tenths
5. 1 tenth = __?__ hundredths
6. 1 hundred = __?__ thousandths
7. 1 hundred = __?__ thousand

8. 1 ten = __?__ hundred
9. 1 unit = __?__ ten
10. 1 tenth = __?__ unit
11. 1 hundredth = __?__ tenth
12. 1 thousandth = __?__ hundredth

Complete this chart to show the ranking of 1 centilitre, 1 decilitre, 1 dekalitre, 1 hectolitre, 1 kilolitre, 1 litre, and 1 millilitre from largest to smallest. Then indicate the equivalent litre measure.

	VOLUME MEASURE FROM LARGEST TO SMALLEST	EQUIVALENCE
13.		__?__ = 1 000 litres
14.		
15.		
16.	1 litre	1 litre = 1 litre
17.		
18.	1 centilitre	
19.		1 millilitre = __?__

Complete this chart to show the ranking of 1 centigram, 1 decigram, 1 dekagram, 1 gram, 1 hectogram, 1 kilogram, and 1 milligram from smallest to largest. Then indicate the equivalent gram measure.

	MASS MEASURE FROM SMALLEST TO LARGEST	EQUIVALENCE
20.		
21.		
22.		
23.	1 gram	1 gram = 1 gram
24.		
25.		
26.		

APPLICATIONS

The metric system is a universal system of measure. In recent years countries such as Canada and the United States have been making the change from other standard units of measure to the metric system. Change is not always easy. Changing the dials on a machine is relatively easy compared to changing the human mind.

The best way to learn a system of measure is to use it. Equivalent measures from one system of measure to another system of measure are discussed in later units. This skill, while useful, is not essential to the effective use of the metric system.

The metric system has standard units which allow the measure of length, volume or capacity, and mass. The standard units of measure are: LENGTH: metre (m); VOLUME: cubic centimetre (cm^3); CAPACITY: litre (L); MASS: kilogram (kg).

12.3 EXERCISES

1. The mass of a patient is determined to be 88.694 kilograms. When recorded it is indicated as 88 694 grams. Is the recorded mass correct?

2. At sea level the mass of 1 millilitre of pure water is equal to 1 gram. Using the equivalent of 1 millilitre equals 1 gram, find the number of grams in a solution containing 925 millilitres of distilled water, 4 grams of NaCl, and 165 grams of KCl.

3. Central supply has 38.654 metres of gauze. A technician is requested to divide the gauze into 150-centimetre lengths. Find the number of 150-centimetre lengths obtained.

4. A graduated pipette is used to measure out these samples.

   Sample **A**:   0.04 mL
   Sample **B**:   0.08 mL
   Sample **C**:   0.10 mL
   Sample **D**:   1.00 mL
   Sample **E**:   1.02 mL

   a. Which sample is the smallest?
   b. Which sample is the largest?

5. A hospital blood bank has 5 units of 0-blood on hand. A trauma patient receives a transfusion of 1.75 units. How many units of 0-blood remain on hand?

unit 13 metric length measure

OBJECTIVES
After studying this unit the student should be able to:
- Express metric length measure in larger or smaller metric units.
- Determine the length measure of a circle.

UNITS OF LENGTH MEASURE

The base unit of metric length measure is the <u>metre</u>. Length measure can also be expressed in kilometres, hectometres, dekametres, decimetres, centimetres, and millimetres. The kilometre, metre, centimetre and millimetre are the most commonly used units. A given metric length measure can be expressed in larger or smaller metric units.

- To express a metric length unit as a smaller metric length unit, multiply by a positive power of ten such as 10, 100, 1 000, 10 000, or 100 000.
- To express a metric length unit as a larger metric length unit, multiply by a negative power of ten such as 0.1, 0.01, 0.001, 0.000 1, or 0.000 01.

This chart summarizes the units of metric length measure, the symbols, the equivalences, and the relationship between the units. The steel rule also shows the relationship between the units.

Unit	kilometre	hectometre	dekametre	metre	decimetre	centimetre	millimetre
Symbol	km	hm	dam	m	dm	cm	mm
Equivalence	1 000 metres	100 metres	10 metres	1 metre	0.1 metre	0.01 metre	0.001 metre
Relationship Between Units	1 km is 10 hm	1 hm is 10 dam	1 dam is 10 m	1 m is 10 dm	1 dm is 10 cm	1 cm is 10 mm	

Section 3 Metric Measure

13.1 EXERCISES

Using the chart, find the relationship between the units.

1. 1 km = __?__ hm
2. 1 hm = __?__ dam
3. 1 dam = __?__ m
4. 1 m = __?__ dm
5. 1 dm = __?__ cm
6. 1 cm = __?__ mm

7. 1 hm = __?__ km
8. 1 dam = __?__ hm
9. 1 m = __?__ dam
10. 1 dm = __?__ m
11. 1 cm = __?__ dm
12. 1 mm = __?__ cm

Expressing metric length measure in larger or smaller units uses the principle of multiplying numbers by powers of ten.

Example: Tim is 1.82 metres tall. How many centimetres is this?
1.82 m = __?__ cm
1 m = 100 cm
1.82 × 100 = 182
1.82 m = 182 cm
Tim is 182 centimetres tall.

Example: Tina is 1 423 mm tall. How many metres is this?
1 423 mm = __?__ m
1 mm = 0.001 m
1 423 × 0.001 = 1.423
1 423 mm = 1.423 m
Tina is 1.423 metres tall.

13.2 EXERCISES

Express each measure in a larger equivalent metric unit or a smaller equivalent metric unit.

1. 1 m = __?__ cm
2. 1 dm = __?__ cm
3. 1 m = __?__ mm
4. 6.5 m = __?__ cm
5. 12 cm = __?__ mm
6. 3.2 km = __?__ m
7. 2.68 hm = __?__ m
8. 4.75 dam = __?__ dm
9. 10 km = __?__ m
10. 0.142 cm = __?__ mm

11. 42 mm = __?__ cm
12. 617 cm = __?__ m
13. 3 275 m = __?__ km
14. 0.753 mm = __?__ dm
15. 15.7 dm = __?__ m
16. 22 dam = __?__ hm
17. 0.32 mm = __?__ m
18. 0.457 cm = __?__ m
19. 823.75 mm = __?__ cm
20. 47.8 dam = __?__ km

21. 712 m = __?__ km
22. 6.2 km = __?__ m
23. 85 cm = __?__ mm
24. 35 cm = __?__ m
25. 25 m = __?__ km
26. 4.8 m = __?__ cm
27. 47 dam = __?__ hm
28. 312 mm = __?__ m
29. 0.625 cm = __?__ mm
30. 48.9 mm = __?__ cm

31. 320 m = 0.32 __?__
32. 3 725 mm = 37.25 __?__
33. 8.71 hm = 8 710 __?__
34. 4 975 cm = 4.975 __?__
35. 18 dm = 1.8 __?__
36. 2 500 __?__ = 2.5 km
37. 17.37 __?__ = 1.737 dam
38. 425 __?__ = 42.5 cm
39. 3.25 __?__ = 3 250 mm
40. 1 500 __?__ = 1.5 km

	kilometres	hectometres	dekametres	metres	decimetres	centimetres	millimetres
41.				37.594			
42.				0.816 3			
43.				407.38			
44.				0.003 57			

Arrange each group of measures from largest to smallest.

45. 14 cm;   14 mm;   14 m
46. 1.62 m;   170 cm;   1 600 mm
47. 0.005 km;   17 m;   2 000 cm
48. 12 m;   1 211 cm;   0.123 km
49. 40 cm;   45 mm;   5 dm
50. 0.25 km;   255 m;   2 560 dm

Solve.

51. If 245 centimetres of cloth are required for a lab coat, how many lab coats could be cut from a 13-metre piece of cloth?

52. Jean walks an average of 1 500 metres per day in the clinic. During one month she works 20 days. How many kilometres does she walk?

53. Craig takes a medical research trip. Craig keeps this record of the distances traveled.

   1st day: 368 km   4th day: 419 km
   2nd day: 279 km   5th day: 317 km
   3rd day: 520 km   6th day: 193 km

   a. Find the total distance driven.
   b. Find the average distance covered per day. Round the answer to the nearer kilometre.
   Note: average = total distance ÷ number of days

54. A rectangular research area, 60 m by 150 m, is to be enclosed with railing that costs $4.60 per metre. Find the cost of the railing.

55. Posts for the rectangular research area, 60 m by 150 m, are to be placed at each corner and 2.5 m apart.

   a. Find how many posts are needed.
   b. If each post costs $1.20, find the cost of all the posts.

LENGTH MEASURE OF A CIRCLE

Length measure of a circle can be found. Before introducing the formula some special terms should be noted.

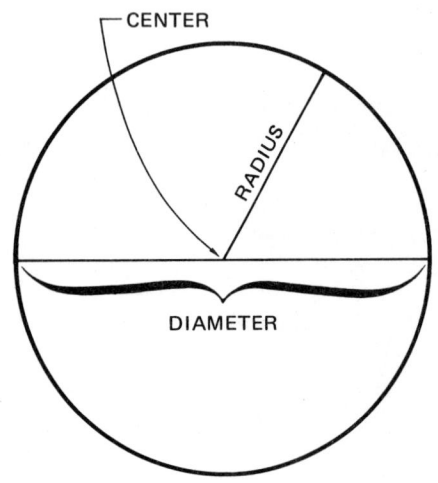

▼ The *center* is the point from which all points on the circle are the same distance.

▼ The *diameter (d)* is the length of the line segment through the center that has both its endpoints on the circle.

▼ The *radius (r)* is the length of the line segment connecting the center to a point on the circle. The radius is one-half the diameter or $r = \frac{1}{2} d$.

▼ The *circumference (C)* is the distance around the circle.

▼ *Pi* (π) is a constant value which compares the circumference and the diameter. The value to four decimal places is 3.141 6.

- The circumference of a circle is:
  $C = \pi d$ or
  $C = 2\pi r$

Example: Find the circumference of a circle with a diameter of 4 cm.

$C = \pi d$	Write the formula.
$C = 3.1416 \times 4$ cm	Substitute the specific value for the unknown.
$C = 12.5664$ cm	Perform the calculations.

Example: Find the circumference of a circle with a radius of 3 cm.

$C = 2\pi r$	Write the formula.
$C = 2 \times 3.1416 \times 3$ cm	Substitute the specific value for the unknown.
$C = 6.2832 \times 3$ cm	Perform the calculations.
$C = 18.8496$ cm	

Note: The circumference of a circle is a little more than 3 times the diameter.

13.3 EXERCISES

Find the circumference of each circle. Use $\pi = 3.1416$.

1. $r = 4$ m
2. $d = 6$ mm
3. $d = 10$ m
4. $r = 2.5$ cm

MEASURING LENGTH

No measurement is exact. The precision of a measurement depends upon the unit of measure that is used. The diameter (distance across the center) of a half-dollar can be measured in centimetres or millimetres.

Unit of Measure — centimetre   Unit of Measure — millimetre

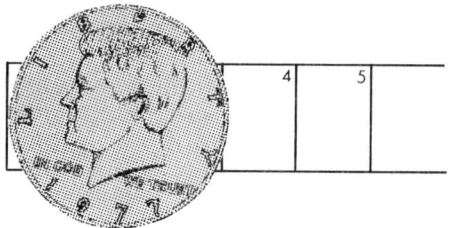   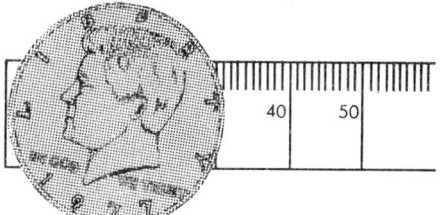

The diameter of the half-dollar, to the nearer centimetre, is 3 centimetres.   The diameter of the half-dollar, to the nearer millimetre is 31 millimetres.

In each case there is some error in the measurement. The error of measurement is the difference between the exact length and the measured length. The error of measurement is less when a smaller unit is used. Since millimetres is a smaller unit of measure, it is more precise than centimetres. In general, the smaller the unit of measure, the more precise the measurement.

13.4 EXERCISES

Measure each item using the given units of measure. Indicate which measure is more precise.

	Item	Unit of Measure	Measurement	More Precise Measurement
1.	length of a dollar bill	centimetre		
		millimetre		
2.	width of a classroom door	metre		
		centimetre		
3.	height of a classroom door	metre		
		centimetre		
4.	diameter of a quarter	decimetre		
		millimetre		

13.5 EXERCISES

Choose the best unit of length (km, m, cm, or mm) for measuring each of these items.

1. Movie film.
2. The diameter of the earth.
3. The height of a tree.
4. The length of a shoelace.
5. The thickness of hair.
6. The length of a car.
7. The height of a mountain.
8. The length of an eyelash.
9. The distance around a person's head.
10. Rainfall.

Place these measures in order from the largest measure to the smallest measure.

11. 15 mm;   16 km;   6 000 m;   50 cm;   6 000 mm
12. 5 km;   25 mm;   2 000 cm;   150 m;   42 km
13. 2 750 cm;   10 km;   5 000 mm;   35 m;   3 025 cm
14. 1.75 m;   200 cm;   0.01 km;   450 mm;   2.75 cm
15. 3.15 km;   52.5 m;   0.31 m;   1.3 mm;   7.38 m

Using the given unit, estimate and then measure the length of each object. Express the measurements in the indicated units.

Object	Estimate (a)	Measurement (b)	Expressing the measurement using other units	
			(c)	(d)
16. A person's right foot.	__?__ mm	__?__ mm	__?__ cm	__?__ m
17. A person's height.	__?__ m	__?__ m	__?__ dm	__?__ cm
18. The width of a ballpoint pen tip.	__?__ mm	__?__ mm	__?__ cm	__?__ dm
19. A person's waist.	__?__ cm	__?__ cm	__?__ mm	__?__ m
20. The length of this room.	__?__ m	__?__ m	__?__ dam	__?__ hm

APPLICATIONS

Length measures have wide applications in health occupations. The height of patients, lengths of cloth supplies, and size of paper supplies are only a few of the situations in which length measure becomes important. Until recent years most health services used the English units of length measure with occasional use of the metric units. Presently, the metric system has progressively replaced other units of measure.

When purchasing glassware or other supplies for the laboratory, a knowledge of metric length measure is valuable. Test tubes are available in various lengths and diameters. Filter paper, chromatography paper, and recording paper are sold in sizes expressed in metric values. When comparing quantities and cost, the ability to determine per unit cost is important to good fiscal management.

13.6 EXERCISES

1. During each 15-minute test, a recording kymograph is geared to use 3.275 m of 12-cm wide paper.

    a. How much paper should be purchased for 500 15-minute tests?
    b. How many tests can be made with 450 m of paper?

2. A baby is 45.750 cm long when born. To determine the growth rate, the baby is measured each week for a five-week period. Calculate the weekly growth rate and the total growth.

	WEEK	LENGTH	GROWTH
	birth	45.750 cm	
a.	1	46.025 cm	__?__
b.	2	46.125 cm	__?__
c.	3	46.475 cm	__?__
d.	4	46.650 cm	__?__
e.	5	46.950 cm	__?__
f.		TOTAL GROWTH	__?__ cm

3. A team of students measures the height of five patients. When the data is compiled the results show this.
   Patient A: 1.896 m
   Patient B: 1 783 mm
   Patient C: 174.6 cm
   Patient D: 2.006 m
   Patient E: 164.8 cm

   a. Find the average height of the patients. Average equals total heights divided by the number of patients. Round the answer to the nearer thousandth.
   b. Which patient is the tallest?
   c. Which patient is the shortest?

4. Brand A of gauze is found to cost $12.60 per 15-metre roll.
   Brand B comes in 25-metre rolls costing $23.90 each.

   a. Find the cost per metre of Brand A.
   b. Find the cost per metre of Brand B.
   c. Assuming the quality is equal, which is the better buy?

5. Chromatography paper is available in 50-metre rolls, 12.5 centimetres wide, at a cost of $37.85. This roll is then cut in lengths 75 centimetres long before using.

   a. How many pieces can be cut from the 50-metre roll?
   b. What is the cost per piece?

6. A patient's room measures 8 metres by 3 metres. If 1 square metre of floor tile requires 75 millilitres of wax, how many litres of wax will be needed to wax ten rooms of this size? NOTE: Area = length times width.

7. A patient's waist measure 105 centimetres. Suppose a role of gauze contains 1.6 metres. Approximately how many times could the gauze be completely wrapped around the patient's waist?

unit 14 metric area measure

OBJECTIVES

After studying this unit the student should be able to:

- Express metric area measures in larger or smaller metric units.
- Determine the area of figures using the appropriate formulas.

MEASURING AREA

The *area* of a region is the number of square units that it takes to cover the region. In the metric system, area measure is a derived unit. It is found by using the base unit of length measure — the metre. One unit of square measure is the square centimetre. To find the area, the number of squares can be counted.

Example: The area of each region is found by counting the number of square centimetres.

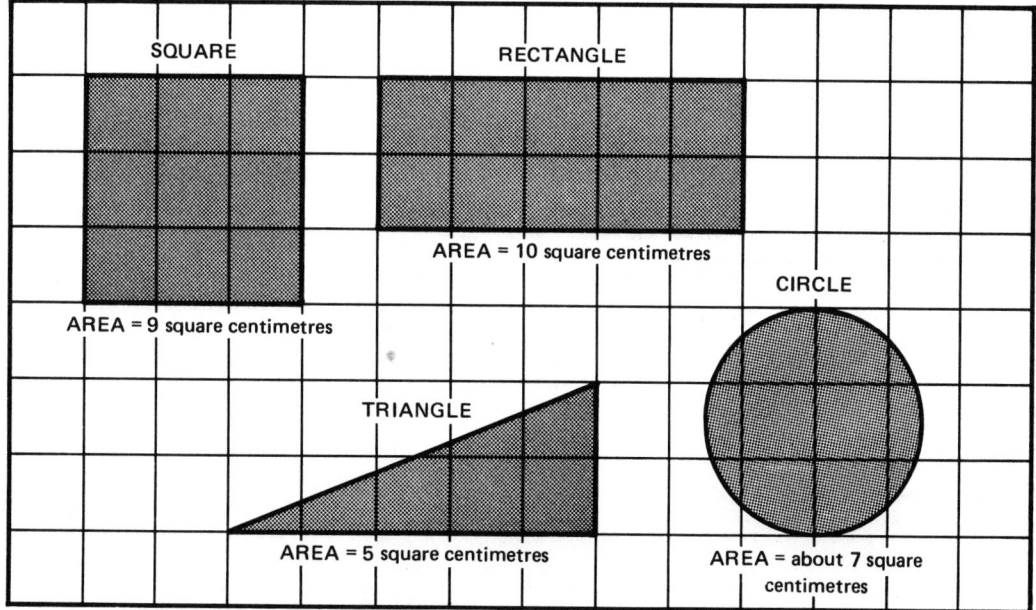

Note: Metric area measures such as 9 square centimetres, 10 square centimetres and 5 square centimetres can be written 9 cm², 10 cm² and 5 cm². The exponent, 2, indicates that the measure consists of 2 dimensions.

In real life, counting squares is impractical. Examining the areas and dimensions more closely leads to the development of formulas for calculating the areas of regions.

FINDING THE AREA OF A SQUARE

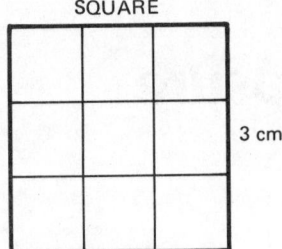

The area of this square is 9 cm².
Each side is 3 cm.
Since 3 cm × 3 cm = 9 cm²,
the area = 3 cm × 3 cm
or area = side × side.

■ The area of a square with sides s units long is:
$$A = s \times s$$
$$or$$
$$A = s^2$$

Note: The symbol for the side, s, includes the unit of measure.

Example: Find the area of a square with sides of 4 metres.

$A = s \times s \; or \; s^2$	Write the formula.
$A = 4 \text{ m} \times 4 \text{ m} \; or \; (4 \text{ m})^2$	Substitute the specific values for the unknowns.
$A = 16 \text{ m}^2$	Perform the calculations.

FINDING THE AREA OF A RECTANGLE

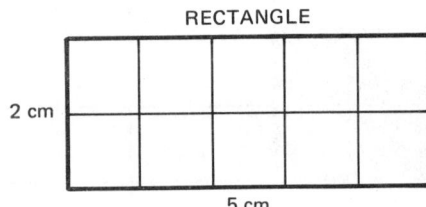

The area of this rectangle is 10 cm².
The length is 5 cm; the width is 2 cm.
Since 5 cm × 2 cm = 10 cm²,
the area = 5 cm × 2 cm or
area = length × width.

■ The area of a rectangle with length l units and width w units is:
$$A = l \times w$$
$$or$$
$$A = lw$$

Note: The symbols l and w include the unit of measure.

Example: Find the area of a rectangle 3 m by 4.5 m.

$A = l \times w$	Write the formula.
$A = 3 \text{ m} \times 4.5 \text{ m}$	Substitute the specific values for the unknowns.
$A = 13.5 \text{ m}^2$	Perform the calculations.

FINDING THE AREA OF A TRIANGLE

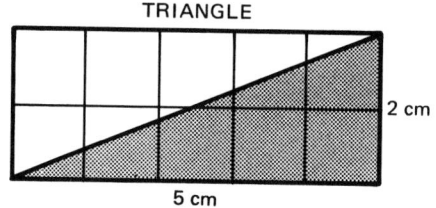

The area of the triangle is 5 cm². The area of the rectangle is 10 cm². Since 5 cm² is $\frac{1}{2}$ (10 cm²), the area of the triangle = $\frac{1}{2}$ (10 cm²) or area = $\frac{1}{2}$ (area of rectangle).

The parts of a triangle have special names.

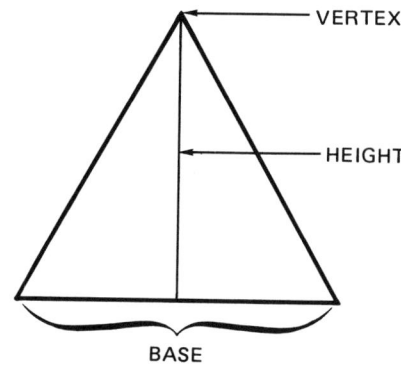

- ▼ The *vertex* is the common endpoint of 2 line segments.
- ▼ The *base* is the length of the side on which the triangle sets.
- ▼ The *height* is the line segment from a vertex intersecting the base at a right angle.

- The area of a triangle with base b units and height h units is:
  $A = \frac{1}{2} \times b \times h$

  or

  $A = \frac{1}{2} bh$

Note: The symbols b and h include the unit of measure. The height is sometimes referred to as the altitude.

Example: Find the area of a triangle with a base of 12 mm and a height (altitude) of 8 mm.

$A = \frac{1}{2} \times b \times h$ — Write the formula.

$A = \frac{1}{2} \times 12 \text{ mm} \times 8 \text{ mm}$ — Substitute the specific values for the unknowns.

$A = 48 \text{ mm}^2$ — Perform the calculations.

FINDING THE AREA OF A CIRCLE

A rectangular region can be used to obtain a very close approximation for the area of a circle. To obtain a "near rectangle," the circle is cut into 16 pie-shaped sections.

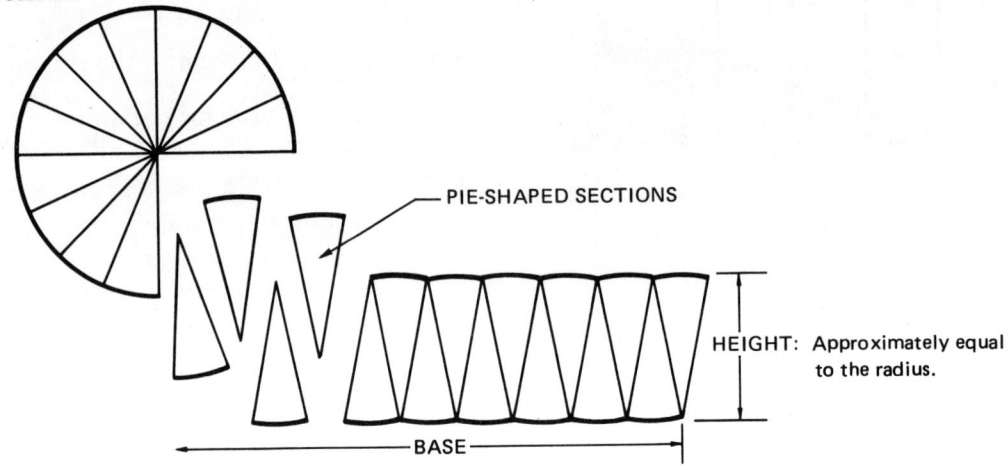

To finish constructing this "near rectangle," the right end pie-shaped section is cut in half. This wedge-shaped piece is then placed on the left side.

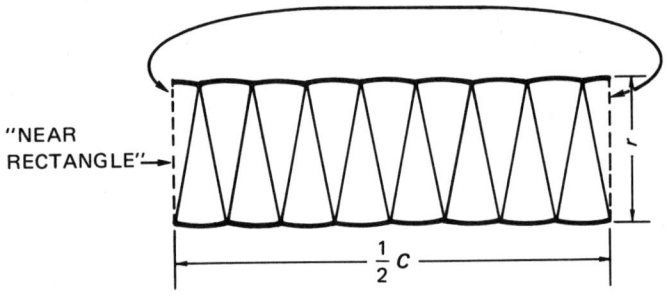

The area of this "near rectangle" is base times the height.

base = $\frac{1}{2} C$; height = r

circumference = πd

diameter = $2r$

$A = b \times h$

$A = \frac{1}{2} \times C \times r$

$A = \frac{1}{2} \times \pi \times d \times r$

$A = \frac{1}{2} \times \pi \times 2 \times r \times r$

$A = \frac{1}{2} \times 2 \times \pi \times r \times r$

$A = \pi r^2$

Simpifying the formula.
- The area of a circle is:
  $A = \pi r^2$ where $\pi \approx 3.141\ 6$

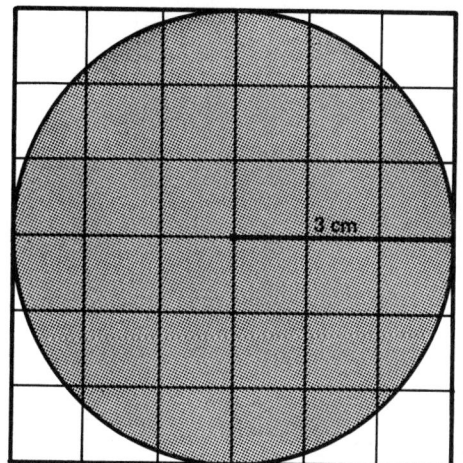

The area of this circle is approximately 28 square centimetres. The radius is 3 cm. Since 3 cm × 3 cm = 9 cm², the area = 9 cm² × 3.141 6 or 28.274 4 cm².

Example: Find the area of a circle with a radius of 4 m.

$A = \pi r^2$ — Write the formula.
$A = (3.141\ 6)(4\ m)^2$ — Substitute the specific value for unknown.
$A = (3.141\ 6)(16\ m^2)$ — Perform the calculations.
$A = (3.141\ 6)(16)\ m^2$
$A = 50.265\ 6\ m^2$

14.1 EXERCISES

Using the grid, estimate the number of square centimetres in each region.

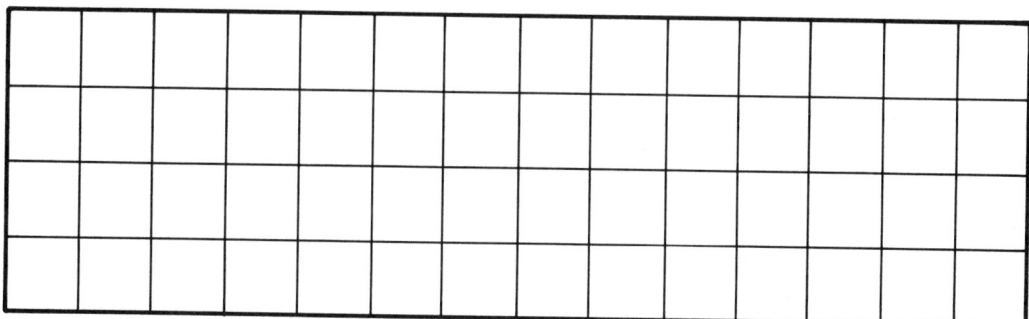

1.    2.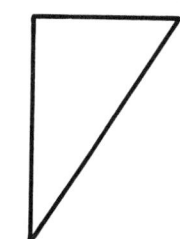

[Grid rectangle figure]

3.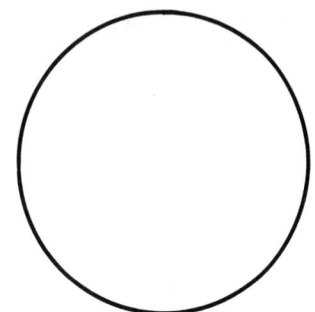

4.

Using the appropriate formula, calculate the area for each region.

5. Square: $s = 25$ cm
6. Rectangle: $l = 10$ cm
   $w = 2.5$ cm
7. Triangle: $b = 6$ mm
   $h = 3$ mm
8. Circle: $r = 8$ cm
9. Square: $s = 6.2$ mm
10. Rectangle: $l = 6$ mm
    $w = 8$ mm
11. Triangle: $b = 5$ m
    $h = 12$ m
12. Circle: $d = 8$ mm
13. Rectangle: $l = 2.5$ cm
    $w = 2.5$ cm
14. Circle: $r = 5$ m
15. Square: $s = 4$ m
16. Triangle: $b = 8$ cm
    $h = 5$ cm

Choose the most appropriate unit of area measure to be used in finding the areas of these objects. Possible choices are: square kilometres, square metres, square centimetres, and square millimetres.

17. A parking lot.
18. This page.
19. A state or province.
20. A fingernail.
21. A floor tile.
22. The laboratory floor.
23. The pupil of an eye.
24. The skin in the palm of the right hand.

UNITS OF AREA MEASURE

The derived unit of metric area measure is the <u>square metre</u>. Area measure can also be expressed in square kilometres, square hectometres, square dekametres, square decimetres, square centimetres, and square millimetres. The square kilometre, square hectometre, square metre, square centimetre, and square millimetre are the most commonly used units. A given metric area measure can be expressed in larger or smaller metric units.

- To express a metric area unit as a smaller metric area unit, multiply by 100, 10 000, 1 000 000, etc.

- To express a metric area unit as a larger metric area unit, multiply by 0.01, 0.000 1, 0.000 001, etc.

Note: Since metric area measure means 10 × 10, all numbers are powers of one hundred such as 100^1, 100^2, 100^3; and 100^{-1}, 100^{-2}, 100^{-3}.

This chart summarizes the units of metric area measure, the symbols, the equivalences, and the relationships between the units.

Unit	square kilometre	square hectometre	square dekametre	square metre	square decimetre	square centimetre	square millimetre
Symbol	km^2	hm^2	dam^2	m^2	dm^2	cm^2	mm^2
Equivalence	1 000 000 m^2	10 000 m^2	100 m^2	1 m^2	0.01 m^2	0.000 1 m^2	0.000 001 m^2
Relationship Between Units	1 km^2 is 100 hm^2	1 hm^2 is 100 dam^2	1 dam^2 is 100 m^2	1 m^2 is 100 dm^2	1 dm^2 is 100 cm^2	1 cm^2 is 100 mm^2	

14.2 EXERCISES

Using the chart, find the relationship between the units.

1. 1 km^2 = _____?_____ hm^2
2. 1 hm^2 = _____?_____ dam^2
3. 1 dam^2 = _____?_____ m^2
4. 1 m^2 = _____?_____ dm^2
5. 1 dm^2 = _____?_____ cm^2
6. 1 cm^2 = _____?_____ mm^2
7. 1 hm^2 = _____?_____ km^2
8. 1 dam^2 = _____?_____ hm^2
9. 1 m^2 = _____?_____ dam^2
10. 1 dm^2 = _____?_____ m^2
11. 1 cm^2 = _____?_____ dm^2
12. 1 mm^2 = _____?_____ cm^2

Expressing area measure in larger or smaller units uses the principle of **multiplying numbers by powers of one hundred**.

Example: A square is 3 cm by 3 cm. Find the area in square millimetres.

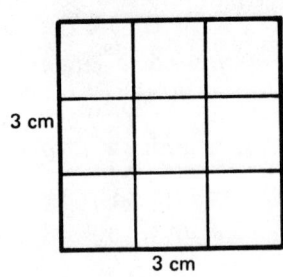
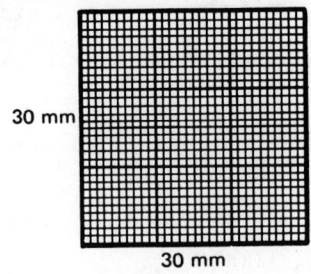

$A = s \times s$
$A = 3 \text{ cm} \times 3 \text{ cm}$
$A = 9 \text{ cm}^2$

$A = s \times s$
$A = 30 \text{ mm} \times 30 \text{ mm}$
$A = 900 \text{ mm}^2$

$1 \text{ cm}^2 = 100 \text{ mm}^2$
$9 \times 100 = 900$
$9 \text{ cm}^2 = 900 \text{ mm}^2$

Example: A rectangle is 20 mm wide and 50 mm long. Find the area in square centimetres.

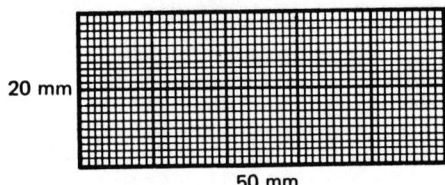
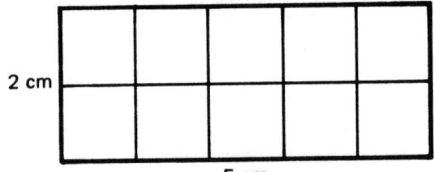

$A = l \times w$
$A = 20 \text{ mm} \times 50 \text{ mm}$
$A = 1\,000 \text{ mm}^2$

$A = l \times w$
$A = 2 \text{ cm} \times 5 \text{ cm}$
$A = 10 \text{ cm}^2$

$1 \text{ mm}^2 = 0.01 \text{ cm}^2$
$1\,000 \times 0.01 = 10$
$1\,000 \text{ mm}^2 = 10 \text{ cm}^2$

Example: Express 2.25 hm² as square metres.
    2.25 hm² = _____?_____ m²
    1 hm² = 10 000 m²
    2.25 × 10 000 = 22 500
    2.25 hm² = 22 500 m²

Example: Express 314 278 mm² as square metres.
    314 278 mm² = _____?_____ m²
    1 mm² = 0.000 001 m²
    314 278 × 0.000 001 = 0.314 278
    314 278 mm² = 0.314 278 m²

14.3 EXERCISES

Express each measure in a larger equivalent metric unit or a smaller equivalent metric unit.

1. 1 km² = _____?_____ m²
2. 1 m² = _____?_____ cm²
3. 1 cm² = _____?_____ mm²
4. 1 m² = _____?_____ mm²
5. 2.31 cm² = _____?_____ mm²
6. 5 m² = _____?_____ mm²
7. 5.25 km² = _____?_____ m²
8. 5.92 dam² = _____?_____ dm²
9. 8.73 hm² = _____?_____ m²
10. 0.318 cm² = _____?_____ mm²
11. 1 375 mm² = _____?_____ cm²
12. 12 750 cm² = _____?_____ m²
13. 3 215 382 m² = _____?_____ km²
14. 13 309 mm² = _____?_____ dm²
15. 450 dm² = _____?_____ m²
16. 2 500 dam² = _____?_____ km²
17. 2 250 000 mm² = _____?_____ m²
18. 9 272 cm² = _____?_____ m²
19. 876.2 mm² = _____?_____ cm²
20. 1 075.73 dam² = _____?_____ km²
21. 184.73 m² = _____?_____ km²
22. 285 719 m² = _____?_____ km²
23. 5 314.62 cm² = _____?_____ m²
24. 13.48 cm² = _____?_____ mm²
25. 1 975 km² = _____?_____ m²
26. 3.17 m² = _____?_____ cm²
27. 497.2 dam² = _____?_____ km²
28. 341 562 mm² = _____?_____ m²
29. 5 219 cm² = _____?_____ mm²
30. 25 mm² = _____?_____ cm²

Using the given unit, estimate and then calculate the area of each object. Express the calculated areas in the indicated units.

Object	Estimate (a)	Area (b)	Expressing the area using other units (c)
31. The classroom floor.	__?__ m²	__?__ m²	__?__ dam²
32. This book cover.	__?__ cm²	__?__ cm²	__?__ mm²
33. The face of a watch.	__?__ mm²	__?__ mm²	__?__ cm²
34. A gum wrapper.	__?__ cm²	__?__ cm²	__?__ mm²
35. A fingernail.	__?__ mm²	__?__ mm²	__?__ cm²

Arrange each group of areas from largest to smallest.

36. 0.029 dam² ;   31 m² ;   3 000 dm²
37. 3.15 dm² ;   31 800 mm² ;   317 cm²
38. 53.6 km² ;   540 000 dam² ;   5 350 hm²

APPLICATIONS

The ability to calculate area of a room, laboratory, or a piece of filter paper may be important in a hospital or clinical assignment. The design of these objects usually allows easy calculation. Irregularly shaped objects create special problems that will not be covered in this text.

The purchasing agent for the clinic calculates the area of a floor when ordering waxes. Laboratory technicians are using metric area measure when determining the number of microorganisms per square millimetre, centimetre, or metre of surface area. The number of viable and nonviable microorganisms in an area requires the knowledge of area measure.

14.4 EXERCISES

1. The surface area of a medical library is determined by the medical data statistician. The measurements show the room to be 6.983 metres long, 5.179 metres wide, and 2.438 metres high.

    a. What is the surface area of the floor to the nearer thousandth square metre?
    b. What is the surface area of the four walls to the nearer thousandth square metre?

2. A study reveals that in a public rest room there are approximately 96 human pinworm eggs present per square metre of floor surface area. At least $\frac{1}{8}$ of the eggs are viable. The rest room of a hospital is 7.6 m X 14.9 m in size.

    a. If 9.7 square metres are deducted for various fixtures in the room, find the area of the floor.
    b. Find the number of viable human pinworm eggs on the floor of this rest room.

3. A glass plate is coated with a thin layer of vaseline. The plate is then placed in an open area outside the clinic for six hours. At the end of this time the plate is returned to the laboratory for microscopic examination. It is discovered that 4 pollen grains are found per square centimetre of surface area. Calculate the surface area for each plate size and determine the number of pollen grains present.

	PLATE SIZE	AREA	TOTAL POLLEN GRAINS
a.	6 cm X 6 cm		
b.	10 cm X 15 cm		
c.	150 mm X 200 mm		
d.	75 mm X 150 mm		
e.	120-mm diameter		
f.	80-mm diameter		
g.	9-cm diameter		

unit 15 metric volume measure

OBJECTIVES

After studying this unit the student should be able to:

- Determine the volume of solids and fluids.
- Express metric volume measures in larger or smaller metric units.
- Express metric capacity measures in larger or smaller metric units.

MEASURING VOLUMES OF SOLIDS

The *volume* of a three-dimensional solid is the number of unit cubes that are required to fill the inside of the figure. In the metric system, volume measure for solids is a derived unit. It is found by using the base unit of length measure — the metre. One common unit of volume measure for solids is the cubic centimetre.

Example: Find the volume of this rectangular solid.

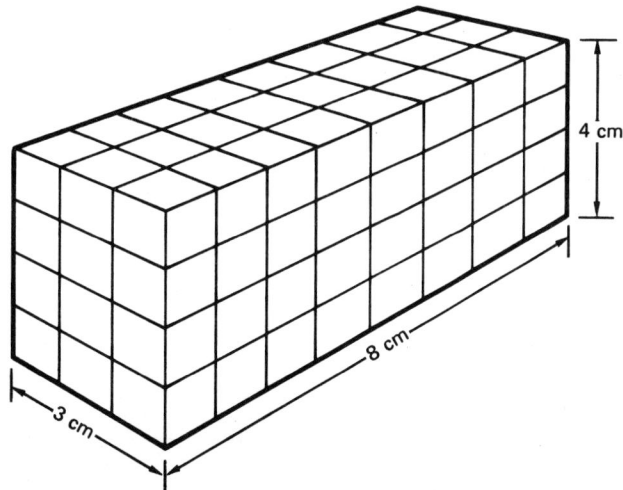

There are 96 cubes in this rectangular solid;
each is a one-centimetre cube.
VOLUME = 96 cubic centimetres

119

Example: This cylindrical solid has 4 π cubes per layer. To find the volume, the number of layers is multiplied by the number of cubes per layer.

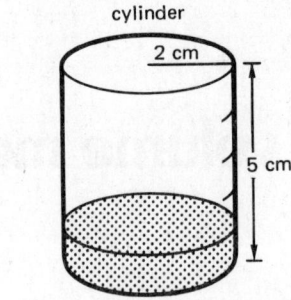

VOLUME = 62.832 cubic centimetres

Note: Metric volume measures for solids, such as 96 cubic centimetres and 62.832 cubic centimetres, can be written 96 cm³ and 62.832 cm³. The exponent, 3, indicates that the measure consists of 3 dimensions.

It may be impractical to determine the number of cubes to find volume. Examining the volume and dimensions more closely leads to the development of a formula for calculating the volume of solids.

FINDING THE VOLUME OF A RECTANGULAR SOLID

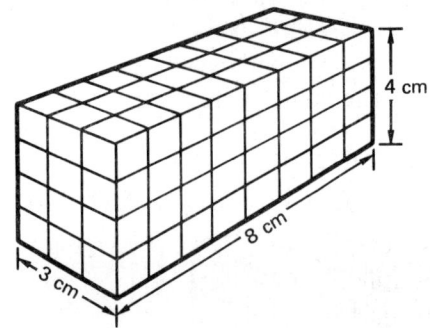

The volume of this rectangular solid is 96 cm³.
The length is 8 cm; the width is 3 cm; the height is 4 cm.
Since 8 cm × 3 cm × 4 cm = 96 cm³, the volume = 8 cm × 3 cm × 4 cm or volume = length × width × height.

- The volume of a rectangular solid is:
  $V = l \times w \times h$
  or
  $V = lwh$

Note: The symbols for l, w, and h include the unit of measure. In order to find the volume, the unit of measure <u>must</u> be the same.

Example: Find the volume of a rectangular solid 3 m by 6 m by 4 m.

$V = l \times w \times h$ Write the formula.
$V = 3 \text{ m} \times 6 \text{ m} \times 4 \text{ m}$ Substitute the specific values for the unknowns.
$V = 18 \text{ m}^2 \times 4 \text{ m}$ Perform the calculations.
$V = 72 \text{ m}^3$

FINDING THE VOLUME OF A CYLINDRICAL SOLID

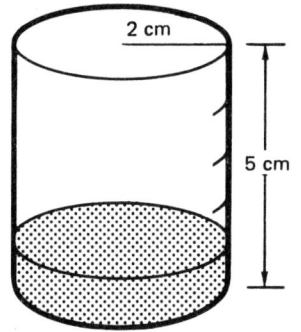

The volume of this cylindrical solid is 62.832 cm³. The height is 5 cm; the radius is 2 cm; the base area is 4π. Since $4\pi = \pi r^2$ and $4\pi \times 5 = 62.832$ cm², the volume = $4\pi \times 5$ or volume = π radius² × height.

- The volume of a cylindrical solid is:
  $V = \pi r^2 \times h$
  or
  $V = \pi r^2 h$

Note: The symbols r and h include the unit of measure. In order to find the volume, the unit of measure <u>must</u> be the same.

Example: Find the volume of a cylindrical solid with a radius of 3 cm and a height of 6 cm.

$V = \pi r^2 h$	Write the formula.
$V = 3.141\,6 \times (3\text{ cm})^2 \times 6\text{ cm}$	Substitute the specific values for the unknowns.
$V = 3.141\,6 \times 9\text{ cm}^2 \times 6\text{ cm}$	Perform the calculations.
$V = 3.141\,6 \times 54\text{ cm}^3$	
$V = 169.646\,4\text{ cm}^3$	

Note: When calculating volumes, it is necessary that all the dimensions be expressed using the same metric unit. When the dimensions have different units, express all the dimensions in the same unit, then find the volume.

15.1 EXERCISES

Find the volume of each rectangular or cylindrical solid.

	Length	Width	Height	Volume
1.	2 cm	2 cm	2 cm	
2.	3 cm	2 cm	2 cm	
3.	3 m	2 m	4 m	
4.	10 mm	20 mm	6 mm	
5.	6 dm	5 dm	4 dm	

	Radius	Height	Volume
6.	2 mm	50 mm	
7.	4 m	10 m	
8.	2 cm	10 cm	
9.	3 cm	4 cm	
10.	1 dm	0.5 dm	

11. Two cylindrical solids have the same height. The radius of the first solid is 2 cm and the radius of the second solid is 4 cm. Does the second solid have a volume exactly twice as much as the first solid?

12. Find the volume in cubic metres.

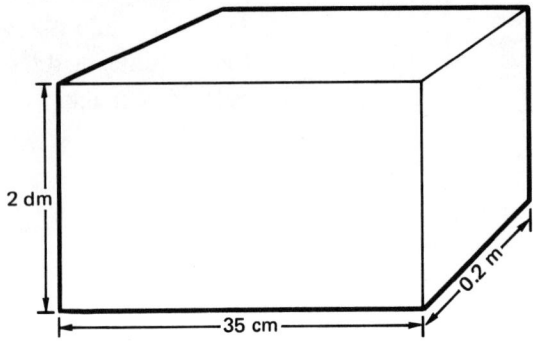

   $V = \underline{\ ?\ }$ m^3

13. Find the volume in cubic decimetres.

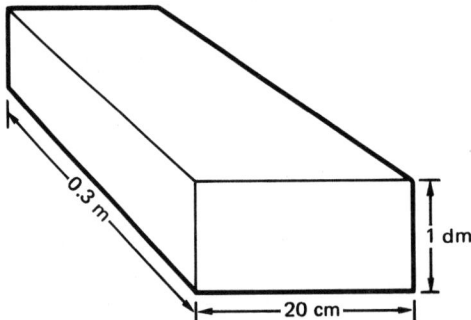

   $V = \underline{\ ?\ }$ dm^3

14. Find the volume in cubic centimetres.

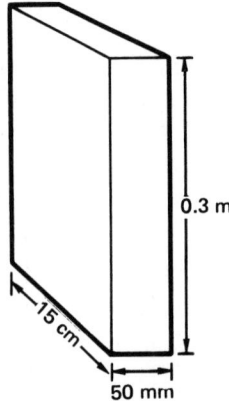

   $V = \underline{\ ?\ }$ cm^3

15. Find the volume in cubic centimetres

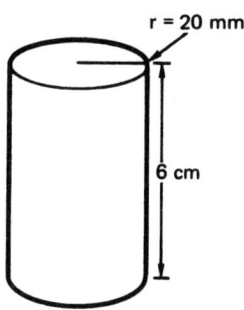

$V =$ ___?___ cm³

16. Find the volume in cubic millimetres.

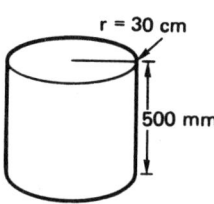

$V =$ ___?___ mm³

17. Find the volume in cubic decimetres.

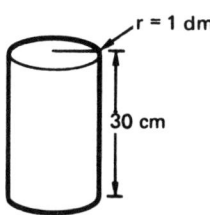

$V =$ ___?___ dm³

The dimensions of a rectangular solid are: length, 5 cm; width, 6 cm; height, 2 cm. Adjust the dimensions as stated, find the new volume, and compare it to the original volume.

18. The volume of the solid is ___?___ cm³.
19. Double one dimension. The new volume is ___?___ times the original volume.
20. Double two dimensions. The new volume is ___?___ times the original volume.
21. Double three dimensions. The new volume is ___?___ times the original volume.
22. Halve one dimension. The new volume is ___?___ times the original volume.
23. Halve two dimensions. The new volume is ___?___ times the original volume.
24. Halve all three dimensions. The new volume is ___?___ times the original volume.

UNITS OF VOLUME FOR SOLIDS

The derived unit of metric volume measure for solids is the <u>cubic metre.</u> Cubic measure for solids can also be expressed in cubic kilometres, cubic hectometres, cubic dekametres, cubic decimetres, cubic centimetres and cubic millimetres. The cubic metre, cubic decimetre, and cubic centimetre are the most commonly used units. A given metric volume measure can be expressed in larger or smaller metric units.

- To express a metric volume unit for solids as a smaller metric volume unit, multiply by 1 000, 1 000 000, 1 000 000 000, etc.
- To express a metric volume unit for solids as a larger metric volume unit, multiply by 0.001, 0.000 001, 0.000 000 001, etc.

Note: Since metric volume measurement means 10 × 10 × 10, all numbers are powers of one thousand such as $1\,000^1$, $1\,000^2$, $1\,000^3$; and $1\,000^{-1}$, $1\,000^{-2}$, $1\,000^{-3}$.

This chart summarizes the units of metric volume measure for solids, the symbols, the equivalences, and the relationships between the units.

Unit	cubic kilometre	cubic hectometre	cubic dekametre	cubic metre	cubic decimetre	cubic centimetre	cubic millimetre
Symbol	km^3	hm^3	dam^3	m^3	dm^3	cm^3	mm^3
Equivalence	$1\,000\,000\,000\ m^3$	$1\,000\,000\ m^3$	$1\,000\ m^3$	$1\ m^3$	$0.001\ m^3$	$0.000\,001\ m^3$	$0.000\,000\,001\ m^3$
Relationship Between Units	$1\ km^3$ is $1\,000\ hm^3$	$1\ hm^3$ is $1\,000\ dam^3$	$1\ dam^3$ is $1\,000\ m^3$	$1\ m^3$ is $1\,000\ dm^3$	$1\ dm^3$ is $1\,000\ cm^3$	$1\ cm^3$ is $1\,000\ mm^3$	

15.2 EXERCISES

Using the chart, find the relationship between the units.

1. $1\ km^3 = $ __?__ hm^3
2. $1\ hm^3 = $ __?__ dam^3
3. $1\ dam^3 = $ __?__ m^3
4. $1\ m^3 = $ __?__ dm^3
5. $1\ dm^3 = $ __?__ cm^3
6. $1\ cm^3 = $ __?__ mm^3
7. $1\ hm^3 = $ __?__ km^3
8. $1\ dam^3 = $ __?__ hm^3
9. $1\ m^3 = $ __?__ dam^3
10. $1\ dm^3 = $ __?__ m^3
11. $1\ cm^3 = $ __?__ dm^3
12. $1\ mm^3 = $ __?__ cm^3

Expressing volume measurements in larger or smaller units uses the principle of multiplying numbers by powers of one thousand.

Example: The volume of a rectangular solid is 30 dm³. Find the volume in cubic centimetres.

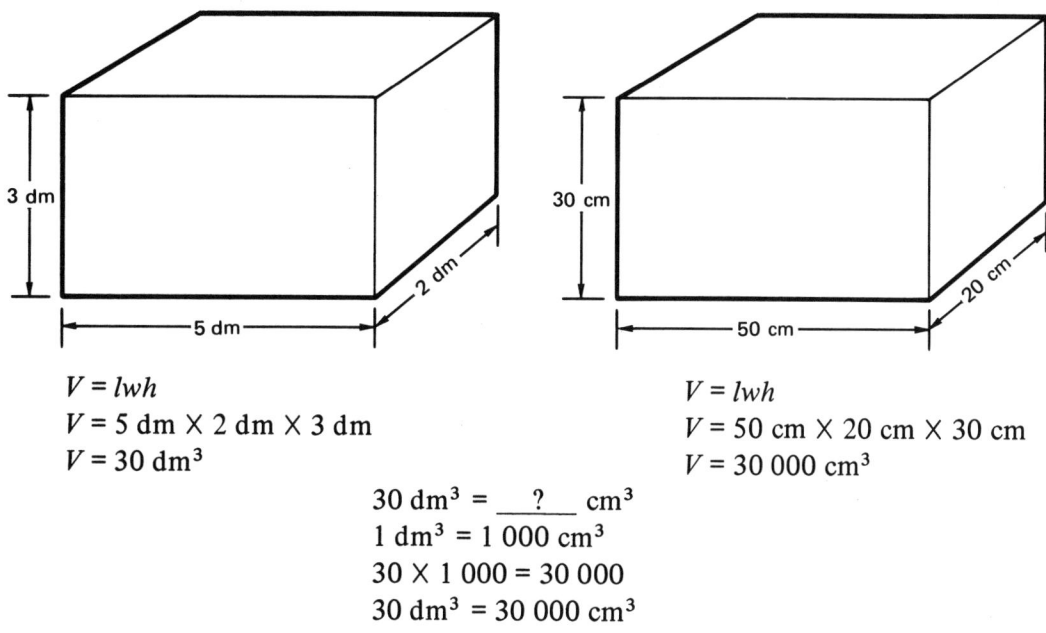

$V = lwh$
$V = 5 \text{ dm} \times 2 \text{ dm} \times 3 \text{ dm}$
$V = 30 \text{ dm}^3$

$V = lwh$
$V = 50 \text{ cm} \times 20 \text{ cm} \times 30 \text{ cm}$
$V = 30\ 000 \text{ cm}^3$

$30 \text{ dm}^3 = \underline{\ \ ?\ \ } \text{ cm}^3$
$1 \text{ dm}^3 = 1\ 000 \text{ cm}^3$
$30 \times 1\ 000 = 30\ 000$
$30 \text{ dm}^3 = 30\ 000 \text{ cm}^3$

Example: The volume of a rectangular solid is 72 000 mm³. Find the volume in cubic centimetres.

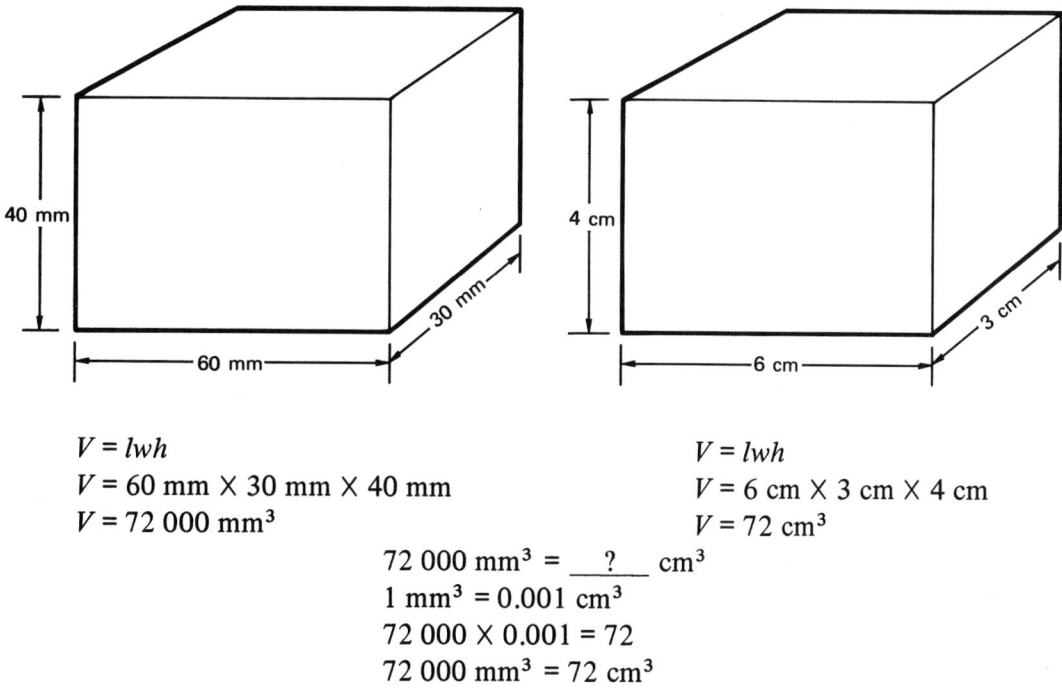

$V = lwh$
$V = 60 \text{ mm} \times 30 \text{ mm} \times 40 \text{ mm}$
$V = 72\ 000 \text{ mm}^3$

$V = lwh$
$V = 6 \text{ cm} \times 3 \text{ cm} \times 4 \text{ cm}$
$V = 72 \text{ cm}^3$

$72\ 000 \text{ mm}^3 = \underline{\ \ ?\ \ } \text{ cm}^3$
$1 \text{ mm}^3 = 0.001 \text{ cm}^3$
$72\ 000 \times 0.001 = 72$
$72\ 000 \text{ mm}^3 = 72 \text{ cm}^3$

15.3 EXERCISES

Express each measure in a larger equivalent metric unit or a smaller equivalent metric unit.

1. 108 dm³ = __?__ m³
2. 286 cm³ = __?__ mm³
3. 3.785 km³ = __?__ m³
4. 3.4 m³ = __?__ km³
5. 0.001 m³ = __?__ dm³
6. 9 km³ = __?__ cm³
7. 7 dm³ = __?__ cm³
8. 858 000 mm³ = __?__ cm³
9. 650 000 mm³ = __?__ m³
10. 380 m³ = __?__ mm³
11. 518 mm³ = __?__ cm³
12. 0.04 dm³ = __?__ m³
13. 12.3 cm³ = __?__ mm³
14. 730 mm³ = __?__ cm³
15. 10 dam³ = __?__ km³
16. 280 000 cm³ = __?__ m³
17. 0.25 m³ = __?__ cm³
18. 132 m³ = __?__ km³
19. 3.58 m³ = __?__ dm³
20. 23 cm³ = __?__ dm³

UNITS OF VOLUME FOR FLUIDS

In the metric system, the volume of a figure that is not a solid is measured by using a derived unit. This derived unit is the <u>litre.</u> The derived unit is used to measure the volume of liquids or gases such as the volume that a test tube will hold or the amount of solution in a container. Volumes of fluids can also be expressed in kilolitres, hectolitres, dekalitres, decilitres, centilitres, and millilitres. The litre, millilitre, and the kilolitre are the most commonly used units.

A given metric volume measure for fluids can be expressed in larger or smaller metric units.

- To express a metric volume unit for fluids as a smaller metric volume unit, multiply by a positive power of ten such as 10, 100, 1 000, 10 000, or 100 000.

- To express a metric volume unit for fluids as a larger metric volume unit, multiply by a negative power of ten such as 0.1, 0.01, 0.001, 0.000 1, or 0.000 01.

This chart summarizes the units of metric volume measure for fluids, the symbols, the equivalences, and the relationships between the units.

Unit	kilolitre	hectolitre	dekalitre	litre	decilitre	centilitre	millilitre
Symbol	kL	hL	daL	L	dL	cL	mL
Equivalence	1 000 litres	100 litres	10 litres	1 litre	0.1 litre	0.01 litre	0.001 litre
Relationship Between Units	1 kL is 10 hL	1 hL is 10 daL	1 daL is 10 L	1 L is 10 dL	1 dL is 10 cL	1 cL is 10 mL	

15.4 EXERCISES

Using the chart, find the relationship between the units.

1. 1 kL = _____?_____ hL
2. 1 hL = _____?_____ daL
3. 1 daL = _____?_____ L
4. 1 L = _____?_____ dL
5. 1 dL = _____?_____ cL
6. 1 cL = _____?_____ mL
7. 1 hL = _____?_____ kL
8. 1 daL = _____?_____ hL
9. 1 L = _____?_____ daL
10. 1 dL = _____?_____ L
11. 1 cL = _____?_____ dL
12. 1 mL = _____?_____ cL

Expressing volume measures for fluids in larger or smaller units uses the principle of multiplying numbers by powers of ten.

Example: Express 0.328 L as millilitres.
0.328 L = __?__ mL
1 L = 1 000 mL
0.328 × 1 000 = 328
0.328 L = 328 mL

Example: Express 2 200 cL as kL.
2 200 cL = __?__ kL
1 cL = 0.000 01 kL
2 200 × 0.000 01 = 0.022 00
2 200 cL = 0.022 00 kL

15.5 EXERCISES

Express each measure in a larger equivalent metric unit or a smaller equivalent metric unit.

1. 2 500 mL = _____?_____ L
2. 1 530 mL = _____?_____ L
3. 8 000 mL = _____?_____ L
4. 3.2 L = _____?_____ mL
5. 0.5 L = _____?_____ mL
6. 0.75 L = _____?_____ mL
7. 250 mL = _____?_____ L
8. 5 L = _____?_____ mL
9. 1 L = _____?_____ mL
10. 10 mL = _____?_____ L

Common objects are listed in Column I. Choose an appropriate measure from Column II and write the letter in the blank.

Column I	Column II	
11. A 3-cm³ syringe.	a. 32 000 L	_____
12. A swimming pool.	b. 82 L	_____
13. A small water glass.	c. 200 mL	_____
14. An automobile gas tank.	d. 8 mL	_____
15. A tablespoon.	e. 3 mL	_____

For each container, choose the most appropriate measure of volume for fluids.

16. GRADUATED FLASK
    40 mL; 1 000 mL; 20 L

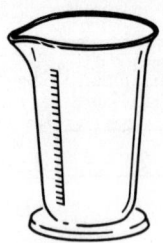

17. TEST TUBE
    15 mL; 1.5 L; 15 L

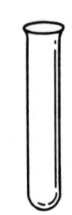

18. PLASTIC STORAGE JUG
    75 L; 7.5 L; 2L

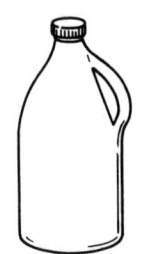

19. METAL STORAGE CAN
    5 L; 5 mL; 50 mL

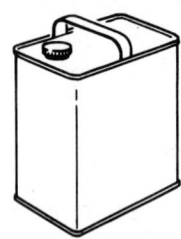

20. UNGRADUATED PIPETTE
    400 mL; 4 mL; 4 L

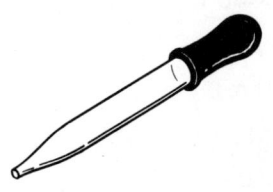

21. GRADUATED PIPETTE
    500 mL; 15 L; 15 mL

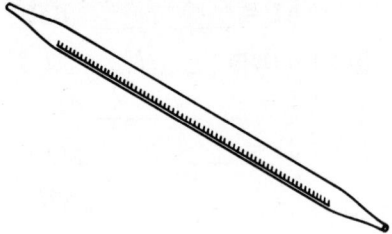

22. CUP
    30 L; 300 mL; 3 L

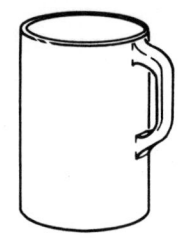

23. LIQUID MEDICINE DISPENSER
    675 mL; 6.75 L; 6.75 mL

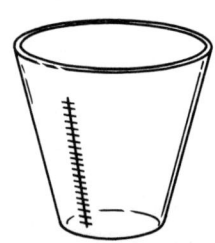

24. ERLENMEYER FLASK
    500 mL; 500 L; 5.00 L

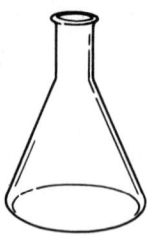

MEASURING VOLUMES OF FLUIDS

The litre and the cubic metre are both derived units for volume measure. Volume measure for fluids cannot be found directly. In order to find the volume measure for fluids, the volume is calculated using units of volume measure for solids. Using equivalences, the volume for fluids can then be found.

- The volume of a container which has a measurement of 1 000 cm³ is 1 L.
  It is written: 1 000 cm³ = 1 L

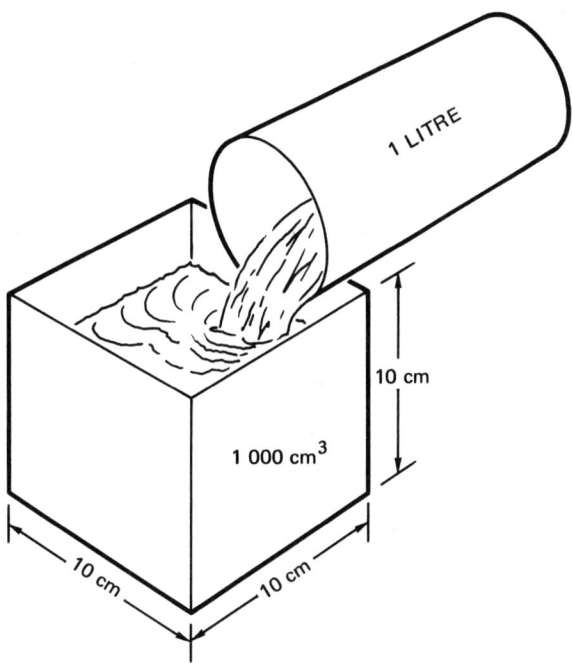

- The volume of a container which has a measurement of 1 cm³ is 0.001 L.
  It is written: 1 cm³ = 0.001 L

  or

  1 cm³ = 1 mL

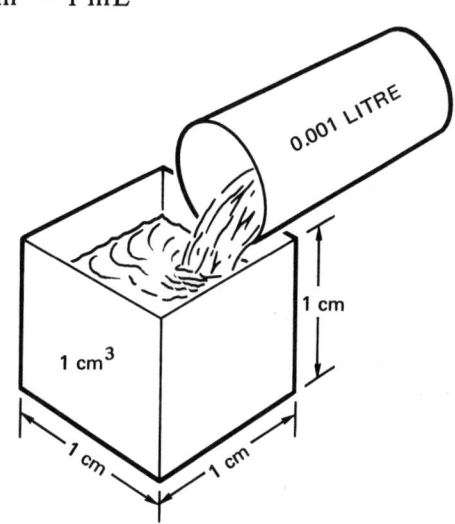

Example: Find the volume, in litres, of this rectangular container.

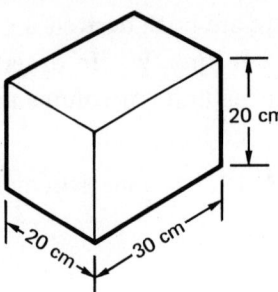

$V = lwh$
$V = 20 \text{ cm} \times 30 \text{ cm} \times 20 \text{ cm}$ Find the volume in cubic centimetres.
$V = 12\,000 \text{ cm}^3$
$12\,000 \text{ cm}^3 = \underline{\ \ ?\ \ } \text{ L}$ Express the volume in litres.
$1 \text{ cm}^3 = 0.001 \text{ L}$
$12\,000 \times 0.001 = 12$
$12\,000 \text{ cm}^3 = 12 \text{ L}$

Example: Find the volume, in millilitres, of the rectangular container.

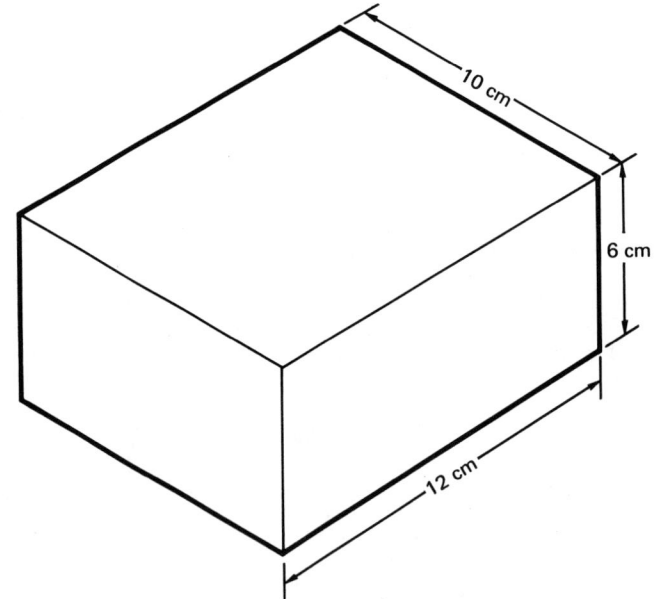

$V = lwh$ Find the volume.
$V = 10 \text{ cm} \times 12 \text{ cm} \times 6 \text{ cm}$
$V = 720 \text{ cm}^3$
$720 \text{ cm}^3 = \underline{\ \ ?\ \ } \text{ mL}$ Express the volume in millilitres.
$1 \text{ cm}^3 = 1 \text{ mL}$
$720 \times 1 = 720$
$720 \text{ cm}^3 = 720 \text{ mL}$

15.6 EXERCISES

For each container:
a. Find the volume in millilitres.
b. Express the volume in litres.

1.
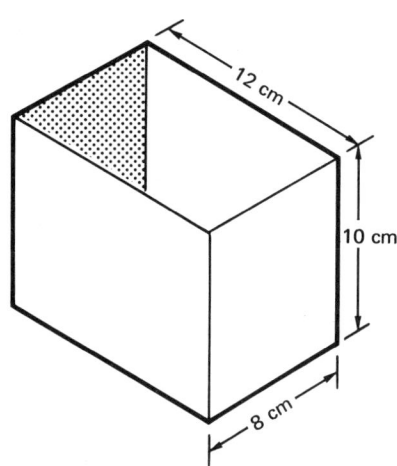

4.
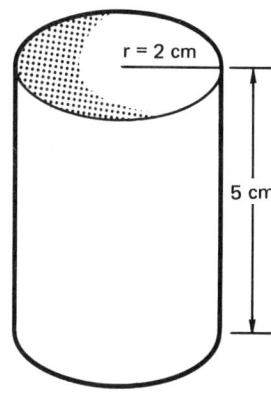

2.
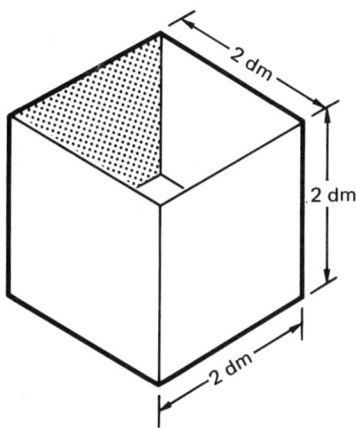

5.
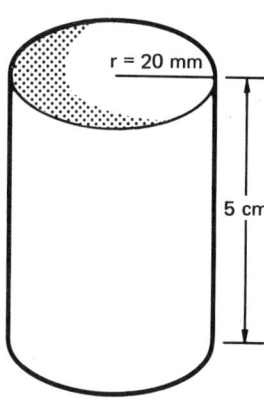

3.
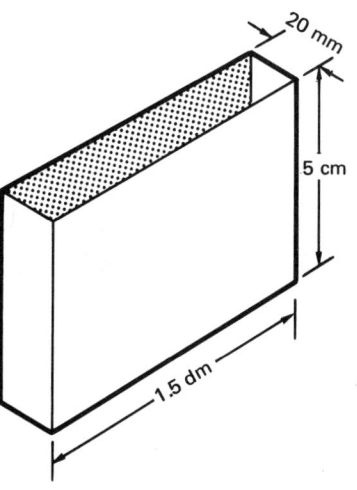

6.
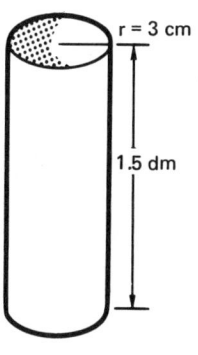

132 Section 3 Metric Measure

Arrange each group of measurements from largest to smallest.
7. 21 L;   0.2 hL;   19 000 mL;   2 000 cm³;   25 000 cm³
8. 628 mL;   0.5 L;   0.3 cL;   1 cm³;   24 m³
9. 250 daL;   50 kL;   49 000 L;   250 dam³;   50 cm³
10. 9L;   12 000 mL; $\frac{1}{10}$ hL; $\frac{1}{100}$ mm³;   90 hm³
11. 1 hL;   200 L;   1 500 mL;   150 cm³;   1 m³

APPLICATIONS

The air in a room and liquid in a container both involve volume measure. These volumes can be calculated. The heating engineer makes calculations to determine the rate at which air is replaced in any given area of the hospital. The laboratory technician must calculate volume when determining the amount of solution required to fill petri dishes. The skill of volume calculation is widely applied in many health areas. Mastering this skill is vital to an effective worker.

15.7 EXERCISES

1. During a specific period of time, the liquid intake and output for a patient are recorded. The intake is 0.250 L, 0.100 L, 0.200 L, 0.350 L, and 0.075 L. The output for the same period of time is 0.465 L.
   a. What is the total intake for this period of time?
   b. How does the output compare with the intake (greater than, equal to, less than)?

2. A graduated cylinder is used to measure the amounts of the same solution to be placed in a beaker and a flask. Determine the total amount of solution needed to fill each beaker and flask with the indicated amounts.

	BEAKER	FLASK	TOTAL
a.	0.750 L	125 mL	?
b.	0.010 L	25 mL	?
c.	0.005 L	10 mL	?

3. Liquid medication is administered to a patient every four hours.
   a. If the dose is 15 mL, how many millilitres are administered in 24 hours?
   b. If the dose is 5 mL, how many millilitres are administered in 16 hours?

4. A 50-mL graduated pipette is used to measure 46 samples, each containing 30 mL.
   a. What is the total volume measured?
   b. How many samples can be taken from a flask containing 750 mL?

5. A patient's room measures 5.750 m by 6.125 m by 3.000 m. A circulating fan can exchange 12.750 m³ of air each hour. How much time is required to exchange all the air in the room?

6. In one section of the hospital, 127 L of dextrose solution are used each day of the week.
   a. How many litres of solution are used in one week?
   b. How many litres of solution are used during the month of June?

unit 16 metric mass and temperature measures

OBJECTIVES

After studying this unit the student should be able to:

- Express metric mass in larger or smaller metric units.
- Determine the relationships between volume, capacity, and mass.
- Express Fahrenheit temperature readings as Celsius temperature readings.
- Express Celsius temperature readings as Fahrenheit temperature readings.

UNITS OF MASS

In order to move an object it is necessary to push, pull, or lift it. When moving the object, the *mass* or quantity of the object is actually being moved. The *weight,* or earth's gravitational pull, is how much the object pushes down on a scale. Two objects containing the same mass have equal weights when weighed at the same place. The kilogram is the base unit of mass in the metric system. Mass measure may also be expressed in hectograms, dekagrams, grams, decigrams, centigrams, and milligrams. The kilogram, gram, and milligram are the most commonly used units. A given metric mass unit can be expressed in larger or smaller metric units.

- To express a metric mass unit as a smaller metric mass unit, multiply by a positive power of ten such as 10, 100, 1 000.
- To express a metric mass unit as a larger metric mass unit, multiply by a negative power of ten such as 0.1, 0.01, 0.001.

This chart summarizes the units of metric mass measure, the symbols, the equivalences, and the relationships between the units.

Unit	kilogram	hectogram	dekagram	gram	decigram	centigram	milligram
Symbol	kg	hg	dag	g	dg	cg	mg
Equivalence	1 000 grams	100 grams	10 grams	1 gram	0.1 gram	0.01 gram	0.001 gram
Relationship Between Units	1 kg is 10 hg	1 hg is 10 dag	1 dag is 10 g	1 g is 10 dg	1 dg is 10 cg	1 cg is 10 mg	

16.1 EXERCISES

Using the chart, find the relationship between the units.

1. 1 kg = _____?_____ hg
2. 1 hg = _____?_____ dag
3. 1 dag = _____?_____ g
4. 1 g = _____?_____ dg
5. 1 dg = _____?_____ cg
6. 1 cg = _____?_____ mg
7. 1 hg = _____?_____ kg
8. 1 dag = _____?_____ hg
9. 1 g = _____?_____ dag
10. 1 dg = _____?_____ g
11. 1 cg = _____?_____ dg
12. 1 mg = _____?_____ cg

Expressing metric mass measure in larger or smaller units uses the principle of multiplying numbers by powers of ten.

Example: Tim has a mass of 86 kg. How many grams is this?
86 kg = __?__ g
1 kg = 1 000 g
86 × 1 000 = 86 000
86 kg = 86 000 g
Tim's mass is 86 000 grams.

Example: Each day Tony takes a vitamin pill containing 18 milligrams of iron. How many grams of iron does he take in 1 year (365 days)?
18 mg = __?__ g
1 mg = 0.001 g
18 × 0.001 = 0.018
18 mg = 0.018 g
0.018 g × 365 = 6.570 g
Tony consumes 6.57 grams of iron in 1 year

16.2 EXERCISES

Express each measure in a larger equivalent metric unit or a smaller equivalent metric unit.

1. 4.5 kg = _____?_____ g
2. 0.32 g = _____?_____ mg
3. 652 g = _____?_____ kg
4. 10 000 mg = _____?_____ kg
5. 0.2 kg = _____?_____ g
6. 3 250 mg = _____?_____ g
7. 2 kg = _____?_____ mg
8. 0.03 g = _____?_____ mg
9. 35 mg = _____?_____ g
10. 89.5 g = 0.895 __?__
11. 375 g = 0.375 __?__
12. 4 750 mg = 4.75 __?__
13. 0.02 kg = 20 __?__
14. 0.005 g = 0.000 005 __?__
15. 3 000 mg = 3 __?__
16. 45 g = 0.045 __?__
17. 4 g = 0.004 __?__
18. 0.002 5 kg = 2.5 __?__

Choose the most appropriate unit of mass to be used in finding the mass of these objects. Possible choices are: kilograms, grams, and milligrams.

19. A teenage girl.
20. A drop of blood.
21. A dime.
22. An eyelash.
23. A cigarette filter.
24. A car.
25. A litre of milk.
26. A tumor.
27. A ballpoint pen.
28. A stick of gum.

Choose the most appropriate mass for each object.

29. SHOE

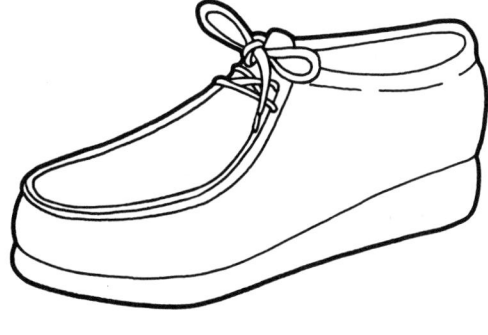

1 kg   1 mg   1 g

30. GLASS OF ORANGE JUICE

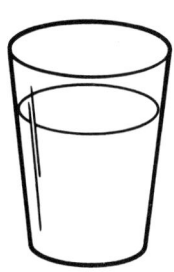

480 mg   480 kg   480 g

31. NICKEL

5 mg   5 g   5 kg

32. SYRINGE

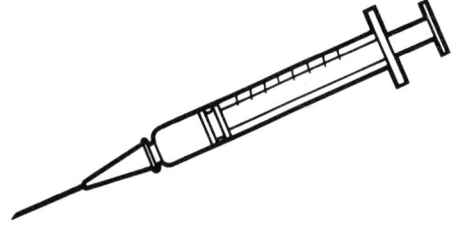

275 mg   275 g   275 kg

33. DRINKING STRAW

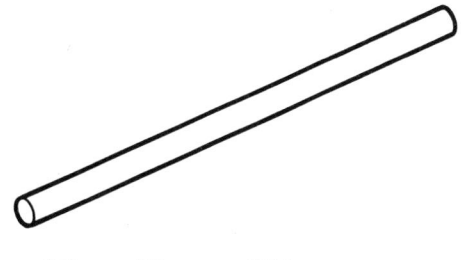

57 g   57 mg   57 kg

34. TELEVISION

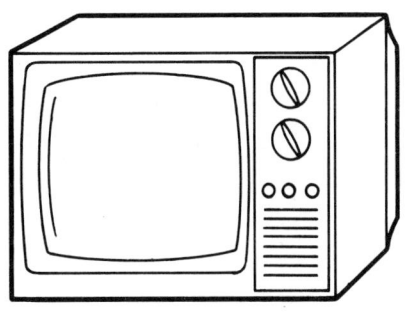

47 g   47 kg   47 mg

Using the given unit estimate and then find the mass of each object. Express the actual mass in the indicated units.

	Object	Estimate (a)	Mass (b)	Expressing the mass using other units (c)
35.	A wallet.	? g	? g	? kg
36.	A shoe.	? kg	? kg	? g
37.	The mass of a student.	? kg	? kg	? g
38.	The change in a wallet or a purse.	? g	? g	? mg

RELATIONSHIP BETWEEN METRIC UNITS

In the metric system, a special relationship exists between the measures of volume and mass for water at 4 degrees Celsius.

At 4 °C, 1 mL of water has a mass of 1 g. This means that 1 000 mL has a mass of 1 000 g.

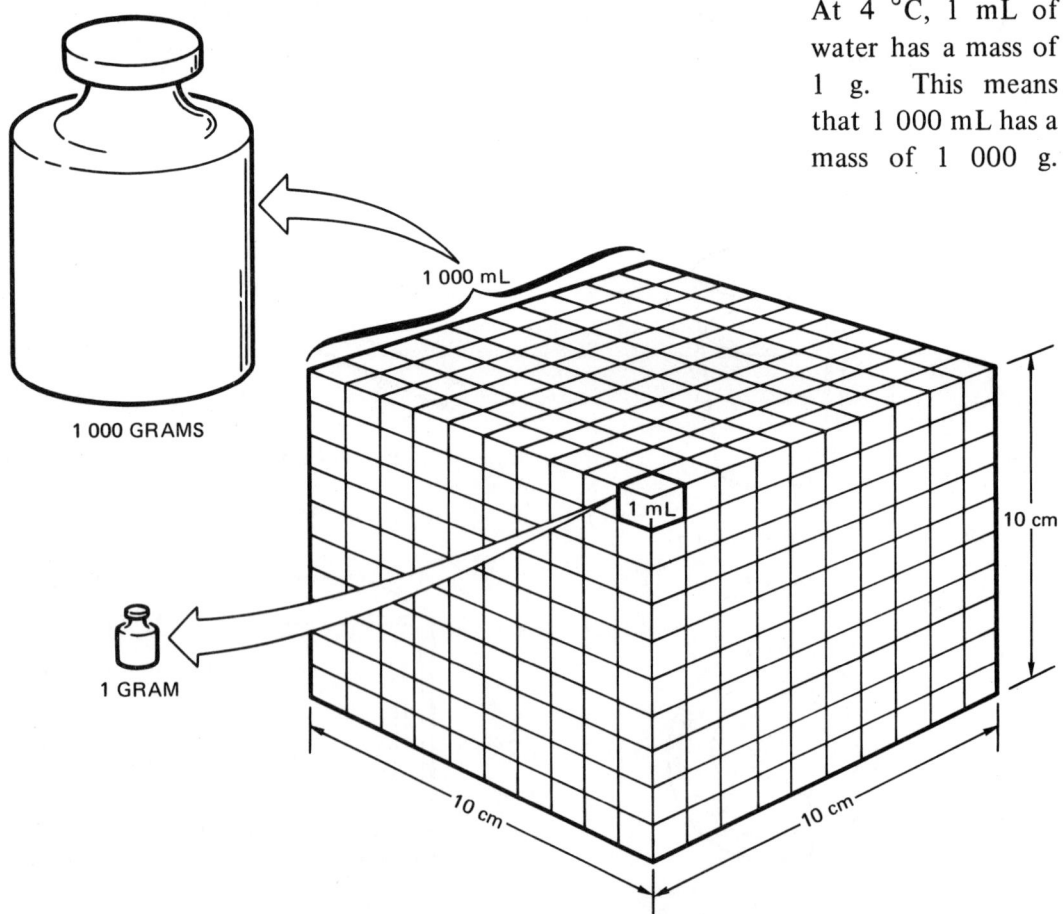

Since the volume of water is found by using cubic units, at 4 °C 1 g of water has a measurement of 1 cm³. This means that 1 000 g of water have a measurement of 1 000 cm³.

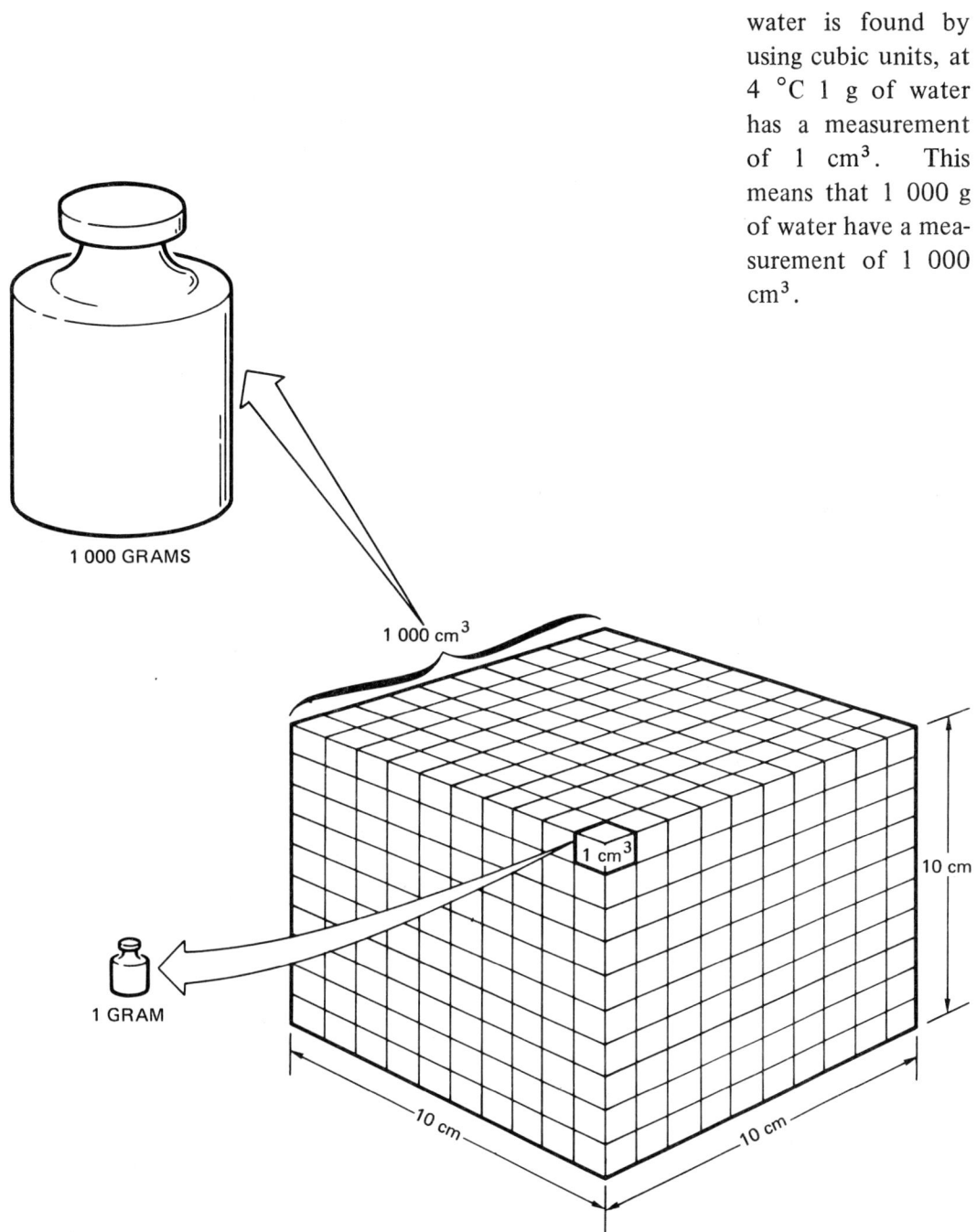

- At 4 degrees Celsius and standard pressure (760 millimetres), the volume and mass of water are equivalent relationships.

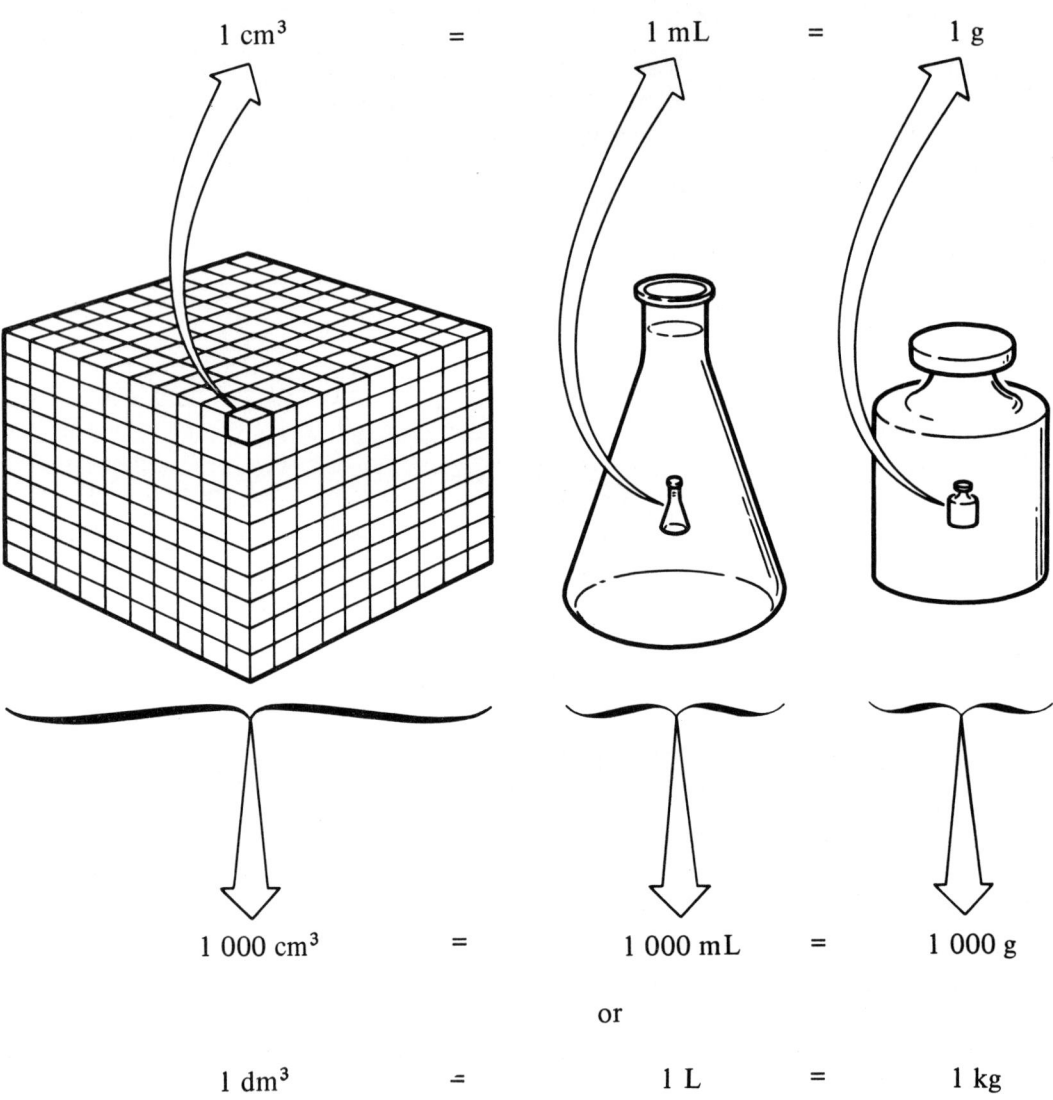

Example: This container of water is at 4 degrees Celsius and standard pressure. Find the volume and mass of the water.

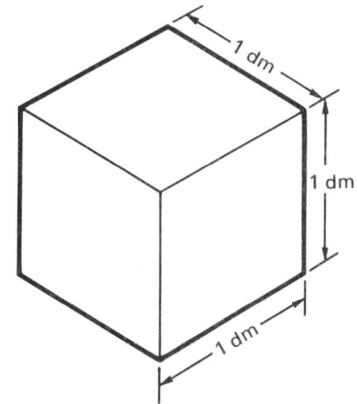

Volume = 1 dm³   *or*   1 000 cm³
Volume = 1 L   *or*   1 000 mL
Mass = 1 000 g   *or*   1 kg

16.3 EXERCISES

Express each measure as an equivalent measure.

1. 5 dm³ = _____?_____ cm³
2. 100 mm = _____?_____ cm
3. 1 500 mL = _____?_____ L
4. 0.20 dm² = _____?_____ m²
5. 625 g = _____?_____ kg
6. 0.175 m³ = _____?_____ cm³
7. 400 m = _____?_____ dm
8. 10 L = _____?_____ daL
9. 0.36 dam² = _____?_____ m²
10. 0.4 g = _____?_____ mg
11. 38 dm³ = _____?_____ m³
12. 425 m³ = _____?_____ dam³
13. 1 500 m = _____?_____ km
14. 0.5 L = _____?_____ mL
15. 375 mg = _____?_____ g
16. 1 dam² = _____?_____ m²
17. 2 km = _____?_____ m
18. 32 L = _____?_____ mL

Complete these relationships for water at 4 degrees Celsius and standard pressure.

	VOLUMES		MASS
19.	12 cm³	12 mL	__?__ g
20.	0.5 cm³	__?__ mL	0.5 g
21.	__?__ dm³	7 L	7 kg
22.	__?__ cm³	20 mL	__?__ g
23.	__?__ dm³	__?__ L	32 kg
24.	37 cm³	__?__ mL	__?__ g
25.	__?__ dm³	0.5 L	__?__ kg
26.	__?__ cm³	__?__ mL	454 g
27.	10 cm³	10 mL	10 __?__
28.	15 dm³	15 __?__	15 kg
29.	0.75 __?__	0.75 L	0.75 kg
30.	18 __?__	18 mL	18 __?__
31.	25 __?__	25 __?__	25 g
32.	0.5 cm³	0.5 __?__	0.5 __?__
33.	17.5 dm³	17.5 __?__	17.5 __?__
34.	82 __?__	82 __?__	82 kg

Find the values which measure the same amount of water at 4 degrees Celsius.

35.	5 L	5 g	5 kg
36.	5 L	5 dm³	5 cm³
37.	30 cm³	30 L	30 mL
38.	30 cm³	30 kg	30 g
39.	17 mL	17 g	17 kg
40.	17 mL	17 dm³	17 cm³

The relationship between units of volume and mass for water at 4 degrees Celsius may require expressing the metric units as equivalent units. Using the indicated units of measure, determine each equivalence.

41. 0.42 cm³ = 420 __?__ (units of volume for solids)

42. 200 cm² = 2 __?__ (units of area)

43. 1.8 dm = 18 __?__ (units of length)

44. 25 mm² = 0.25 __?__ (units of area)

45. 8.5 m = 0.008 5 __?__ (units of length)

46. 1 250 dm² = 12.5 ___?___ (units of area)
47. 125 cm = 1.25 ___?___ (units of length)
48. 15 dam² = 1 500 ___?___ (units of area)
49. 2.75 m = 275 ___?___ (units of length)
50. 50 g = 50 000 ___?___ (units of mass)
51. 0.5 kg = 500 ___?___
    a. units of volume for fluids
    b. units of mass
52. 1 mL = 1 ___?___
    a. units of volume for solids
    b. units of mass
53. 825 mL = 0.825 ___?___
    a. units of volume for solids
    b. units of volume for fluids
    c. units of mass
54. 2.5 L = 2 500 ___?___
    a. units of mass
    b. units of volume for solids
    c. units of volume for fluids
55. 1 500 cm³ = 1.5 ___?___
    a. units of volume for solids
    b. units of mass
    c. units of volume for fluids
56. 3.2 kg = 3 200 ___?___
    a. units of volume for mass
    b. units of volume for fluids
    c. units of volume for solids
57. 0.36 L = 360 ___?___
    a. units of volume for fluids
    b. units of mass
    c. units of volume for solids
58. 1 750 mm³ = 1.750 ___?___
    a. units of mass
    b. units of volume for fluids
    c. units of volume for solids
59. 2.5 mg = 0.002 5 ___?___
    a. units of volume for solids
    b. units of volume for fluids
    c. units of mass
60. 5 dm³ = 5 000 ___?___
    a. units of mass
    b. units of volume for solids
    c. units of volume for fluids

MEASURING METRIC TEMPERATURE

Temperature can be measured in degrees Celsius or in degrees Fahrenheit. On the Celsius scale, water boils at 100 °C and freezes at 0 °C.

On the Fahrenheit scale, water boils at 212 °F and freezes at 32 °F.

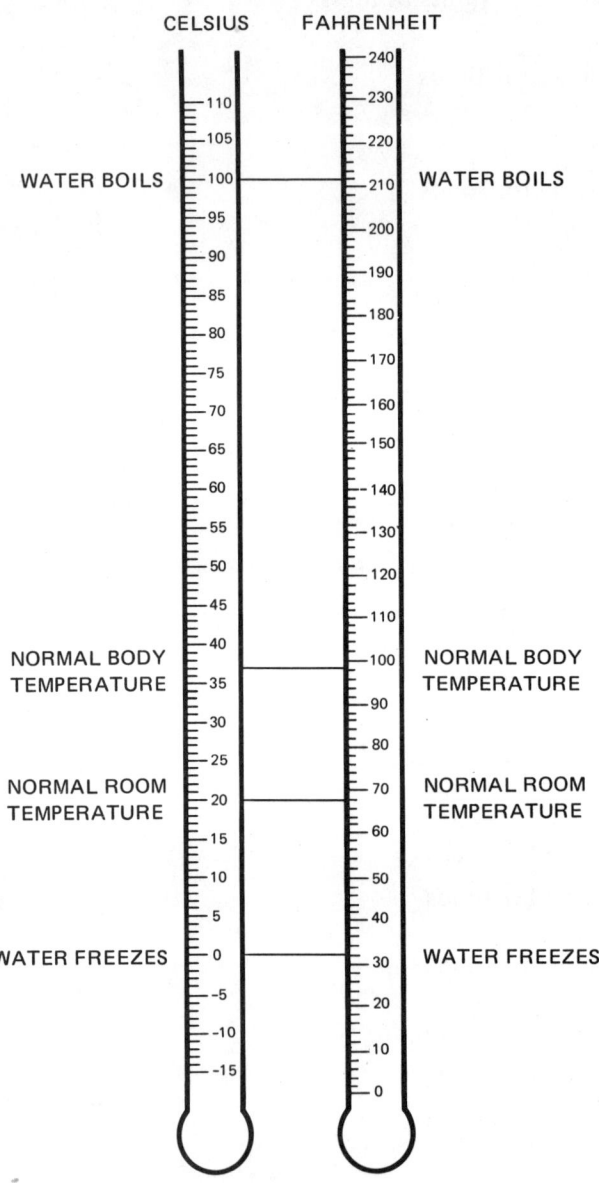

- To express degrees Fahrenheit as degrees Celsius use the relationship:
$$°C = \frac{5}{9}(°F - 32)$$

- To express degrees Celsius as degrees Fahrenheit use the relationship:
$$°F = \frac{9}{5}°C + 32$$

Example: Express 68 °F as degrees Celsius.

$$°C = \frac{5}{9}(°F - 32)$$ Write the formula.

$$°C = \frac{5}{9}(68 - 32)$$ Substitute the specific values for the unknowns.

$$°C = \frac{5}{\cancel{9}_1}(\cancel{36}^4)$$ Perform the calculations.

$$°C = 20$$

$$68 °F = 20 °C$$

Example: Express 35 °C as degrees Fahrenheit.

$$°F = \frac{9}{5}°C + 32$$ Write the formula.

$$°F = \frac{9}{5}(35) + 32$$ Substitute the specific values for the unknown.

$$°F = \frac{9}{\cancel{5}_1}(\cancel{35}^7) + 32$$ Perform the calculations.

$$°F = 63 + 32$$

$$°F = 95°$$

$$35 °C = 95 °F$$

16.4 EXERCISES

Express each Celsius temperature as an equivalent Fahrenheit temperature and each Fahrenheit temperature as an equivalent Celsius temperature.

1. 113 °F
2. 50 °F
3. 14 °F
4. −13 °F
5. −10 °C
6. 25 °C
7. 70 °C
8. 110 °C

Choose the more appropriate Celsius temperature for each activity.

9. Having a fever.   20 °C   38.5 °C
10. Air on a summer day.   26 °C   45 °C
11. Sunbathing.   10 °C   28 °C
12. Raining.   0 °C   3 °C
13. Building a snowman.   −5 °C   10 °C
14. Mowing the grass.   27 °C   8 °C

APPLICATIONS

All health care workers are involved in measuring mass. The health care assistant, the LPN and the RN may be involved in determining the mass of patients. The pharmacist is involved with measuring medication. Laboratory personnel measure the mass of substances to be used in cultures or in laboratory tests. The dietitian measures the mass of the food that is to be administered. Different health care workers use different types of instruments to measure mass. The instrument that is used must be accurate and the health care worker must read the measurements correctly and must record the measurements promptly and correctly.

Health care workers are also involved in measuring temperature. Temperature is measured in units termed degrees Celsius (°C). The freezing temperature of pure water at 760 mm pressure is 0 °C and the boiling temperature is 100 °C. The temperature of the human body serves as an indicator of a person's well being. Normal body temperature is 36.99 °C or 37 °C. The Celsius scale is and has been the common unit of measure in laboratories for many years.

16.5 EXERCISES

1. To determine the total daily medication that each patient receives, daily records are kept. This record shows the medication administered to three patients.

Mrs. Larson	Mr. Davonport	Miss Juliet
2.5 g	1.6 g	9.6 g
1.6 g	1.6 g	0.250 g
0.4 g	1.6 g	7.5 g
0.25 g	0.6 g	0.3 g

   a. How much medication does Mrs. Larson receive?
   b. How much medication does Mr. Davonport receive?
   c. How much medication does Miss Juliet receive?

2. The mass loss of a patient is recorded over a five-day period. The initial mass of the patient is 68.500 kg. Determine the patient's new mass for each day and the total mass loss.

	DAY	MASS LOSS	NEW MASS
a.	1	250 g	?
b.	2	750 g	?
c.	3	80 g	?
d.	4	500 g	?
e.	5	250 g	?
f.		TOTAL	?

3. Mrs. Judson receives 250 grams of meat for each meal. Miss Keebler receives 0.56 times as much meat as Mrs. Judson does. How much meat does Miss Keebler receive?

4. To produce 1 000 millilitres of a liquid medium suitable for culturing bacteria, 21 grams of a dehydrated culture medium are needed.

   a. How many litres can be prepared from 975 grams of dehydrated culture medium? Round the answer to the nearer thousandth litre.
   b. How many grams are required to prepare 5.750 L of solution?

5. An analytical balance is used to obtain these measurements: 1.250 grams, 16 milligrams, 46 milligrams, and 0.750 gram.

   a. What is the total mass in grams?
   b. What is the total mass in milligrams?

6. A triple beam balance is used to measure amounts of bacto-dextrose agar used for the culture of bacteria. The amounts measured are: 16.00 g, 4.25 g, 12.75 g, and 22.12 g. A preparation of 10.5 L requires 453.59 g of bacto-dextrose agar.

   a. What is the total mass of the bacto-dextrose agar?
   b. How many grams of bacto-dextrose agar are required per litre of preparation? Round the answer to the nearer tenth gram.
   c. How many litres can be prepared from the measured amounts of bacto-dextrose agar? Round the answer to the nearer thousandth litre.
   d. How many litres can be prepared from 1 000 grams of bacto-dextrose agar? Round the answer to the nearer thousandth litre.

7. A solution is formed when a granular material is placed in water and is heated to 100 °C. A solution condition continues to exist until the temperature drops to 45 °C. A laboratory has only a Fahrenheit thermometer.

   a. Find the Fahrenheit value of 100 °C.
   b. Find the Fahrenheit value of 45 °C.

8. A normal temperature for a human is considered to be 98.6 °F. A fever condition exists for a body temperature that is over 98.6 °F.

   a. Determine the degree Celsius value for normal body temperature.
   b. Determine the degree Celsius value for a fever condition of 102.5 °F. Round the answer to the nearer tenth degree.
   c. Determine the degree Celsius value for a fever condition of 100 °F. Round the answer to the nearer tenth degree.

9. The temperature of several rooms are recorded with a Fahrenheit thermometer. What are the degree Celsius readings for each temperature measure? Round the answers to the nearer tenth degree.

   a. 75 °F
   b. 78 °F
   c. 81 °F
   d. 86 °F

unit 17 section three applications to health work

OBJECTIVES

After studying this unit the student should be able to:

- Use the various units of metric measure to solve health work problems.

Measurement is an important component in all health work. Health care workers are concerned with how much patients eat, the amount of medication they take, the weight they gain or lose, the amount of liquid gained or lost, and the temperature at which the body is functioning. Some form of measurement is taken for each patient every day. The units of measure most commonly used are metric.

- The height of the patient or length of gauze is measured using the metre as the base unit. This unit of measure is convenient for measuring large units such as height, room size, or parking lot dimensions. Centimetres and millimetres are commonly used to measure smaller objects that are still detectable by the human eye. The size of this page, the length of a pin, and the width of a pen may be expressed in centimetres or millimetres. The micrometre is used to measure small objects such as fungi spores and bacterial cells.

- The mass of a patient or the amount of a dry substance is measured using the kilogram as the base unit. For large masses, such as the human body, the kilogram is the most practical unit of measure. The gram is the most common unit of measure in weighing out dry substances in the laboratory. Very small units are measured in milligrams.

- The volume of water taken in by a patient or the volume of water given off may be measured in either litres or millilitres. Large volumes are most commonly measured in litres. The millilitre is the common unit of measure for liquids in the laboratory.

- The temperature of a patient above or below an accepted norm is a concern of the health care staff. The Celsius scale is the unit of measure for determining this variation. This unit of measure is used in the laboratory as well as in the patient's room.

17.1 EXERCISES

1. A patient is weighed once a month over a period of five months. Find the change in the patient's mass between each weighing.

	MONTH	MASS	CHANGE
	Beginning Mass	75.125 kg	— — —
a.	1	75.052 kg	
b.	2	74.983 kg	
c.	3	75.005 kg	
d.	4	77.015 kg	
e.	5	79.250 kg	

2. Several samples are weighed and the average mass is determined. Find the average mass of these samples. Average equals total divided by the number of samples. Round the answer to the nearer thousandth gram.

SAMPLE	MASS
A	0.125 g
B	1.750 g
C	2.015 g
D	6.835 g
E	4.321 g
F	3.895 g
G	7.396 g
H	3.425 g

3. A roll of gauze is 35 metres in length. How many 50-centimetre lengths can be obtained from the roll?

4. A piece of circular filter paper has a diameter of 16 centimetres. Calculate the surface area for one side of the paper.

5. The liquid intake measured for a patient during a specified period of time is 1.275 litres. During the same period the liquid given off is 0.498 litre. Find the difference between these two measures.

6. A storage tank of distilled water has a capacity of 2 000 litres.
    a. If the storage tank contains 1 256.025 litres, how many litres are required to fill the tank?
    b. If 37.850 litres are used from the tank each day, how many litres are left in the tank after seven days of use? The tank is full at the start and not filled during the seven-day period.

7. Agar-agar, a solidifying agent used in bacteriological and mycological study, melts when heated in water to 100 °C. When allowed to cool it solidifies at about 45 °C. What is the temperature difference between melting and solidification?

148   Section 3 Metric Measure

8. The temperature of a bacteriological culture is measured each hour for six hours. What is the average temperature during the six hour period?

   1st hour: 23.8 °C   4th hour: 25 °C
   2nd hour: 24.0 °C   5th hour: 25 °C
   3rd hour: 23.7 °C   6th hour: 25.8 °C

9. The diameter of a capillary tube is 0.025 mm. Calculate the area of a circle this size.

10. A Petri dish has a diameter of 9 centimetres. Find the surface area on the floor of the Petri dish.

11. A nutrient agar is inoculated with a pathogenic microorganism. At the end of 24 hours it is discovered that one colony is present per 9 square millimetres. How many colonies are present in a Petri dish which is —

   a. 9 centimetres in diameter?
   b. 120 millimetres in diameter?
   c. 10 centimetres in diameter?

12. A medication is provided in container quantities of 50 mL. How many times can a 15-mL syringe be filled from this single container?

13. A one-litre graduated cylinder contains 942 mL of distilled water. A total of 127 mL is removed. What is the amount remaining in the cylinder?

14. A hemacytometer is used to measure the number of cells in 0.1 mL of solution. The population is determined to be 15 cells. How many cells can be predicted in these volumes of the same solution?

	VOLUME	NUMBER OF CELLS
a.	5 mL	
b.	50 mL	
c.	1 000 mL	
d.	1 L	

15. An analytical balance is used to measure the mass of four different tissue masses. The masses are determined to be:

   Specimen A: 1.059 grams
   Specimen B: 0.984 grams
   Specimen C: 1.001 grams
   Specimen D: 0.493 grams

   a. What is the combined mass of the tissue masses?
   b. What is the average mass per tissue mass? Round the answer to the nearer thousandth.

16. A laboratory technician is requested to prepare 25 Petri dishes for a bacteriological study. The dishes are 9 cm in diameter. A nutrient solution is to be prepared and poured to a depth of 0.5 cm. How much nutrient solution is required to fill all 25 dishes?

17. A manometer is used to measure the amount of oxygen used by a culture of microorganisms.

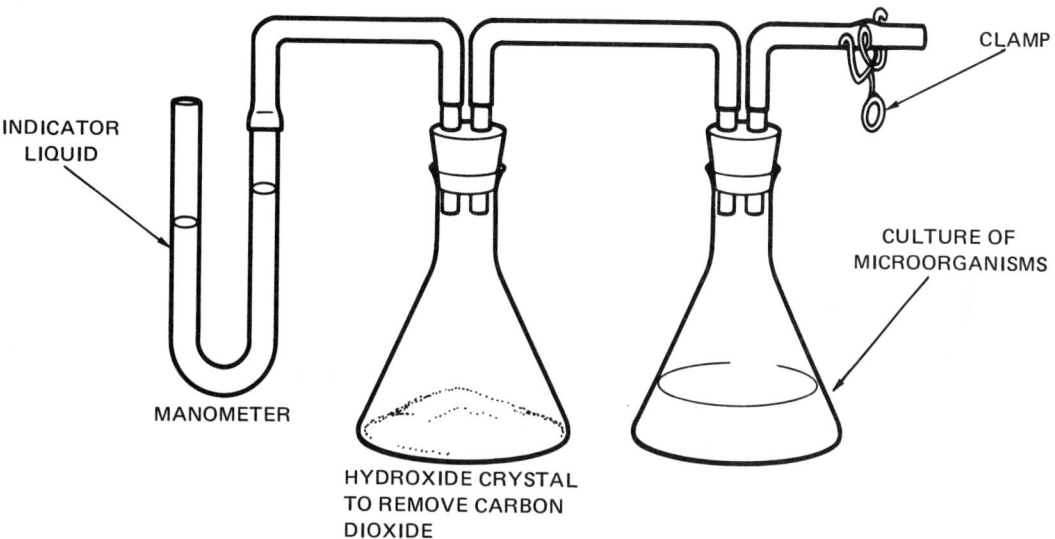

The liquid in the manometer changes level as the oxygen is used. The diameter of the manometer tube is 0.5 mm. During one ten-minute period the indicator liquid moves 43 mm. Find the volume of gas change in the system.

18. A system requiring a measure of liquid is constructed. One section requires a graduated manometer. It is necessary to calibrate a section of the glass tubed manometer into 2-cubic millimetre units. If the diameter of the glass tubing is 0.75 mm, what is the distance between each graduation?

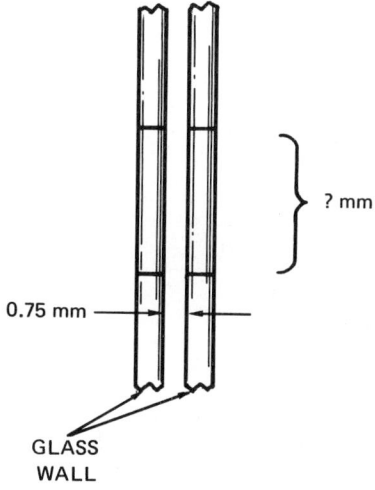

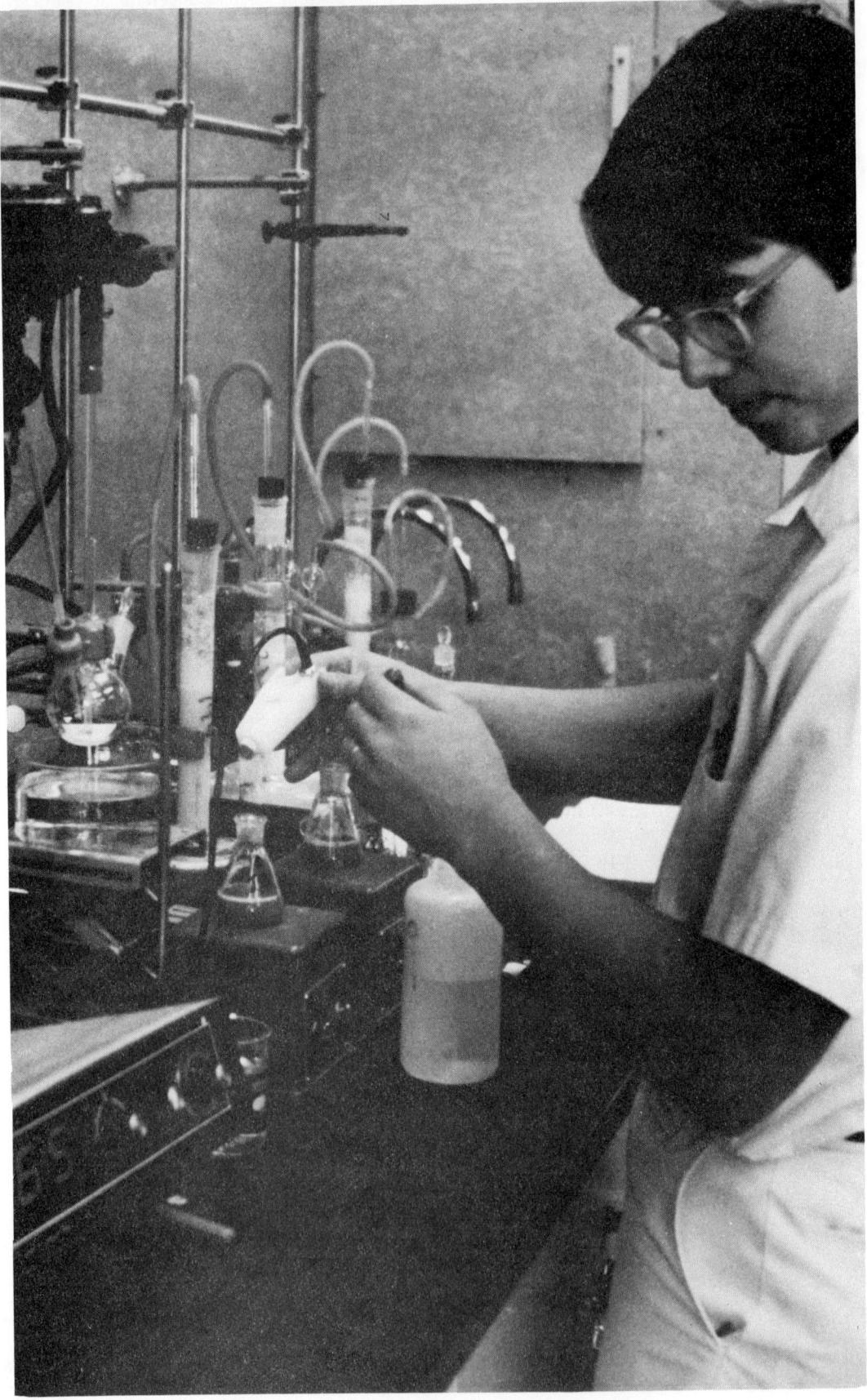

SECTION 4 RATIO, PROPORTION, AND PERCENTS

unit 18 introduction to ratio and proportion

OBJECTIVES

After studying this unit the student should be able to:
- Compare quantities using ratios.
- Identify mean terms and extreme terms in a proportion.
- Determine if a proportion is an equality using the means and extremes.
- Determine the unknown component in a simple proportion.

The ability to accurately compare numbers of quantities is a skill used by many people. Ratios and proportions are one method of comparison.

RATIO

Quantities can be compared in different ways. A comparison between numbers by division is a *ratio*. The numbers that are compared are the *terms*, or *components*, of the ratio.

Example: This diagram can be used to illustrate several comparisons, *or* ratios.

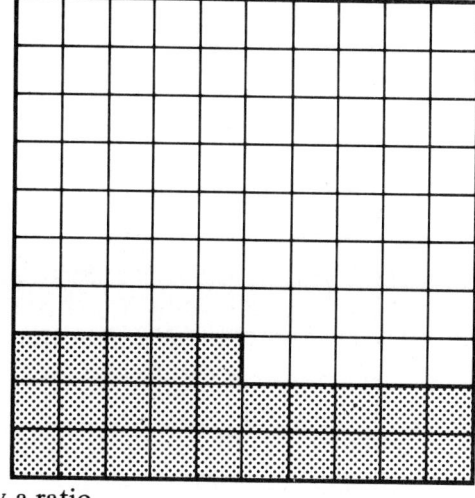

There are 25 shaded squares compared to 75 unshaded squares.
The ratio can be written 25 to 75 *or* 1 to 3.
There are 25 shaded squares compared to 100 total squares.
The ratio can be written 25 to 100 *or* 1 to 4.
The ratio of the unshaded squares compared to the shaded squares is $\frac{75}{25}$ *or* $\frac{3}{1}$.
The ratio of the unshaded squares to the total squares is 75:100 *or* 3:4.

The three notations, "to,":, and —, all identify a ratio.

152 Section 4 Ratio, Proportion, and Percents

■ In general, the ratio of a to b can be written as:

$$a \text{ to } b; \quad a:b; \quad \frac{a}{b}$$

As in fractions, the components or terms of a ratio can be expressed in lowest terms.

▼ A *simplest-term ratio* is a ratio in which the terms or components contain no common factors other than 1.

A ratio can compare like measurements or unlike measurements. When the ratio is a comparison of unlike measurements, this is classified as a *rate*.

Example: 35 kilometres per hour
This compares kilometres and hours, two unlike measurements. Since <u>per</u> means <u>to</u>, the ratio can be read "35 kilometres to 1 hour."

Example: $1.50 per kilogram
This compares the unlike measurements of dollars and kilograms. The ratio can be read "$1.50 to 1 kilogram."

PROPORTION

Ratios can be used to form proportions. A *proportion* is an equation which states that two ratios are equal.

■ In general, the proportion formed by using the ratios *a:b* and *c:d* is:

$$a:b = c:d; \quad \text{or} \quad \frac{a}{b} = \frac{c}{d}$$

It is read "*a* is to *b* as *c* is to *d*."

▼ In a proportion the middle terms or components are the *means* and the end components are the *extremes*.

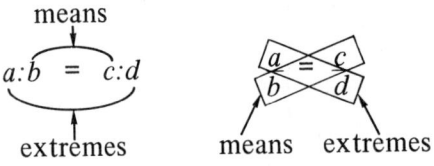

The equality of a proportion may be verified by using the means and extremes. The product of the means is calculated. The product of the extremes is also calculated. If the product of the means equals the product of the extremes, the proportion is an equality. Conversely, if the proportion is an equality, then the product of the means equals the product of the extremes.

■ Generally, if $\frac{a}{b} = \frac{c}{d}$, then $ad = bc$ and
if $ad = bc$, then $\frac{a}{b} = \frac{c}{d}$.

Example: Using the product of the means and the product of the extremes, prove that $\frac{8}{12} = \frac{2}{3}$.

$\frac{8}{12} \stackrel{?}{=} \frac{2}{3}$ $\frac{8}{12} \stackrel{?}{=} \frac{2}{3}$

$8 \times 3 = 24$ $12 \times 2 = 24$

Since $24 = 24$, $\frac{8}{12} = \frac{2}{3}$.

Example: Using the product of the means and the product of the extremes, determine if $\frac{2}{5} = \frac{8}{15}$.

$\frac{2}{5} \stackrel{?}{=} \frac{8}{15}$ $\frac{2}{5} \stackrel{?}{=} \frac{8}{15}$

$2 \times 15 = 30$ $5 \times 8 = 40$

Since $30 \neq 40$, $\frac{2}{5} \neq \frac{8}{15}$.

As in ratios, proportions may use unlike measurements. The comparison of the unlike measurement is the rate. The proportional relationships between ratios of unlike measurements are *rate pairs*.

18.1 EXERCISES

Express each ratio in simplest terms.

1. 8:6
2. $\frac{10}{12}$
3. 9 to 12
4. 30:50
5. $\frac{85}{40}$

6. The ratio of the number of men in the class to the number of women in the class.

7. The ratio comparing the number of students in the class to the total number of desks in the room.

Identify the mean terms and extreme terms in each proportion.

8. $\frac{3}{5} = \frac{12}{20}$
9. $\frac{20}{3} = \frac{N}{6}$
10. $\frac{1}{x} = \frac{33}{100}$

Using the product of the means equals the product of the extremes, determine if each proportion is an equality or inequality.

11. $\frac{3}{10} \stackrel{?}{=} \frac{30}{100}$
12. $\frac{2}{3} \stackrel{?}{=} \frac{3}{4}$
13. $\frac{8}{4} \stackrel{?}{=} \frac{1}{2}$
14. $\frac{9}{12} \stackrel{?}{=} \frac{18}{24}$
15. $\frac{5}{3} \stackrel{?}{=} \frac{50}{30}$

PROPORTIONAL COMPUTATIONS

A proportion is an equation which states that two ratios are equal. Generally, if $\frac{a}{b} = \frac{c}{d}$, then $ad = bc$ or if $ad = bc$, then $\frac{a}{b} = \frac{c}{d}$. Many times a component of a proportion is unknown. By using the product of the means and the product of the extremes, the unknown component may be determined.

Example: Find the unknown component, X, for which $\frac{8}{X} = \frac{2}{3}$ will be an equality.

$$\frac{8}{X} = \frac{2}{3}$$
$$2(X) = 8(3)$$
$$2X = 24$$
$$\frac{2X}{2} = \frac{24}{2} \quad \text{(\underline{Divide} both sides of the equation by 2, the number in front of the unknown component.)}$$
$$X = 12$$

Since $\frac{8}{12} = \frac{2}{3}$, 12 is the correct answer.

Note: Since 1 times any number is that number, the 1 in front of the X need not be shown. In actuality, $1X = X$. The expression $2(X)$ means $2X$. The parenthesis may be shown or not shown.

Example: Find the unknown term, X, for which $\frac{2}{5} = \frac{X}{20}$ will be an equality.

$$\frac{2}{5} = \frac{X}{20}$$
$$5(X) = 2(20)$$
$$5X = 40$$
$$\frac{5X}{5} = \frac{40}{5} \quad \text{(\underline{Divide} both sides of the equation by 5, the number in front of the unknown term.)}$$
$$X = 8$$

Since $\frac{2}{5} = \frac{8}{20}$, 8 is the correct answer.

18.2 EXERCISES

Find the unknown component for which each proportion will be an equality.

1. $\frac{1}{2} = \frac{3}{X}$
2. $\frac{4}{1} = \frac{X}{4}$
3. $\frac{X}{8} = \frac{8}{1}$
4. $\frac{2}{X} = \frac{1}{10}$
5. $\frac{6}{5} = \frac{X}{10}$
6. $\frac{3}{4} = \frac{30}{X}$
7. $\frac{X}{100} = \frac{3}{10}$
8. $\frac{2}{X} = \frac{5}{15}$
9. $\frac{0.7}{10} = \frac{X}{100}$
10. $\frac{\frac{1}{2}}{5} = \frac{X}{100}$

APPLICATIONS

Many health care workers prepare solutions. A *solution* is a liquid preparation of one or more substances dissolved in a liquid, usually water. Pharmacists prepare solutions of medication to be administered to patients. Registered nurses (RN) may prepare solutions to be administered orally; licensed practical nurses (LPN) may prepare solutions to be administered topically. Medical technologists (4 years of postsecondary training), medical laboratory technicians (2 years of postsecondary training), and medical laboratory assistants (1 year of postsecondary training) prepare solutions to be used in chemical microscopic and bacteriological tests.

A solution consists of a solvent and a solute.

▼ The *solvent* is the liquid in which the substance or substances are dissolved. It is usually water.

▼ The *solute* is the substance that is dissolved in the liquid. The solute is the drug.

The ratio between the solute (drug) and the solution is the *ratio strength of the solution.* That is:

amount of drug:amount of solution
is the ratio strength of the solution

or

$$\frac{\text{amount of drug}}{\text{amount of solution}} = \frac{\text{ratio strength}}{\text{of the solution}}$$

A 1:5 solution means $\frac{1}{5}$ or 1 part solute (drug) to 5 parts solution. This may mean that there is 1 millilitre of the drug in 5 millilitres of solution. Since the ratio 1:5 is in lowest terms, it may also be 2 millilitres of the drug in 10 millilitres of solution or even 25 millilitres of the drug in 125 millilitres of solution.

18.3 EXERCISES

1. Drugs may be in many forms. One form is crystals. There are 3 parts boric acid in 12 parts of solution. Express the strength of the solution as a ratio.

2. Glycerin is a liquid. There are 8 millilitres of glycerin in 24 millilitres of solution. Express the strength of a solution as a ratio.

3. The ratio strength of a certain solution is 1:5. There are 15 millilitres of the drug. How many millilitres of solution are there? (Use the proportion $\frac{1}{5} = \frac{15}{x}$.)

4. The ratio strength of a lysol solution is 1:20. If there are 1 000 millilitres of solution, how many millilitres of lysol are there? (Use the proportion $\frac{1}{20} = \frac{y}{1\,000}$.)

5. Doses of a 2:50 solution are to be administered to a patient. Each dose is 0.5 millilitre.

    a. How much medication is needed to administer 5 doses?

    b. Using the proportion $\frac{2}{50} = \frac{\text{amount of drug}}{\text{total amount of medication}}$, find the amount of drug.

unit 19 computations with proportions

OBJECTIVES

After studying this unit the student should be able to:
- Determine the unknown component in a rate pair.
- Determine the unknown component in a proportion which contains an implied component.
- Determine the unknown component in a proportion which contains fractional components.

RATE PAIR COMPUTATIONS

Rate pairs express proportional relationships between ratios. The ratios are comparisons, in the same order, of unlike measurements. Determining unknown components in rate pairs uses the same procedure as in proportions.

Example: A medical supplier sells 4 tongue depressors for 24 cents. What is the cost of 1 tongue depressor?

The rate is depressors:cost.

The rate pair is $\frac{\text{depressors}}{\text{cost}} = \frac{\text{depressor}}{\text{cost}}$.

$$\frac{\text{depressors}}{\text{cost}} = \frac{\text{depressors}}{\text{cost}}$$

$\frac{4}{24} = \frac{1}{N}$ (This is read 4 depressors are to 24 cents as 1 depressor is to N cents.)

$4(N) = 1(24)$

$4N = 24$

$\frac{4N}{4} = 24$ (Divide both sides of the equation by 4, the number in front of the unknown component.)

$N = 6$ or $N = 6$ cents

One tongue depressor costs 6 cents.

Note: The answer is a descriptive quantity. It describes what type of measurement the unknown component is.

Example: An ambulance travels an average speed of 70 kilometres per hour. The ambulance is on the road 21 hours in a three-day period. How many kilometres are traveled?

The rate is kilometres:hours.

$$\frac{\text{kilometres}}{\text{hour}} = \frac{\text{kilometres}}{\text{hours}}$$

$$\frac{70}{1} = \frac{X}{21}$$ (This is read 70 kilometres is to one hour as X kilometres is to 21 hours.)

$$1(X) = 70(21)$$

$$X = 1\ 470 \text{ or } X = 1\ 470 \text{ kilometres}$$

In 21 hours, the ambulance travels 1 470 kilometres.

19.1 EXERCISES

An incorrect rate pair is written in each proportion. Write the correct rate pairs. Determine the value of each unknown component.

RATES	INCORRECT RATE PAIRS	CORRECT RATE PAIRS	ANSWER
1. 400 metres in 80 seconds N metres in 10 seconds	$\frac{400}{80} \neq \frac{10}{N}$		
2. 8 kilograms lost in 4 weeks 2 kilograms lost in x weeks	$\frac{8}{4} \neq \frac{x}{2}$		
3. 12 cents per y stirring rods 144 cents for 12 stirring rods	$\frac{y}{0.12} \neq \frac{1.44}{12}$		
4. $6 for 1 hour of work $Z for 100 hours of work	$\frac{Z}{100} \neq \frac{1}{6}$		
5. 1 centimetre for 80 kilometres q centimetres for 360 kilometres	$\frac{80}{1} \neq \frac{q}{360}$		

Express each rate pair. Determine the unknown component. Express the answer as a descriptive quantity.

6. During a rainstorm, the rain falls at a rate of 0.4 centimetres per hour. At this rate, how much rain will fall in 4 hours?

7. At a price of 2 test tubes for $0.99, how many test tubes can Peg buy for $9.00?

8. A compact car travels 10 kilometres on 1 litre of gasoline. How many litres are needed to travel 485 kilometres?

9. To make a salt solution John uses 0.5 teaspoon of salt for each 0.75 litre of water. How much salt is used in 15 litres of water?

10. It is found that $5 worth of rock salt keeps a section of the hospital walk clear of ice. What is the cost if this amount is used fifty times during a winter season?

11. The ratio of kilometres driven to litres of gasoline used is 15 to 2. The gas tank holds 8 litres. How many kilometres can be driven on a tank of gas?

12. An automatic washer can wash 100 large flasks in 60 minutes. At this rate, how many flasks can be washed in 15 minutes?

13. A 150-page book is 1 centimetre thick. A different book, printed on the same kind of paper, has 450 pages. How thick is the second book?

14. Jerry can move his wheel chair 25 metres in 18.5 seconds. How long would it take Jerry to move 200 metres?

15. The clinic buys material and uses $\frac{3}{4}$ of it to make draperies. If $4\frac{1}{4}$ metres are used for the draperies, how many metres are bought?

IMPLIED COMPONENTS

Many situations in everyday life use proportions. Sometimes the components are implied. The number 1 is often an implied component.

Examples: *Three times faster* is a ratio of 3:1. The number 1 is an implied component.

Fifty miles per hour is a ratio of 50:1. The number 1 is implied to mean 1 hour.

In using implied components form the ratios, then determine the unknown component.

Example: Joan's drive to the hospital is 5 times as far as Betty's. Betty drives 1 440 kilometres. How far does Joan drive?

The ratio between Joan's and Betty's driving is $\frac{5}{1}$.

The ratio between Joan's kilometres traveled and Betty's kilometres traveled is $\frac{X}{1\ 440}$.

$$\frac{5}{1} = \frac{X}{1\ 440}$$

$$1(X) = 5(1\ 440)$$

$$X = 7\ 200 \text{ or } X = 7\ 200 \text{ kilometres}$$

Joan drives 7 200 kilometres.

Example: Ted purchases 18 metres of material for $72. How much does he pay per metre?

$$\underrightarrow{\text{metres purchased}} \quad \frac{18}{72} = \frac{1}{X} \quad \underleftarrow{\begin{array}{l}\text{1 metre}\\\text{unknown cost per metre}\end{array}}$$

$$18(X) = 72(1)$$

$$18X = 72$$

$$\frac{18X}{18} = \frac{72}{18}$$

$$X = 4 \text{ or } X = \$4$$

Ted pays $4 for 1 metre of material.

FRACTIONAL COMPONENTS

Many times, proportions have fractions as components. The method used when working with fractions is the same as the method used when working with whole numbers.

Example: A prescription calls for $\frac{1}{2}$ tablet every 3 hours. How many tablets will be taken in 15 hours?

$$\frac{\text{tablets}}{\text{hours}} \longrightarrow \frac{\frac{1}{2}}{3} = \frac{X}{15} \longleftarrow \text{unknown number of tablets} \atop \longleftarrow \text{known number of hours}$$

$$3(X) = \frac{1}{2}(15)$$

$$3X = \frac{15}{2}$$

$$\frac{3X}{3} = \frac{\frac{15}{2}}{3}$$

$$X = \frac{15}{2} \div \frac{3}{1}$$

$$X = \frac{\cancel{15}^{5}}{2} \times \frac{1}{\cancel{3}_{1}}$$

$$X = \frac{5}{2} \text{ or } 2\frac{1}{2} \text{ tablets}$$

In 15 hours, $2\frac{1}{2}$ tablets will be taken.

Example: In an experiment, Tom uses $\frac{1}{3}$ gram of sugar for $\frac{3}{4}$ litre of water. How much sugar does he use for 5 litres of water?

$$\frac{\text{grams of sugar}}{\text{litres of water}} \longrightarrow \frac{\frac{1}{3}}{\frac{3}{4}} = \frac{X}{5} \longleftarrow \text{unknown grams of sugar used} \atop \longleftarrow \text{litres of water used}$$

$$\frac{3}{4}X = \frac{1}{3}(5)$$

$$\frac{3}{4}X = \frac{5}{3}$$

$$\frac{\frac{3}{4}X}{\frac{3}{4}} = \frac{\frac{5}{3}}{\frac{3}{4}}$$

$$X = \frac{5}{3} \div \frac{3}{4}$$

$$X = \frac{5}{3} \times \frac{4}{3}$$

$$X = \frac{20}{9} \text{ or } 2\frac{2}{9} \text{ grams}$$

Tom uses $2\frac{2}{9}$ grams of sugar.

19.2 EXERCISES

Find each unknown term.

1. $\dfrac{X}{\frac{1}{3}} = \dfrac{9}{16}$

2. $\dfrac{\frac{1}{2}}{X} = \dfrac{4}{9}$

3. $\dfrac{\frac{1}{3}}{1} = \dfrac{X}{5}$

4. $\dfrac{\frac{1}{2}}{\frac{5}{8}} = \dfrac{2}{X}$

5. $\dfrac{\frac{3}{4}}{X} = \dfrac{1\frac{1}{4}}{5}$

6. $\dfrac{\frac{1}{5}}{\frac{2}{3}} = \dfrac{X}{\frac{1}{3}}$

Form each proportion. Determine the unknown components as descriptive quantities.

7. The clinic charges 12 cents for each page run on the copier. A total of 53 pages are copied in one day. How much is the total charge?

8. Brenda's yearly salary is $14,048. What is her monthly salary?

9. The staff in clinic **A** treats 152 patients in one day. The staff in clinic **B** treats 38 patients. How many times more patients are treated in clinic **A** than clinic **B**?

10. During one day the clinic staff writes 27 checks. The total bank service charge is $2.97. What is the service charge per check?

11. Joan is a nurse earning $5.25 per hour. How much does she earn for a 40-hour work week?

12. A replacement valve on an autoclave costs 7 times as much today as it did 10 years ago. If the valve cost $28.00 ten years ago, how much does it cost today?

13. Distilled water costs 25¢ per litre. How many litres can be purchased for $10.00?

14. Sally makes a salt solution using 64 millilitres of water and 10 milligrams of salt. She wants to make more solution of the same strength. If she uses 45 milligrams of salt, how much water should be used?

15. If 4 glasses of lemonade can be made from 1 lemon, how many lemons of the same size are needed to make 48 glasses of lemonade?

16. Washington D.C. is 7.5 metres above sea level. The elevation of St. Louis is 18.5 times the elevation of Washington D.C. What is the elevation of St. Louis?

17. A recipe for making 15 cookies calls for $2\frac{3}{4}$ cups of flour. How much flour is needed to make 24 cookies?

18. If 2.5 centimetres represents 40 kilometres, what distance does 1 centimetre represent?

19. Lisa travels 4 kilometres per litre with her new car. At this rate, how many litres of gasoline will she need for a trip of 300 kilometres?

20. On a map, 0.5 centimetre represents 50 kilometres. What distance does 4.5 centimetres represent?

APPLICATIONS

Proportions are used in calculating the amount of solvent and solute to be used in a solution. The ratio compares the amount of solute to the amount of solution. The proportion equates two ratios formed when comparing different amounts of a solution. Remember that for calculation purposes, 1 gram is equal to 1 millilitre.

Example: In 100 millilitres of a solution there are 15 millilitres of solute. How much solute is required to prepare 325 millilitres of this solution?

$$\frac{\text{amount of solute}}{\text{amount of first solution}} = \frac{\text{amount of solute}}{\text{amount of second solution}}$$

$$\frac{15 \text{ millilitres}}{100 \text{ millilitres}} = \frac{X \text{ millilitres}}{325 \text{ millilitres}}$$

$$100(X) = 15(325)$$
$$100(X) = 4\,875$$
$$\frac{100(X)}{100} = \frac{4\,875}{100}$$
$$X = 48.75 \text{ millilitres}$$

19.3 EXERCISES

1. A total of 62 grams of sodium chloride is present in 950 millilitres of solution. How many grams are in 125 millilitres of a solution with the same strength?

2. Solution **A** of Fehling's solution is prepared from copper sulfate and distilled water. There are 69.30 grams of copper sulfate in 1 000 millilitres of solution. How much copper sulfate is used in 125 millilitres of solution to obtain a solution with the same strength?

3. Solution **B** of Fehling's solution contains potassium hydroxide, potassium sodium tartrate and distilled water. There are 250 grams of potassium hydroxide and 346 grams of potassium sodium tartrate in 1 000 millilitres of solution. This means that there are 250 parts potassium hydroxide in 1 000 parts of solution and 346 parts potassium sodium tartrate in 1 000 parts of solution.

   a. How many grams of potassium hydroxide are needed to prepare 125 millilitres of this solution?

   b. How many grams of sodium tartrate are needed to prepare 125 millilitres of this solution?

4. In 115 millilitres of Lugol's solution there are 10 grams of potassium iodide and 5 grams of iodine. How much of each solute is in 750 millilitres of Lugol's solution?

    a. potassium iodide
    b. iodine

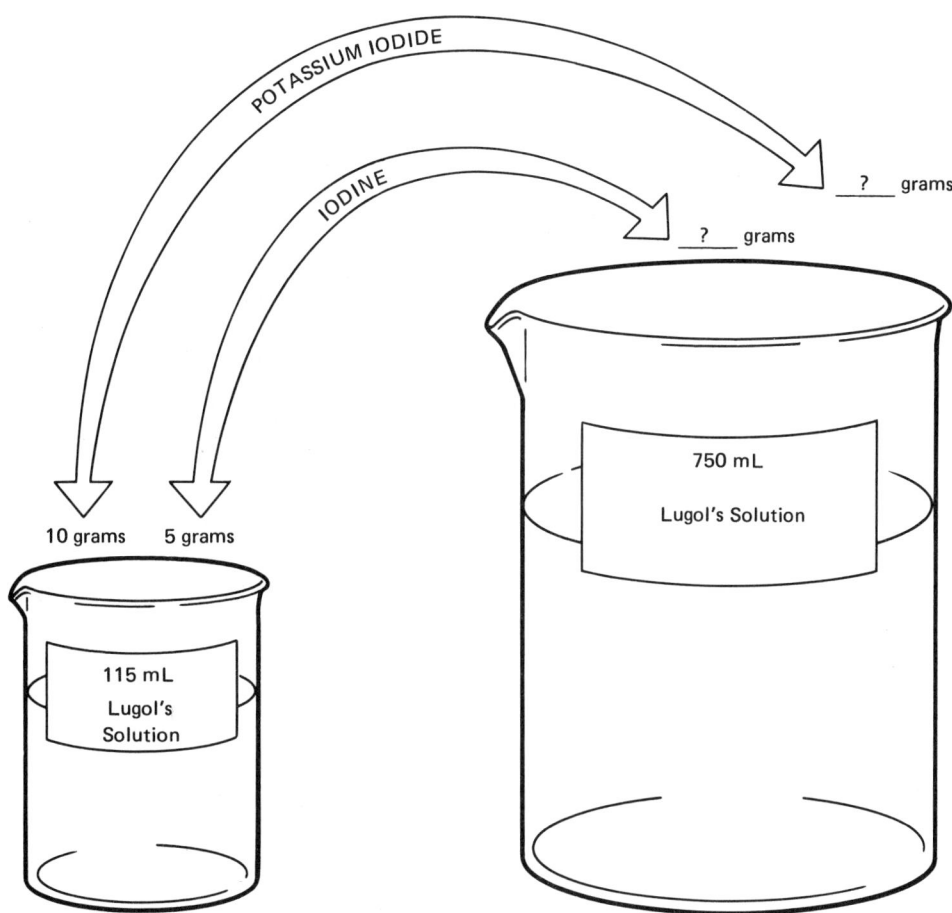

5. A five percent solution is prepared by dissolving five grams of crystals in 100 mL of distilled water. How many grams would be required to prepare a five percent solution with only 30 mL of distilled water?

6. The case load in one ward is determined to be 12 patients for each 2 nurses. To have an equal case load, how many nurses would be required for a 50-patient ward?

7. The case load in one ward is determined to be 12 patients for reach 16 hours of nursing time in an 8-hour shift. To have an equal case load, how many nursing hours in an 8-hour shift would be required for a 50-patient ward?

8. A local school district uses birth rates in the county hospitals to predict kindergarten enrollment. For example, the number of births in 1985 would be used to determine kindergarten enrollment for the 1990-91 school year. Fifteen years of data analysis reveals 27 children enroll for each 100 births five year earlier. In 1987 a total of 2,347 births were recorded for the county. How many children can be predicted to enroll in kindergarten for the 1992-93 school year?

9. During a one-week period it is found that 21 new patients are admitted to the hospital and 63 previously admitted patients are dismissed.
   a. What is the ratio of those admitted compared to those dismissed during this period of time?
   b. What is the ratio of those admitted compared to all patients admitted and dismissed during this period of time?
   c. What is the ratio of those dismissed compared to all patients admitted and dismissed during this period of time?

10. The mortality rate, as determined by a nationwide survey, for a particular surgical procedure has been stated to be one death for each 125 operations.
    a. In one year a total of 2,000 operations using this surgical procedure are conducted. What is the anticipated number of deaths relating to this type of surgery for this period of time?
    b. If the research indicated 29 deaths resulted during a given period of time for this type of surgery, how many operations would you determine have taken place?

11. Medical service cost for each patient treated at a clinic averaged $27.00 per visit.
    a. If the clinic must recover its monthly operational cost of $67,500, how many patients must be served during the month for the clinic to break even?
    b. What is the ratio of one patient's cost compared to the cost of operating the clinc?

12. Instructions to prepare a disinfectant requires 1000 mL of distilled water for each 20 mL of stock disinfectant.
    a. What is the ratio of disinfectant to distilled water?
    b. How many 2 500 mL capacity disinfectant containers can be prepared from 1 500 mL of stock disinfectant?

13. The number of patients served in two separate wards of the hospital varies due to the type of service provided. WARD A requires three nurses each eight-hour shift to serve 21 patients. WARD B requires three nurses each eight-hour shift to serve 12 patients.
    a. Express the nurse/patient ratio for WARD A.
    b. Express the nurse/patient ratio for WARD B.

14. Daily processing of patient records requires 20 minutes of computer-operator time per patient.
    a. Using this ratio, calculate the amount of time required to process 125 patient records in one day.
    b. At a cost of $9.50 per hour for record processing, what is the per patient cost?
    c. Each operator can process three records per hour. How many computer operators would be required to process these records?

15. The per patient bed space in a hospital has been calculated to be 180 square feet.
    a. Express the ratio of patient per square foot.
    b. A ward in the hospital has 5,760 square feet of bed space. Calculate the number of patients that can be housed at any one time.

unit 20 introduction to percents

OBJECTIVES

After studying this unit the student should be able to:
- Express ratios, fractions, and decimals as percents.
- Express percents as equivalent fractions or decimals.
- Express fractional, decimal, and percent equivalents.

PERCENT

The constant use of ratio comparisons has led to a special percent notation for ratios. This compares a quantity to one hundred.

Example: Determine the ratio of coverage for each figure compared to the total region.

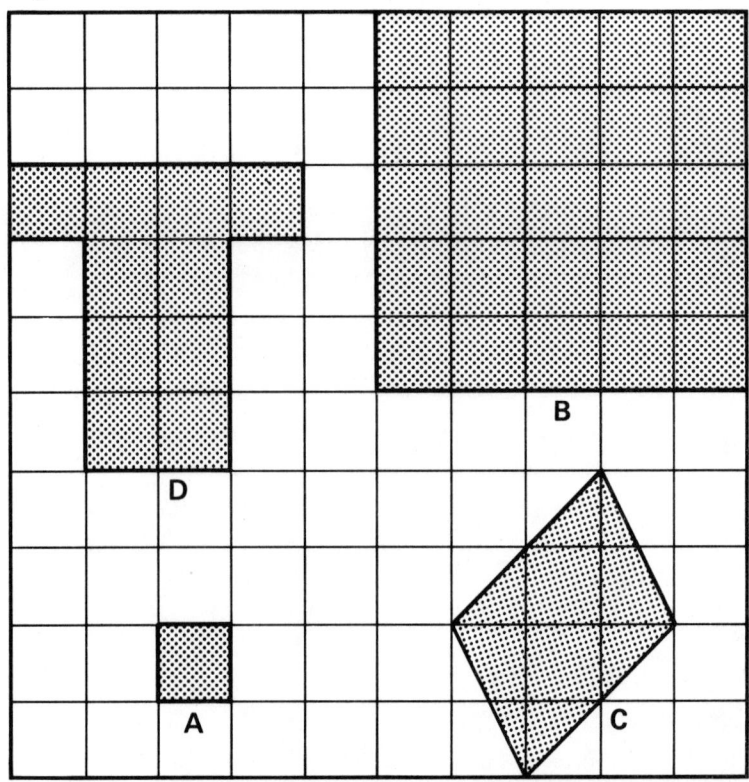

Figure **A** covers $\frac{1}{100}$ of the total region.
Figure **B** covers $\frac{25}{100}$ of the total region.
Figure **C** covers $\frac{6}{100}$ of the total region.
Figure **D** covers $\frac{10}{100}$ of the total region.

Each of these figures is compared to 100.

- If n is any number, then $\frac{n}{100}$ can be expressed using the symbol $n\%$. Rather than using fractions to express the ratios, equivalent decimal or percent notation can be used.

FIGURE	RATIO	FRACTION (hundredths)	DECIMAL	PERCENT
A	1:100	$\frac{1}{100}$	0.01	1%
B	25:100	$\frac{25}{100}$	0.25	25%
C	6:100	$\frac{6}{100}$	0.06	6%
D	10:100	$\frac{10}{100}$	0.10	10%

Note: The percent symbol, %, is always written to the right and has a decimal and fractional equivalent.

- Generally $n\% = n\,(0.01) = n\,(\frac{1}{100})$ or $\frac{n}{100}$.

Example: Use the percent notation to express the ratio 3:20.

$3:20 = \frac{3}{20}$

$\frac{3}{20} = \frac{15}{100} = 15\%$

Example: Express the fractions $\frac{1}{5}$ and $\frac{36}{200}$ using percent notation.

$\frac{1}{5} = \frac{20}{100} = 20\%$

$\frac{36}{200} = \frac{18}{100} = 18\%$

Example: Express the decimals 0.32 and 2.75 using percent notation.

$0.32 = \frac{32}{100} = 32\%$

$2.75 = 2\frac{75}{100} = 275\%$

Note: In actual use the percent symbol % is only a reference and is replaced by a ratio, a fraction, or a decimal for computational purposes.

20.1 EXERCISES

Use the percent notation to express each ratio, fraction, or decimal.

1. 23 to 100
2. 13:100
3. 40 to 50
4. 3:25
5. 200 to 100
6. 135:100
7. 200 to 200
8. 150:50
9. $\frac{1}{4}$ to 100
10. $\frac{1}{2}$ to 100
11. 0.5 to 100
12. 0.75:100
13. 120 to 1,000
14. 500 to 1,000
15. 1,200 to 1,000
16. $\frac{3}{10}$
17. $\frac{2}{5}$
18. $\frac{23}{25}$
19. $\frac{13}{20}$
20. $\frac{1}{2}$
21. $\frac{3}{4}$
22. $\frac{10}{10}$
23. $\frac{0}{3}$
24. $\frac{25}{10}$
25. $\frac{3}{50}$
26. $\frac{27}{20}$
27. $\frac{80}{200}$
28. $\frac{150}{1,000}$
29. $\frac{12}{600}$
30. $\frac{7}{200}$
31. 0.02
32. 0.25
33. 0.10
34. 0.55
35. 0.09
36. 0.99
37. 1.00
38. 1.25
39. 3.50
40. 4.75

Percent means out of one hundred; one hundred is a power of ten. Finding decimal equivalents is simplified since the decimal system is also based on powers of ten. In finding an equivalent fraction, the denominator of one hundred is used and then the fraction is expressed in lowest terms.

EXPRESSING PERCENTS AS EQUIVALENT FRACTIONS

Example: Express 35% as a fraction.

$35\% = \frac{35}{100}$ Express 35% as a fraction with a denominator of one hundred.

$35\% = \frac{5 \times 7}{5 \times 20}$

$35\% = \frac{7}{20}$ Express the fraction in lowest terms.

Example: Express 146% as a mixed number.

$146\% = \frac{146}{100}$

$146\% = \frac{2 \times 73}{2 \times 50}$

$146\% = \frac{73}{50}$ or $1\frac{23}{50}$

Example: Express $66\frac{2}{3}\%$ as an equivalent fraction.

$$66\frac{2}{3}\% = \frac{66\frac{2}{3}}{100} = \frac{\frac{200}{3}}{100}$$

$$66\frac{2}{3}\% = \frac{\frac{200}{3}}{100} = \frac{200}{3} \div \frac{100}{1}$$

$$66\frac{2}{3}\% = \frac{200}{3} \div \frac{100}{1} \text{ or } \frac{200}{3} \times \frac{1}{100}$$

$$66\frac{2}{3}\% = \frac{200 \times 1}{3 \times 100} \text{ or } \frac{200}{300}$$

$$66\frac{2}{3}\% = \frac{2 \times 100}{3 \times 100} \text{ or } \frac{2}{3}$$

EXPRESSING PERCENTS AS EQUIVALENT DECIMALS

Example: Express 8% as a decimal.

$8\% = \frac{8}{100}$ — Express 8% as a fraction with a denominator of one hundred.

$8\% = 100 \overline{)8.00}^{\,0.08}$ — Using the concept that a fraction bar indicates division, divide.

$8\% = 0.08$

Example: Express 12.5% as an equivalent decimal.

$12.5\% = \frac{12.5}{100}$

$12.5\% = 100 \overline{)12.500}^{\,0.125}$

$12.5\% = 0.125$

Example: Express 130.5% as a decimal number.

$130.5\% = \frac{130.5}{100}$

$130.5\% = 100 \overline{)130.500}^{\,1.305}$

$130.5\% = 1.305$

The basic meaning of percents, decimals, and fractions is adhered to when expressing decimals and fractions as percents. Decimals are expressed as equivalent fractions with a denominator of 100. Then the fraction is expressed as a percent. Proportions may be used to express a fraction as an equivalent fraction with a denominator of 100.

EXPRESSING DECIMALS AS EQUIVALENT PERCENTS

Example: Express 0.75 as a percent.

$0.75 = \dfrac{0.75 \times 100}{100}$ Express the decimal as an equivalent fraction with a denominator of 100.

$0.75 = \dfrac{75}{100}$

$0.75 = 75\%$ Express the fraction as an equivalent percent.

Example: Express 0.005 using percent notation.

$0.005 = \dfrac{0.005 \times 100}{100}$

$0.005 = \dfrac{0.5}{100}$

$0.005 = 0.5\%$ or $\tfrac{1}{2}\%$

Example: Express the decimal number 3.61 as an equivalent percent.

$3.61 = \dfrac{3.61 \times 100}{100}$

$3.16 = \dfrac{361}{100}$

$3.61 = 361\%$

EXPRESSING FRACTIONS AS EQUIVALENT PERCENTS

Example: Express $\tfrac{1}{3}$ as a percent.

$\dfrac{1}{3} = \dfrac{X}{100}$ Using proportions, express the fraction as an equivalent fraction with a denominator of 100.

$3(X) = 1(100)$

$3X = 100$

$X = \dfrac{100}{3} = 33\tfrac{1}{3}$ or $33.\overline{3}$

$\dfrac{33\tfrac{1}{3}}{100} = 33\tfrac{1}{3}\%$ or $\dfrac{33.\overline{3}}{100} = 33.\overline{3}\%$ Express the equivalent fraction as a percent.

$\dfrac{1}{3} = 33\tfrac{1}{3}\%$ or $33.\overline{3}\%$

Example: Express $\frac{3}{2}$ as an equivalent percent.

$$\frac{3}{2} = \frac{X}{100}$$
$$2(X) = 3(100)$$
$$2X = 300$$
$$\frac{2X}{2} = \frac{300}{2}$$
$$X = 150$$
$$\frac{150}{100} = 150\%$$
$$\frac{3}{2} = 150\%$$

Example: Express $\frac{1}{400}$ using percent notation.

$$\frac{1}{400} = \frac{X}{100}$$
$$400(X) = 1(100)$$
$$400X = 100$$
$$\frac{400X}{400} = \frac{100}{400}$$
$$X = \frac{1}{4}$$
$$\frac{\frac{1}{4}}{100} = \frac{1}{4}\% \text{ or } 0.25\%$$
$$\frac{1}{400} = \frac{1}{4}\% \text{ or } 0.25\%$$

20.2 EXERCISES

Express each percent as indicated.

Fraction in Lowest Terms

1. 20%
2. 60%
3. $33\frac{1}{3}\%$
4. 5%
5. 0.2%
6. 7.5%
7. 6.25%
8. 120%
9. 150.5%
10. 210%

Decimal

11. 35%
12. 81%
13. 16.25%
14. $\frac{1}{2}\%$
15. 0.05%
16. 0.5%
17. 0.125%
18. 225%
19. 300%
20. 250.65%

172 Section 4 Ratio, Proportion, and Percents

Express each decimal or fraction as a percent. Round where indicated.

21. 0.47   23. 0.293   25. 0.078   27. 0.0502   29. 6.82
22. 0.76   24. 0.926   26. 0.001   28. 0.00064 30. 51.9

Round to the Nearer Whole Percent

31. $\frac{5}{8}$ 33. $\frac{5}{12}$ 35. $\frac{95}{100}$ 37. $\frac{4}{7}$ 39. $\frac{13}{4}$
32. $\frac{1}{6}$ 34. $\frac{4}{8}$ 36. $\frac{17}{20}$ 38. $\frac{7}{6}$ 40. $\frac{11}{9}$

Round to the Nearer Tenth Percent

41. $\frac{5}{12}$ 43. $\frac{5}{6}$ 45. $\frac{1}{9}$ 47. $\frac{13}{8}$ 49. $\frac{14}{5}$
42. $\frac{3}{8}$ 44. $\frac{3}{13}$ 46. $\frac{7}{16}$ 48. $\frac{28}{7}$ 50. $\frac{16}{11}$

20.3 EXERCISES

Complete the chart of fractional, decimal, and percent equivalents.

	Mixed Number or Fraction	Decimal	Percent
1.		$0.33\overline{3}$	$33\frac{1}{3}\%$
2.			30%
3.	$\frac{1}{4}$		
4.	$\frac{1}{10}$		
5.			75%
6.	$\frac{1}{5}$		
7.			50%
8.		0.875	
9.			60%
10.	$1\frac{1}{4}$		
11.		0.4	

	Mixed Number or Fraction	Decimal	Percent
12.	$\frac{1}{8}$		$12\frac{1}{2}\%$
13.		2.5	
14.			$\frac{1}{2}\%$
15.	$\frac{2}{1}$		
16.	$\frac{4}{5}$		
17.			$62\frac{1}{2}\%$
18.	$1\frac{1}{2}$		
19.			$66\frac{2}{3}\%$
20.	$\frac{3}{8}$		
21.		0.0025	
22.			85%

APPLICATIONS

The strength of a solution is usually expressed as a percent. A 5% solution of lugol means that there are 5 parts lugol in 100 parts of solution. Since 5% represents the ratio 5:100 or 1:20, it may also mean 1 part lugol in 20 parts of solution or 100 parts lugol in 2 000 parts of solution.

In determining percent of solution strength, the units of measure must be the same for the solution and the solute. A 5% solution of lugol means 1 millilitre lugol in 20 millilitres water or 100 ounces lugol in 2,000 ounces lugol. Ratios such as 1 millilitre lugol in 20 litres water or 100 litres lugol in 2,000 ounces water will not provide a correct percent of solution strength.

For liquid solutes, the strength of the solution is a *percent by volume*. It is the percent of the final solution volume represented by the volume of the solute used to make the solution. It is determined by $\frac{\text{volume of solute}}{\text{volume of solution}} \times 100$. A 12% alcohol solution (by volume) would be a solution made from 12 parts (usually millilitres) of alcohol and enough solvent to bring the total volume up to 100 parts (usually millilitres).

For solid solutes, the strength of the solution is a *percent by weight (mass)*. It is the percent of the total solution mass contributed by the solute. It is determined by $\frac{\text{mass of solute}}{\text{volume of solution}} \times 100$. A 4% boric acid solution (by weight) would be 4 parts (usually grams) of boric acid per 100 parts (usually millilitres) of solution. Remember that for computational purposes, 1 gram is equal to 1 millilitre.

▼ A *pure solution* is a substance with a strength of 100%. This means that the substance has not been mixed with any other substance.

▼ A *stock solution* is a solution which is kept on hand. The component has been mixed in solution form and has a strength less than 100%. The strength of stock solutions may greatly exceed that required for safe use. In these instances the stock solution is used to form a new solution with a lower strength. For example, a 15% stock solution of alcohol may be used to form a 5% alcohol solution.

20.4 EXERCISES

1. Express each solution strength as a ratio.
    a. 4% boric acid solution
    b. 50% stock hydrochloric acid solution
    c. 75% stock glycerin solution
    d. 95% stock lysol solution
    e. $\frac{1}{10}$% silver nitrate solution
    f. $\frac{2}{5}$% sodium bicarbonate solution
    g. 7.5% sodium phosphate solution
    h. $\frac{3}{4}$% phenylephrine solution
    i. 100% magnesium sulfate

2. The amount of solute in a solution is often expressed as a percent. It may also be expressed as a fraction or a decimal. Express each percent of solute as a fraction and a decimal.

	PERCENT OF SOLUTE	FRACTIONAL VALUE	DECIMAL VALUE
a.	1% sodium chloride		
b.	5% glucose		
c.	20% lactose		
d.	25% sodium chloride		
e.	50% ethyl alcohol		
f.	60% methyl alcohol		
g.	95% ethyl alcohol		

3. Determine the strength of each solution.

   a. 7 parts sodium chloride and 50 parts of solution
   b. 7 grams sodium chloride and 50 millilitres of solution
   c. 30 millilitres pure ethyl alcohol and 75 millilitres of solution
   d. 50 grams of glucose in 1 litre (1 000 millilitres) of solution
   e. 5 tablets each containing 6 grains dissolved in 100 millilitres of solution
      Note: 1 gram = 15 grains

4. What percent solution is obtained when 7 grams of boric acid crystals are in a 500-millilitre solution.

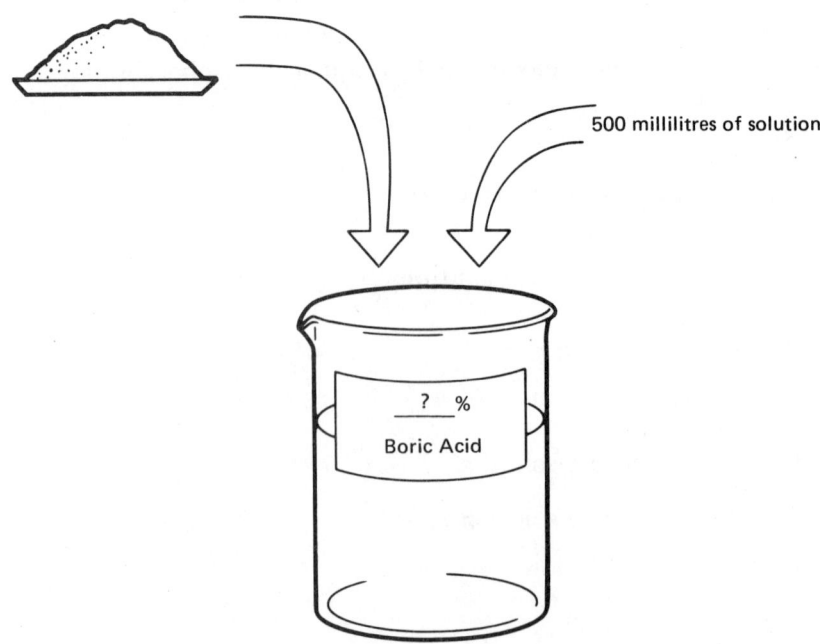

unit 21 equations involving percents

OBJECTIVES

After studying this unit the student should be able to:

- Determine unknown quantities involving percents by using proportions.
- Determine unknown quantities involving percents by using percent equation.

USING PERCENTS

In real life three types of percent problems are encountered. Notice that in any problems involving percent all that is required is a proportion.

Example: 25% of 200 is what number?

$25\% = \dfrac{25}{100}$ Express 25% as an equivalent fraction.

$\dfrac{X}{200}$ Express as a ratio the comparison of the unknown number to 200.

$\dfrac{25}{100} = \dfrac{X}{200}$

$100(X) = 25(200)$

$100X = 5{,}000$

$\dfrac{100X}{100} = \dfrac{5{,}000}{100}$

$X = 50$

25% of 200 is 50.

Example: 40 is what percent of 400?

$\dfrac{40}{400}$ — Express the comparison of the two given numbers.

$\dfrac{n}{100}$ — Express as a ratio the unknown number compared to 100. This comparison represents a percent.

$\dfrac{40}{400} = \dfrac{n}{100}$

$400(n) = 40(100)$

$400n = 4{,}000$

$\dfrac{400n}{400} = \dfrac{4{,}000}{400}$

$n = 10;\ \dfrac{n}{100} = \dfrac{10}{100}\ \text{or}\ 10\%$

40 is 10% of 400.

Example: 75 is 25% of what number?

$25\% = \dfrac{25}{100}$ — Express 25% as a ratio.

$\dfrac{75}{y}$ — Express the ratio of 75 to the unknown number.

$\dfrac{25}{100} = \dfrac{75}{y}$

$25(y) = 100(75)$

$25y = 7{,}500$

$\dfrac{25y}{25} = \dfrac{7{,}500}{25}$

$y = 300$

75 is 25% of 300.

21.1 EXERCISES

Find each unknown quantity. Round the answer to the nearer tenth if necessary.

1. 50% of 80 is what number?
2. 75% of 120 is what number?
3. 33.3% of 90 is what number?
4. 30% of 43.5 is what number?
5. 5% of 130 is what number?
6. 2.5% of 80 is what number?
7. 0% of 38 is what number?
8. 120% of 50 is what number?
9. 200% of 145 is what number?
10. 500% of 30 is what number?
11. 20 is what percent of 80?
12. 15 is what percent of 75?
13. 15 is what percent of 45?
14. 35 is what percent of 45?
15. 3 is what percent of 42?
16. 28 is what percent of 81?
17. 17 is what percent of 102?
18. 50 is what percent of 25?
19. 300 is what percent of 160?
20. 163 is what percent of 42?
21. 82 is 50% of what number?
22. 76 is 40% of what number?
23. 48 is 15.5% of what number?
24. 4.23 is 1% of what number?
25. 13 is 40% of what number?
26. 121 is 55% of what number?
27. 65 is 10% of what number?
28. 42 is 80% of what number?
29. 50 is 200% of what number?
30. 32 is 350% of what number?
31. 15 is what percent of 300?
32. 27% of 130 is what number?
33. 110 is 30% of what number?
34. 12.5% of 80 is what number?
35. 2.2 is 10% of what number?
36. 22.5 is what percent of 180?
37. 45 is 50% of what number?
38. 12 is what percent of 2,400?
39. 32% of 8 is what number?
40. $1\frac{1}{2}$ is 200% of what number?

21.2 EXERCISES

Complete the chart by determining the value of the unknown quantity. Round the answer to the nearer tenth if necessary.

	Known Quantity	Known Quantity	Unknown Quantity	Answer
1.	The regular price is $50.	The amount of discount is $10.	What is the percent of discount?	
2.	Earned: $400	Spent: 40%	Amount spent	
3.	Paid: $42	This is 25% of total amount owed.	Total amount owed	
4.	Recommended shots: 30	Shots taken: 21	Percent of shots taken	
5.	Regular Price: $200	Rate of discount: 25%	Amount of discount	
6.	8 hours sleep each night	24 hours in each day	Percent of day spent sleeping	
7.	Paid: $25	This is 50% of the total amount owed.	Total amount owed	
8.	An account has $650 to be paid.	The interest rate is 6% per year.	What is the interest charged in one year?	
9.	Food: $150 per month	Salary: $1,000 per month	What percent is spent on food?	
10.	Paid: $84	This is 20% of the total amount owed.	Total amount owed	

ANOTHER METHOD OF CALCULATING WITH PERCENTS

Although proportional rate pairs will solve every type of percent problem, there are quicker methods. In this method the word "of" is expressed by using the times sign ($\times$). Similarly, the equal sign (=) is used to express the word "is."

Example: 25% of 200 is what number?

25% of 200 is what number?

$25\% \cdot 200 = X$

$0.25 \cdot 200 = X$

$50 = X$

25% of 200 is 50.

Example: 40 is what percent of 400?

40 is what percent of 400?

$40 = n\% \cdot 400$

$$\frac{40}{400} = \frac{n\% \cdot 400}{400}$$

$$\frac{10}{100} = n\%$$

$10\% = n$

40 is 10% of 400.

Example: 75 is 25% of what number?

75 is 25% of what number?

$75 = 25\% \cdot y$

$75 = 0.25 \cdot y$

$$\frac{75}{0.25} = \frac{0.25\, y}{0.25}$$

$300 = y$

75 is 25% of 300.

21.3 EXERCISES

Find each unknown quantity. Round the answer to the nearer tenth if necessary.

1. 20% of 63 is what number?
2. 65% of 90 is what number?
3. 66.6% of 120 is what number?
4. 25% of 39.3 is what number?
5. 14.4% of 100 is what number?
6. $1\frac{1}{2}$% of 40 is what number?
7. 0.5% of 900 is what number?
8. 15% of 80 is what number?
9. 25% of 30 is what number?
10. 400% of 65 is what number?
11. 15 is what percent of 60?
12. 84 is what percent of 126?
13. 16.6 is what percent of 33.2?
14. 22.3 is what percent of 111.5?
15. 2 is what percent of 21?
16. 1.5 is what percent of 90?
17. 15.21 is what percent of 121.68?
18. 100 is what percent of 75?
19. 220 is what percent of 180?
20. 68.5 is what percent of 13.7?
21. 40 is 20% of what number?
22. 92 is 55% of what number?
23. 32 is 28% of what number?
24. 0.5 is 2% of what number?
25. 18 is $\frac{1}{2}$% of what number?
26. 1.5 is 1.5% of what number?
27. 235 is 25% of what number?
28. 16.7 is 0% of what number?
29. 300 is 150% of what number?
30. 85 is 250% of what number?
31. 25 is what percent of 400?
32. 16% of 320 is what number?
33. 52 is 50% of what number?
34. 9.5% of 145 is what number?
35. 1.5 is 20% of what number?
36. 14 is what percent of 70?
37. 150 is 75% of what number?
38. 5 is what percent of 6,000?
39. 85% of 9 is what number?
40. 3.5 is 400% of what number?

21.4 EXERCISES

Complete the chart by determining the value of the unknown quantity. Round the answer to the nearer tenth if necessary.

	Known Quantity	Known Quantity	Unknown Quantity	Answer
1.	Normal weight: 98 kilograms	Weight after illness: 80 kilograms	Percent of normal weight	
2.	Regular price: $67	Amount of discount: $15	Percent discount	
3.	Test: 100 questions	Incorrect: 15	Percent correct	
4.	World population: 4 billion	Starving: 460,000,000	Percent starving	
5.	Patients admitted: 30	Patients released: 70%	Patients remaining	
6.	Paid: $90	This is 25% of the total amount owed.	Total amount owed	
7.	25 shots recommended	20 shots given	Percent of shots not given	
8.	Earned: $10,500	Spent: $9,000	Percent spent	
9.	An autoclave is bought for $3,000.	The purchase price was marked up 15%.	Price after mark up	
10.	Owed: $120	This is 30% of the original amount owed.	Original amount owed	
11.	9 hours sleep per night	Total hours in one day	What percent of one day are the non-sleeping hours?	
12.	World population: 4 billion	Farmers: $\frac{1}{10}$%	How many are farmers?	
13.	An account has $5,200 remaining to be paid.	The interest rate is $6\frac{1}{4}$% per year.	What is the interest for one year?	
14.	Earned: $18,500	Spent: 93%	Amount saved	
15.	Regular price: $350	Rate of discount: 10%	Sale price	

APPLICATIONS

Solutions may be prepared in various strengths. The strength of the solution is indicated by the amount of solute that is in the solution. This amount may be expressed as a percent. A 5% glucose solution means that 5% of the solution consists of the glucose. Since solid solutes are measured in grams and 1 gram is equal to 1 millilitre, the amount of solute is the product of the percent strength times the amount of solution.

Example: Determine the number of grams of glucose that are present in 100 millilitres of 5% glucose solution.

5% of 100 millilitres is what number?

$$\frac{5}{100} = \frac{x}{100}$$

$$100(x) = 5(100)$$

$$100x = 500$$

$$\frac{100x}{100} = \frac{500}{100}$$

$$x = 5 \text{ grams glucose}$$

21.5 EXERCISES

1. Determine the number of grams of solute present in each solution.

   a. 45 millilitres of a 7% procaine solution
   b. 125 millilitres of a 13% glucose solution
   c. 275 millilitres of a 5% potassium permanganate solution
   d. 750 millilitres of a 2% tyrothricin solution
   e. 900 millilitres of a 0.9% saline solution
   f. 2.750 litres (2 750 millilitres) of a 12% sodium bicarbonate solution

2. Calculate the quantity of glucose required to prepare 1 litre of a 27% solution.

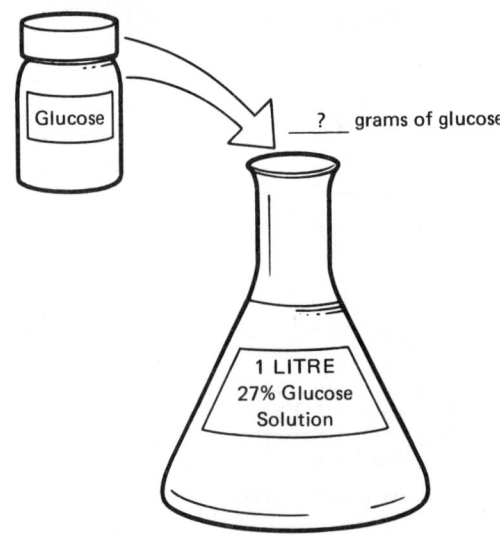

3. A physiological solution is a solution which matches a person's body chemistry. A 0.9% physiological saline solution is prepared. How many grams of sodium chloride are needed to prepare 500 millilitres of this solution?

4. Using tablets, a health care worker prepares 300 millilitres of a $\frac{1}{2}$% solution. Each tablet weighs 15 milligrams or 0.015 gram.

   a. Find the amount of solute needed to prepare the solution.
   b. Find the number of tablets needed to prepare the solution.

   Note: number of tablets = $\dfrac{\text{amount (mass) of solute}}{\text{mass of one tablet}}$ or

   $\dfrac{\text{amount (mass) of solute}}{0.015 \text{ gram}}$

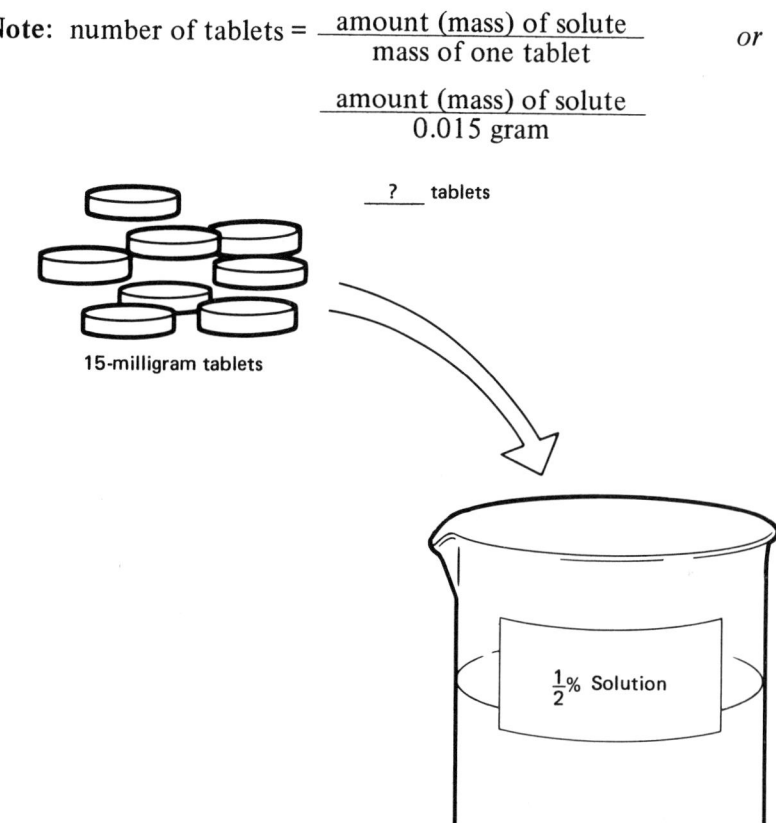

unit 22 computations with percents

OBJECTIVES

After studying this unit the student should be able to:
- Find the percent of increase and the percent of decrease.
- Perform calculations using two or more percents.
- Estimate answers using percents.

PERCENT OF INCREASE OR DECREASE

When a measurement increases or decreases it is often convenient to use a percent to compare this increase or decrease to the original measurement.

- To find the percent of increase or decrease:
  - Find the difference between the original and the new quantity.
  - Set up a ratio comparing to amount of increase or decrease and the original quantity.

  $$\frac{\text{amount of increase or decrease}}{\text{original quantity}}$$

  - Express the ratio as a percent.

Example: The percent of increase is illustrated by using pulse rates.

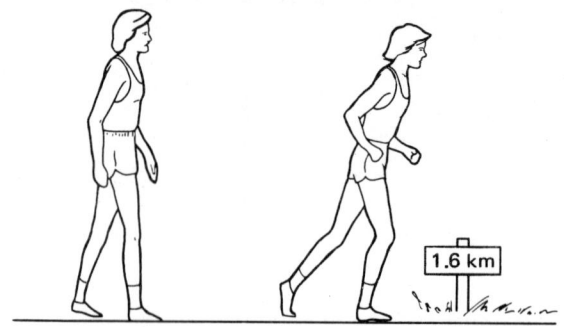

Normal pulse rate: (original quantity)	50	Increase: (change)	30
Pulse rate after running 1.6 kilometres: (new quantity)	80	Percent of increase: $\frac{30}{50} = 0.60$	60%

Example: The percent of decrease is also illustrated by using pulse rates.

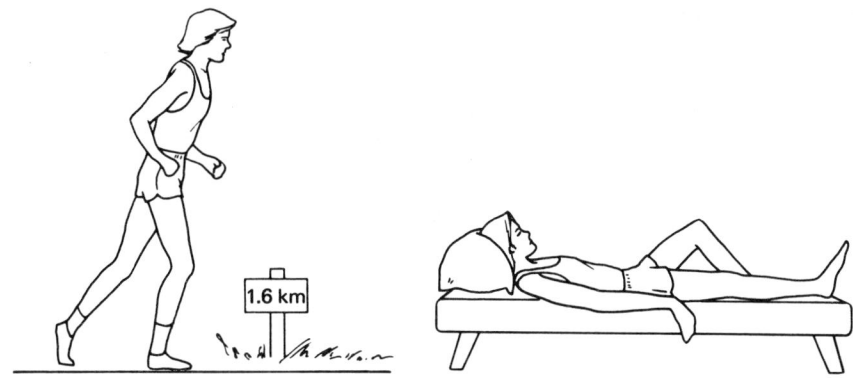

Pulse rate after running
  1.6 kilometres   80
  (original quantity)
Pulse rate after two
  minutes rest: 60
  (new quantity)

Decrease: 20
  (change)
Percent of decrease:
  $\frac{20}{80} = 0.25$ 25%

22.1 EXERCISES

Calculate the percent of increase or decrease by completing the tables.

	Normal Pulse Rate	Pulse Rate After Running	Increase	Increase ÷ Normal Pulse Rate	Percent of Increase (Nearer Tenth)
1.	60	90			
2.	54	78			
3.	80	100			
4.	70	120			
5.	65	88			

	Pulse Rate After Running	Pulse Rate After Two Minutes Rest	Decrease	Decrease ÷ Pulse Rate After Running	Percent of Decrease (Nearer Tenth)
6.	90	75			
7.	78	65			
8.	100	90			
9.	120	100			
10.	88	77			

Using percents of increase or decrease, determine each answer. Round the answer to the nearer tenth when necessary.

11. Marilee earns $205 per week. She receives a raise to $225 per week. What percent increase does Marilee get?

12. Ivan earns $750 per month. He receives a 12% raise. What is Ivan's new monthly earning?

13. During a recent six month period, the average daily cost of a hospital stay jumped from $111.66 to $131.20. If the percent of increase is the same for the next six months, how much will it then cost to spend a day in the hospital?

14. In 1952, manufacturers used 1.2 kilograms of tobacco to make 1,000 cigarettes. Today they use 0.8 kilogram to make the same number. What is the percent decrease?

15. Joyce said, "Last year I was in school so I had no salary. This year I am earning $14,500. This is an increase of $14,500 or a 100% increase." Is Joyce's statement correct?

16. After George pays $4,500 on his account he still has $500 remaining to be paid. He concludes that the decrease is more than 100%. Is he correct?

COMBINING PERCENTS

Using percents, this circle graph shows how Jan spends her day. This information can be used to determine how many hours Jan spends in various activities.

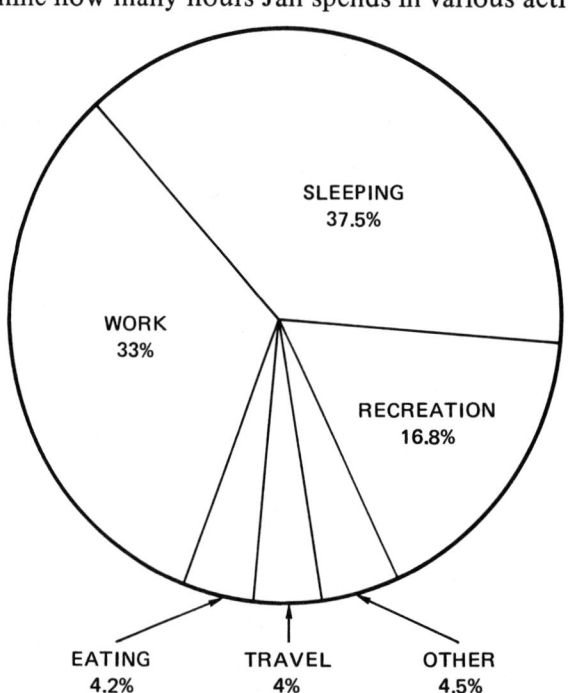

Unit 22 Computations With Percents

Example: Using this graph, determine, to the nearer whole number, how many hours a day Jan spends working and sleeping.

Hours working:	33% of 24	=	0.33 × 24	≈	8 hours
Hours sleeping:	37.5% of 24	=	0.375 × 24	or	9 hours
Total hours working and sleeping:	70.5% of 24	=	0.705 × 24	≈	17 hours

The computations can also be illustrated by using this diagram.

HOURS WORKING:
33% of 24 = 0.33 × 24 ≈ ⑧ hours

HOURS SLEEPING:
37.5% of 24 = 0.375 × 24 ≈ ⑨ hours

TOTAL HOURS
WORKING AND SLEEPING

0.33 (24) + 0.375 (24)

(0.33 + 0.375) (24) =
(0.705) (24) ≈
17 hours

Example: Using the graph, find, to the nearer whole number, the number of hours a day Jan spends eating and at recreation.

Hours eating:	4.2% of 24	=	0.042 × 24	≈	1 hour
Hours in recreation:	16.8% of 24	=	0.168 × 24	≈	4 hours
Total hours eating and in recreation:	21% of 24	=	0.210 × 24	≈	5 hours

This diagram illustrates another method that may be used.

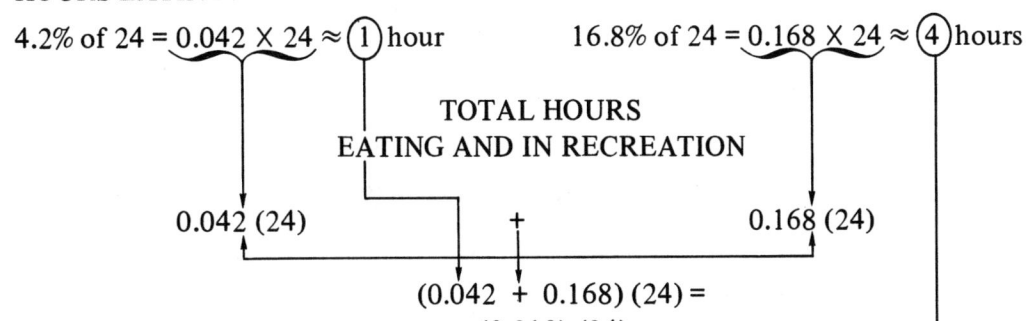

HOURS EATING:
4.2% of 24 = 0.042 × 24 ≈ ① hour

HOURS IN RECREATION:
16.8% of 24 = 0.168 × 24 ≈ ④ hours

TOTAL HOURS
EATING AND IN RECREATION

0.042 (24) + 0.168 (24)

(0.042 + 0.168) (24) =
(0.210) (24) ≈
5 hours

188   Section 4 Ratio, Proportion, and Percents

- The diagrams illustrate that since the percents refer to the same quantity, the percents may be combined. The addition may be performed before the multiplication.

Example: Sue has 2 part-time jobs. She saves 60% of the $500 she earns at the clinic and 20% of the $250 she earns as a waitress. Find the amount she saves.

Clinic:	60% of $500 = 0.60 × $500 *or* $300
Waitress:	20% of $250 = 0.20 × $250 *or* $ 50
Total savings:	$350

Note: The percents cannot be combined since each percent refers to a different quantity.

Example: A new copier costs $5,000. The first year the copier will depreciate (decrease in value) 25%. The second year the copier will depreciate 20%. What is the value of the copier after the second year?

First year's depreciation:	25% of $5,000	=	0.25 × $5,000 *or* $1,250
Value of the copier at the end of one year:	$5,000 − $1,250	=	$3,750
Second year's depreciation:	20% of $3,750	=	0.20 × $3,750 *or* $750
Value of the copier at the end of the second year:	$3,750 − $750	=	$3,000

This method involves finding the amount of depreciation and then finding the value of the copier. Another method is to express the value as a percent and then find the amount of value.

First year:	100% − 25%	=	75%
	75% of $5,000	=	0.75 × $5,000 *or* $3,750
Second year:	100% − 20%	=	80%
	80% of $3,750	=	0.80 × $3,750 *or* $3,000

Note: The percents 75% and 80% represent the percent of value.

22.2 EXERCISES

Use this graph for 1-5.

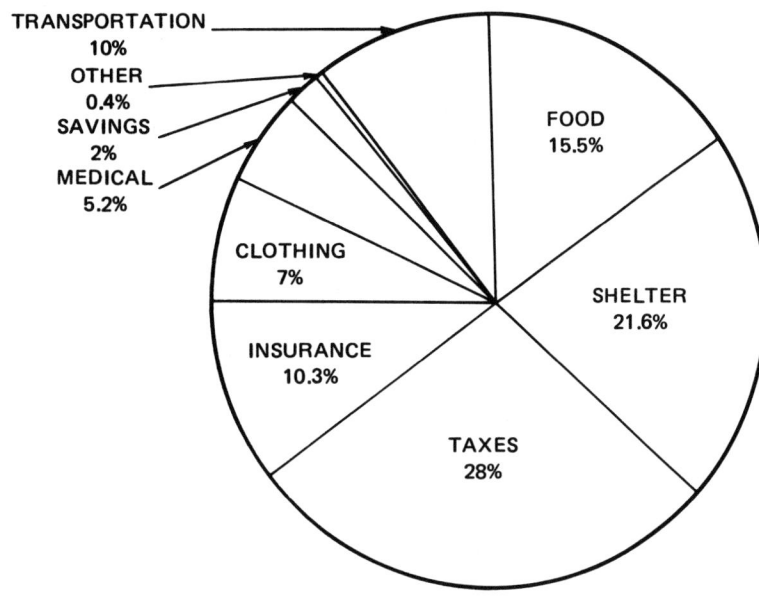

Income: $24,250

1. What percent of their income does the James family spend on food and shelter?

2. How much money do they spend on food and shelter?

3. They spend approximately how many times as much money on shelter as on insurance?

4. What percent of their income is classified as "other?"

5. How much money do they spend on medical, taxes, and insurance?

6. Sue had two part-time jobs. She saves 60% of the $500 she earns at the clothing store and 20% of the $300 she earns as a worker in a clinic.
   a. How much money does Sue save?
   b. What percent of her total earnings is this?

7. A new piece of laboratory equipment costs $7,325. It depreciates 28% the first year, 22% the second year, and 17% the third year. What is the value of the equipment after 3 years?

8. A strip of land costing $620 appreciates or increases in value 15% the first year and 13% the second year. What is the value of the land after two years?

9. A store discounts a $120 mattress 20% for a sale. One week later the sale price is discounted another 15%. At what price can the mattress now be purchased?

10. Paula earns $800 per month plus a 6% commission on her sales in the pharmacy. One month her sales are $4,350. What are her monthly earnings?

11. During the first quarter Les receives these grades in math. Using these grades, complete the chart. Round the answers to the nearer tenth.

	Item	A Points Received	B Points Possible	A ÷ B Individual Item %	C Total Points	D Total Points Possible	C ÷ D Accumulated Grades %
a.	Quiz 1	25	30	83.3%	25	30	83.3%
b.	Quiz 2	44	45		69	75	92%
c.	Quiz 3	15	25				
d.	Test 1	85	100				
e.	Quiz 4	8	20				
f.	Quiz 5	42	50				
g.	Quiz 6	13	30				
h.	Test 2	67	100				
i.	Take Home Test	95	100				
j.	Test 3	80	100				

ESTIMATING WITH PERCENTS

Estimation affords the opportunity to perform calculation mentally without the aid of pencils, paper, or a calculator. Mental images and calculations should be utilized in the examples.

Example: Visualize what percent of the diamond is shaded.

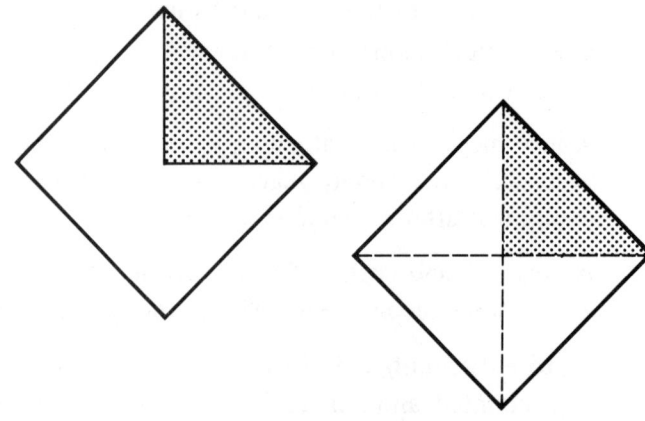

Mentally, "draw in the diagonals" (segments connecting opposite angles). There is 1 out of 4 regions shaded. This is 25%.

Example: Mentally calculate 250% of 50.

Think: 100% of 50 = 50 so, 200% of 50 = 100
50% of 50 = 25

250% of 50 is 125.

Example: Estimate 29.7% of 448.02.

Think: 29.7% is rounded to 30%.
448.02 is rounded to 450.
30% of 450 is 135.

29.7% of 448.02 is about 135.

Example: Mentally determine if 2% of 600 is less than, equal to, or greater than 4% of 300.

Think: 2% of 600 is 12.
4% of 300 is 12.

2% of 600 = 4% of 300.

22.3 EXERCISES

Estimate what percent of each region is shaded.

1.

2.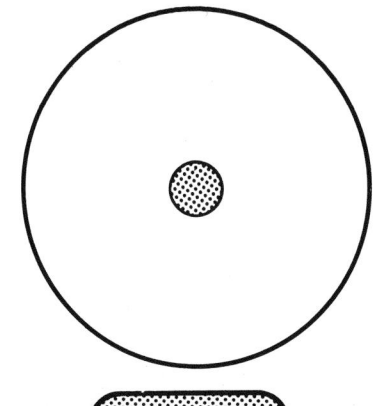

3.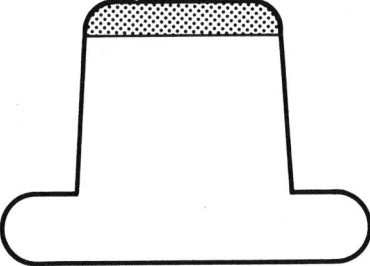

4.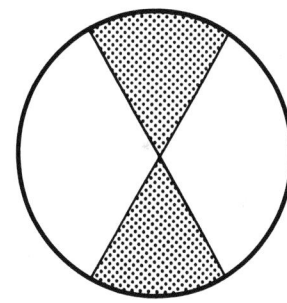

5.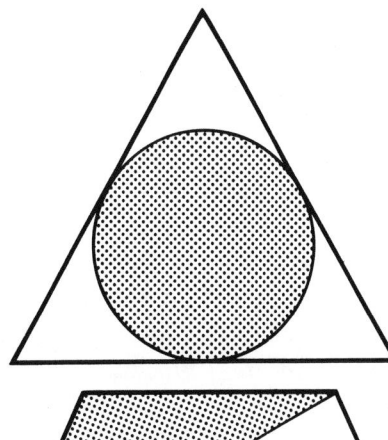

6.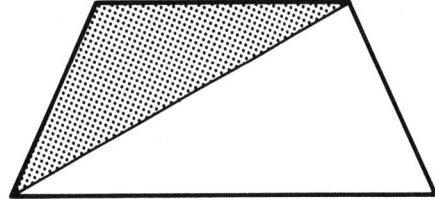

Estimate the sales tax to the nearer dollar.

	ITEM	COST	RATES				
			2%	3%	4%	5%	6%
7.	Car	$4,995					
8.	Washer-Dryer	$ 899					
9.	Refrigerator	$ 530					
10.	Furniture	$2,419					

Using rounded numbers, estimate each product.

11. 14.2% of 39.6
12. $1\frac{1}{10}$% of 278.89
13. 0.03% of 7,239.93
14. 98% of 135.79
15. 132.1% of 203.14

Using estimation and mental calculations, determine each relationship. Use the symbols $<, >, =$.

16. 3% of 600 ___?___ 5% of 300
17. $\frac{1}{4}$% of 400 ___?___ $\frac{1}{2}$% of 600
18. 0.05% of 2,500 ___?___ 0.1% of 1,500
19. 0.25% of 12,000 ___?___ 0.75% of 4,000
20. 150% of 800 ___?___ 200% of 600

APPLICATIONS

In determining the amount of an available drug that is to be administered, the strength of the drug does not change. For this reason, a direct ratio and proportion can be used. When preparing many other solutions, especially ones desired for topical use, the strength of the solution may be changed to a weaker strength or to the strength ordered to be used. Determining the new strength and the amount of solute to be used requires a different type of proportion. This proportion is:

smaller % strength:larger % strength = smaller volume:larger volume

or

weaker:stronger = solute:solvent

- ▼ The *smaller % strength (weaker)* is the strength of the solution ordered or desired.
- ▼ The *larger % strength (stronger)* is the strength of the drug or solution that is available.
- ▼ The *smaller volume (solute)* is the amount of solute of stock solution to be used.
- ▼ The *larger volume (solvent)* is the amount of solution to be prepared.

In preparing solutions from tablets, powders, or crystals, the amount of solution (larger volume) to be prepared may be considered to be the amount of solvent. Although the drug to be added to the solvent will increase the total volume of the solution, the increase is not appreciable when preparing large amounts of solutions. Measuring instruments used in preparing large amounts of solutions make it difficult to account for the volume increase, or displacement, of the drugs in tablet, crystal, or powder form. Caution must be taken not to generalize this concept. Displacement is an important factor when preparing many drugs for administration. Adding 2 millilitres of a solvent to 1 gram of a solute will yield more than 2 millilitres of solution; the exact amount will depend upon the displacement of the drug. Always adding the solvent to the solute—and not the solute to the solvent—will account for the displacement of the drug.

Example: A 5% boric acid solution is needed in the laboratory. A total of 750 millilitres are required. Calculate the amount of boric acid crystals required to prepare this solution.

smaller % strength : larger % strength = smaller volume : larger volume

$$5\% : 100\% = x \text{ millilitres} : 750 \text{ millilitres}$$
$$5 : 100 = x : 750$$
$$100(x) = 750(5)$$
$$100x = 3\ 750$$
$$\frac{100x}{100} = \frac{3\ 750}{100}$$
$$x = 37.5 \text{ grams of boric acid}$$

Note: Boric acid is in crystal form and is measured in grams. For computational purposes, 1 millilitre = 1 gram.

When preparing solutions from a stock solution, the amount of solvent must be considered. The amount of solvent is the difference between the amount of solute and the amount of solution. This is written:

$$\text{solvent} = \text{solution} - \text{solute}$$

Notice that this is not simply the solvent. A stock solution (solute) is a liquid and displaces approximately the same volume. This displacement is reflected in the formula: solvent = solution – solute.

Example: A laboratory technician prepares 100 millilitres of 25% ethyl alcohol from a 95% ethyl alcohol stock solution.

    a. Determine, to the nearer millilitre, the amount of 95% ethyl alcohol that is needed.

    b. Determine, to the nearer millilitre, the amount of distilled water that is added.

a. smaller % strength : larger % strength = smaller volume : larger volume

$$25\% : 95\% = x \text{ millilitres} : 100 \text{ millilitres}$$
$$25 : 95 = x : 100$$
$$95(x) = 25(100)$$
$$95x = 2\,500$$
$$\frac{95x}{95} = \frac{2\,500}{95}$$
$$x = 26 \text{ millilitres of 95\% ethyl alcohol}$$

b. solvent = solution – solute
   solvent = 100 millilitres – 26 millilitres
   solvent = 74 millilitres of distilled water

22.4 EXERCISES

1. Calculate the number of grams of iodine crystals that are required to prepare 250 millilitres of a 4% iodine solution.

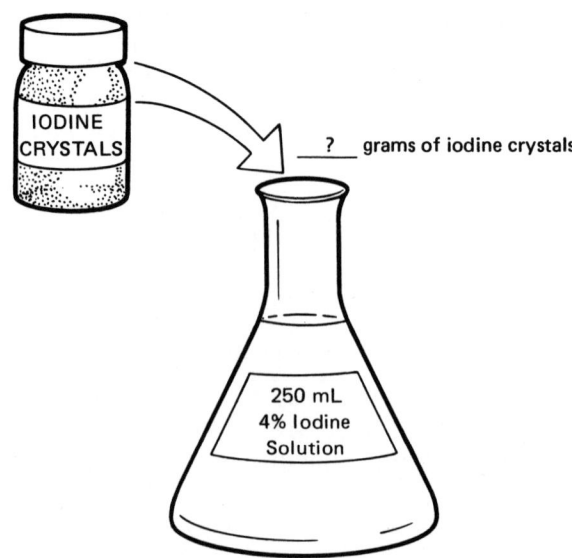

2. A 0.5% boric acid solution is to be prepared from a 5% boric acid stock solution.
   a. How much of the 5% boric acid solution is needed to prepare 750 millilitres of the 0.5% boric acid solution?
   b. How much distilled water must be added to obtain 750 millilitres of the 0.5% boric acid solution?

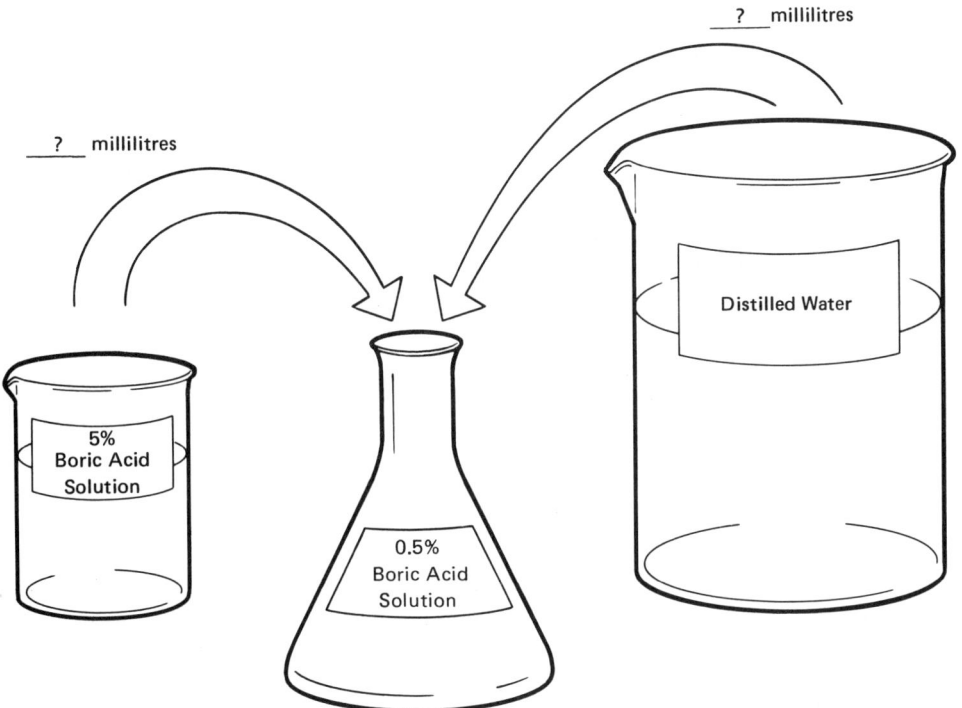

3. How many millilitres of 40% ethyl alcohol can be prepared from 135 millilitres of 95% ethyl alcohol?

4. Using a 40% ethyl alcohol solution, 250 millilitres of a 1:10 ethyl alcohol solution is made.
   a. By expressing the 1:10 ratio as a percent, determine the amount of 40% ethyl alcohol to be used.
   b. Determine the amount of distilled water to be used.

5. A stock solution of boric acid contains 1 part boric acid in 200 parts solution. A 1:500 solution is to be prepared. How much of the stock solution must be used to prepare 600 millilitres of the 1:500 solution?

6. A stock solution of 25% ethyl alcohol is available. A total of 250 millilitres of this solution is present in the storage flask. How many 100-millilitre containers of 5% ethyl alcohol can be made from the stock solution?

   Note: Find the amount of 25% ethyl alcohol needed to prepare 100 millilitres of the solution.

unit 23 section four applications to health work

OBJECTIVES

After studying this unit the student should be able to:
- Use the basic principles of ratios, proportions and percents to solve health work problems.

Solutions are prepared for many uses. A solution consists of a solute—the drug—and the solvent—the liquid used to dissolve the drug. Solutions are prepared from pure drugs and from stock solutions.

▼ Pure drugs are in either a solid form, such as tablets, powders, or crystals, or a liquid form. Pure drugs are 100% strength.

▼ Stock solutions are solutions that are "on hand" and usually are of a strong strength. The stock solutions are used to make weaker solutions. Stock solutions, as the words imply, are always in a liquid form.

- Preparing solutions from crystals or powders
  - The drug is usually measured in grams. For purposes of calculation, 1 gram is considered equal to 1 millilitre.
  - Weigh the amount of drug desired. Place the drug in a graduated container and add the solvent to obtain the desired amount of solution.
  - Since a solid drug does not displace an appreciable volume of liquid, the amount of liquid that is added is considered to be the same as the amount of solution when making large volumes of solutions.

- Preparing solutions from liquids or stock solutions
  - The drug is usually measured in millilitres.
  - Measure the amount of drug desired. Place the drug in a graduated container and add a sufficient amount of liquid to obtain the desired amount of solution.
  - Since a liquid drug displaces approximately the same volume as the liquid, the amount of liquid that is added is the difference between the solution and the solute (drug). That is, for liquids:

$$\text{solution} = \text{solvent} + \text{solute}$$

- Preparing solutions from tablets

  • Tablets come in a pre-measured form.

  • Determine the number of tablets to be used. Dissolve the desired number of tablets in the amount of solution that is needed.

  • The drug (solute) is dissolved in the solvent rather than the solvent being added to the solute. The volume of the solution is not increased appreciably by the solute.

Any solution which is to be sterilized is poured or filtered into a glass flask and sterilized according to prescribed or accepted techniques. Solutions that are used for intravenous or injections, such as glucose or saline solutions, are made from distilled water, are filtered, and then are sterilized.

23.1 EXERCISES

1. Determine the number of grams of solute that are required to prepare each solution.

   a. 500 millilitres of a 0.9% sodium chloride solution

   b. 750 millilitres of a 0.2% bichloride of mercury solution

   c. 600 millilitres of a 4.5% magnesium sulfate solution

   d. 250 millilitres of a 0.75% sodium chloride solution

   e. 1 litre of a 0.5% potassium permanganate solution

   f. 8 litres of a 35% glucose solution

2. When using 20-milligram (0.020-gram) tablets to prepare 500 millilitres of a 0.75% solution, how many tablets would be required?

   Note: number of tablets = $\dfrac{\text{amount (mass) of solute}}{\text{mass of one tablet}}$

3. Drugs in solution are expressed as weight (mass)/volume. Vistaril 100 milligrams/2 millilitres means 100 milligrams of the drug in 2 millilitres of solution. The doctor orders the medication in units of weight (mass) measure. To administer the drug, the prescription must be expressed in units of volume measure. The doctor orders Vistaril 37.5 milligrams. How many millilitres of the Vistaril 100 milligrams/2 millilitres must be administered?

Section 4 Ratio, Proportion, and Percents

4. The doctor orders scopalomine 0.2 milligram. The ampul contains 0.6 milligram of scopalomine in 1 millilitre of solution. How many millilitres are required to supply this dosage?

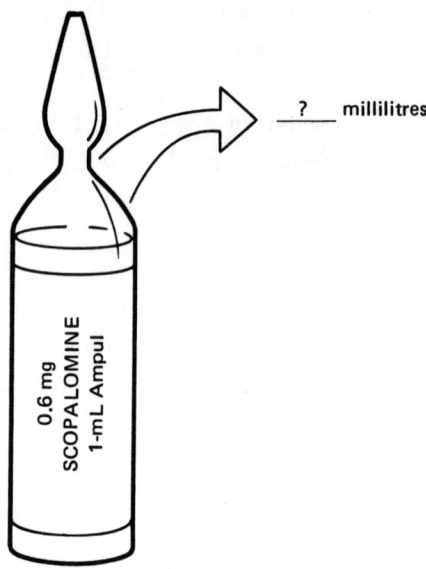

5. Tincture of iodine is prepared by dissolving 70 grams of iodine and 50 grams of potassium iodide in 50 millilitres of solution. This is then diluted with 95% ethyl alcohol to make 1 000 millilitres (1 litre) of solution.

   a. What percent of the final solution does the iodine constitute?
   b. What percent of the final solution does the potassium iodide constitute?
   c. What percent of the final solution does the alcohol constitute?
   d. How many grams of potassium iodide are present in 625 millilitres of tincture of iodine?
   e. How many millilitres of water are present in 1 000 millilitres of solution?

   Note: It can be assumed that in the 50-millilitre solution of iodine, potassium iodide, and solvent, the solvent is 50 millilitres of water. In 95% ethyl alcohol there is 5% water.

6. A sodium chloride solution is prepared using 1.5 drams of sodium chloride in 750 millilitres of solution. What is the percent strength?

   Note: 1 dram = 4 grams

7. Give the percent strength for each chemical in the solutions.

   a. 1.5 grams of merthiolate crystals in 135 millilitres of solution
   b. 50 grams of glucose in 625 millilitres of solution
   c. 0.9 grams of cocaine in 175 millilitres of solution
   d. 3 grams of sodium bromide in 4 fluid ounces of solution

   Note: 1 fluid ounce = 31.10 grams

8. A 0.9% physiological saline solution means that there are 9 grams of sodium chloride in 1 000 millilitres of solution. How many grams are present in 15 millilitres of solution?

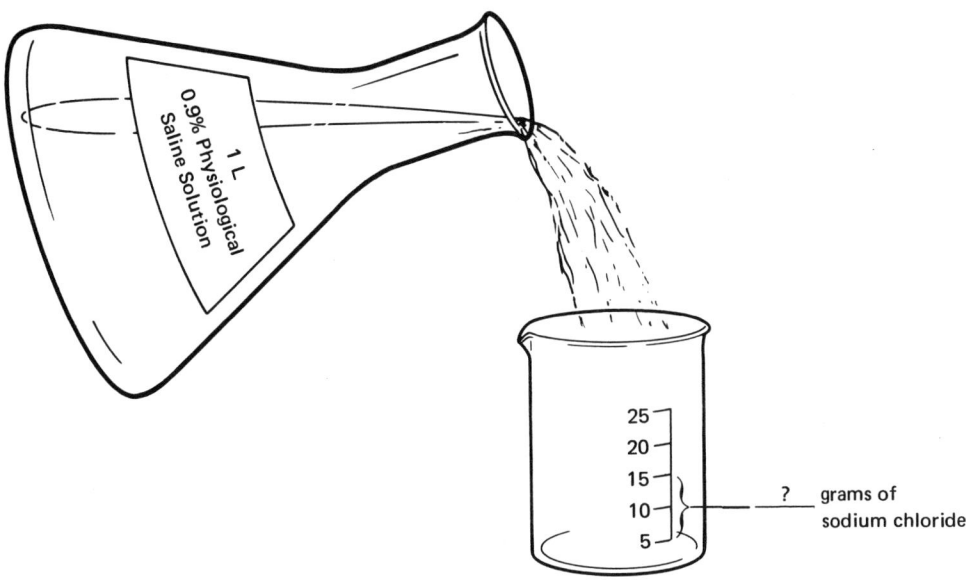

9. Hayem's solution contains 0.25 grams of mercuric chloride, 2.5 grams of sodium sulfate, and 0.5 grams of sodium chloride in 100 millilitres of solution. Find the amount of each solute in 375 millilitres of an identical solution.

   a. mercuric chloride
   b. sodium sulfate
   c. sodium chloride

10. Gram's iodine solution is prepared by using iodine crystals and potassium iodide. A 300-millilitre solution contains 1 gram of iodine crystals and 2 grams of potassium iodide.

    a. How many grams of iodine crystals are in 1 000 millilitres of this solution?
    b. How many grams of potassium iodide are in 1 000 millilitres of this solution?

11. It takes 1 gram of iodine crystals and 2 grams of potassium iodide to make 300 millilitres of Gram's iodine solution. An inventory of the laboratory indicates that there are 135 grams of potassium iodide and 450 grams of iodine crystals. What is the maximum amount of Gram's iodine solution that can be prepared from the chemicals not in inventory?

12. A 0.3% zephiran chloride solution is made from a 15% zephiran chloride stock solution.

   a. How many millilitres of solute are required to make 750 millilitres of the 0.3% zephiran chloride solution?
   b. How many millilitres of solvent are required?

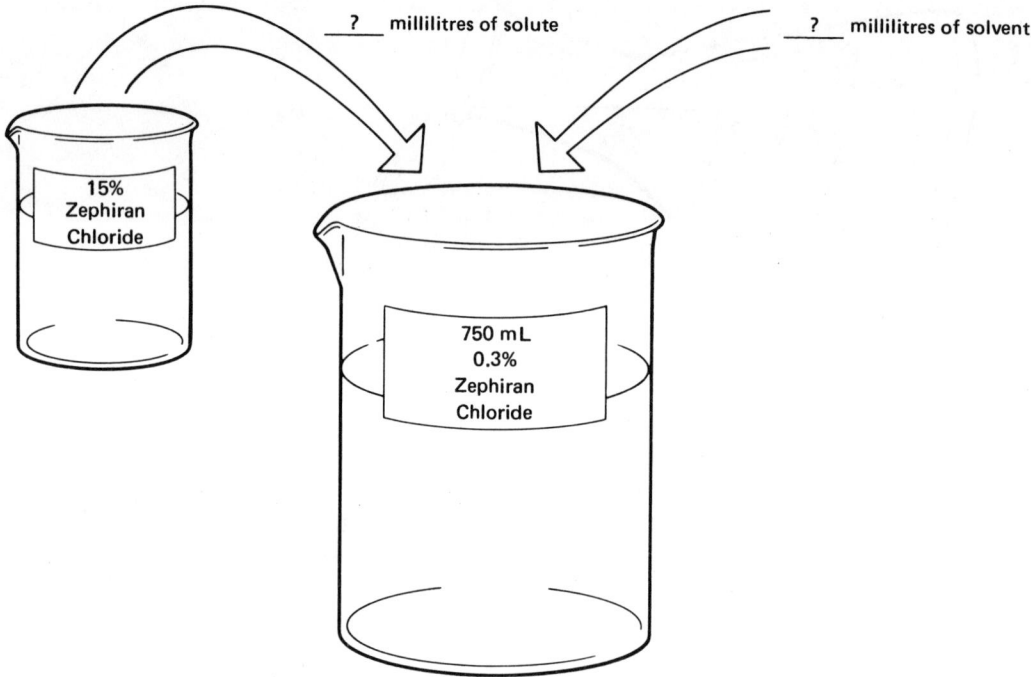

13. A 40% ethyl alcohol preparation is available in the laboratory.

   a. Calculate the amount of stock solution needed to prepare 100 millilitres of a 15% ethyl alcohol solution.
   b. Calculate the amount of distilled water needed.

14. A 30% ethyl alcohol solution is available in the laboratory. How much stock solution is required to prepare 50 millilitres of each dilution?

   a. 25% ethyl alcohol
   b. 10% ethyl alcohol
   c. 5% ethyl alcohol

15. Absolute (100%) ethyl alcohol is available as a stock solution. How much stock solution is required to prepare 125 millilitres of each dilution?

   a. 25% ethyl alcohol solution
   b. 65% ethyl alcohol solution
   c. 95% ethyl alcohol solution

16. A 40% magnesium sulfate solution is available. How much water must be added to 60 millilitres of this solution to prepare a 2% solution?

17. A flask contains 57 millilitres of 6% potassium permanganate. How many millilitres of 4% solution can be prepared from 57 millilitres of 6% potassium permanganate?

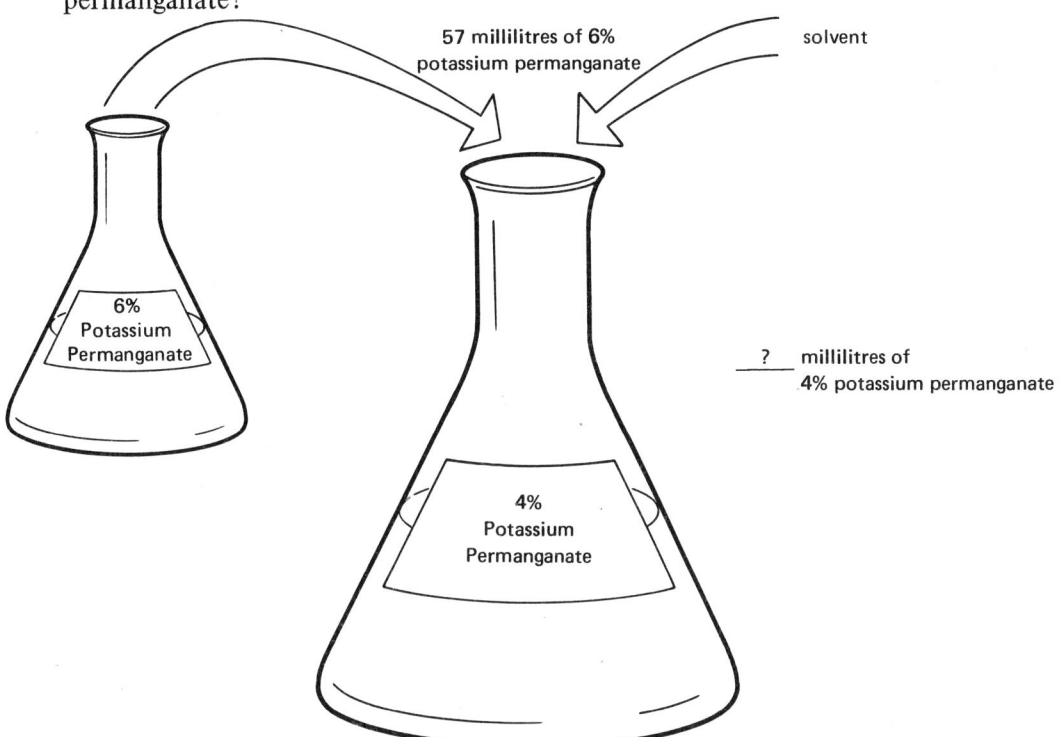

18. How many millilitres of 35% ethyl alcohol can be prepared from 250 millilitres of 40% ethyl alcohol?

19. A total of 4.750 litres of 95% ethyl alcohol is available in the laboratory. For a series of tests, several dilutions are required. The allocation of the alcohol is: 1.500 litres for 50% ethyl alcohol; 1.250 litres for 25% ethyl alcohol; 0.75 litres for 20% ethyl alcohol; and 1.250 litres for 12% ethyl alcohol. How many millilitres, or litres, will each of the designated amounts prepare when added to distilled water?

 a. 50% ethyl alcohol
 b. 25% ethyl alcohol
 c. 20% ethyl alcohol
 d. 12% ethyl alcohol

20. There are 62 grams of sodium chloride in 950 millilitres of a solution. How many grams are in 125 millilitres of the same solution?

21. Using distilled water, boric acid may be dissolved in various dilutions.

 a. A boric acid solution is prepared by using 57 grams of boric acid in 10 litres of solution. What is the ratio strength of the solution?
 b. A bottle contains a boric acid in a dilution of 1:400 (1 part boric acid to 400 parts solution). How much boric acid is present in 150 millilitres of the solution?

22. Ethyl alcohol may be used in various dilutions for a variety of purposes. The stock solution of 95% ethyl alcohol and 5% water is a 95:100 or 19:20 ethyl alcohol solution.

   a. A laboratory technician is requested to prepare 100 millilitres of a 1:4 ethyl alcohol solution (25 parts ethyl alcohol to 100 parts water). How much 95% ethyl alcohol is needed?
   b. How much 95% ethyl alcohol is needed to prepare 125 millilitres of a 1:10 ethyl alcohol solution?
   c. How much distilled water is needed to prepare 125 millilitres of a 1:10 ethyl alcohol solution?

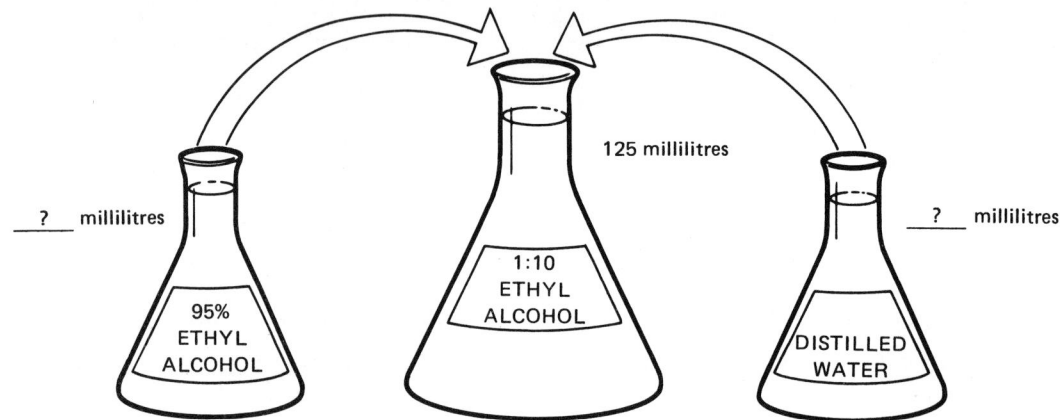

23. Methylene blue contains 0.3 grams of methylene blue in 30.0 millilitres of 95% ethyl alcohol.

   a. What percent of the solution is methylene blue?
   b. What percent of the solution is ethyl alcohol?
   c. How much methylene blue is present in 125 millilitres of solution?
   d. How much ethyl alcohol is present in 125 millilitres of solution?

24. One litre of Ringer's solution contains 0.42 gram of potassium chloride, 9.0 grams of sodium chloride, 0.24 gram of calcium chloride, 0.20 gram of sodium carbonate, and distilled water.

   a. What percent of the solution is composed of potassium chloride?
   b. What percent of the solution is composed of sodium chloride?
   c. What percent of the solution is composed of calcium chloride?
   d. Determine the amount of potassium chloride needed for 750 millilitres of solution.
   e. Determine the amount of sodium chloride needed for 750 millilitres of solution.
   f. Determine the amount of calcium chloride needed for 750 millilitres of solution.

25. A physiological saline solution is composed of 0.9% sodium chloride and 99.1% distilled water.

   a. How much sodium chloride is present in 125 millilitres of solution?
   b. How much distilled water is present in 750 millilitres of solution?

26. A clinic consists of 47 full-time and 6 part-time employees.
    a. What percent of the individuals are part-time employees?
    b. Laboratory technicians make up 16.98% of the staff. How many staff members are laboratory technicians?

27. In one month a clinic treats 1,262 patients. The cost of operating the clinic (expenditures) is $102,467. The clinic sent out bills (revenue) totalling $127,472. A study reveals that 67% of these bills are paid within 30 days. Insurance payments account for 27% of the money received within the 30 days.
    a. How much money is received within 30 days following the billing?
    b. How much of the money received is paid by insurance?
    c. Salaries account for 78% of the operating cost. How much is spent on salaries?
    d. For the month, insurance premiums are $3,894. What percent of the operating cost is represented by this figure?
    e. By what percent do the operating costs exceed the amount of money received within the 30 days from the billing?
    f. If all the revenue (total billing) is received, what is the percent of the excess of revenue over expenditure?

28. During a one month period, the clinic treats a total of 1,262 patients. The illnesses and conditions are grouped into categories and are placed on a circle graph.

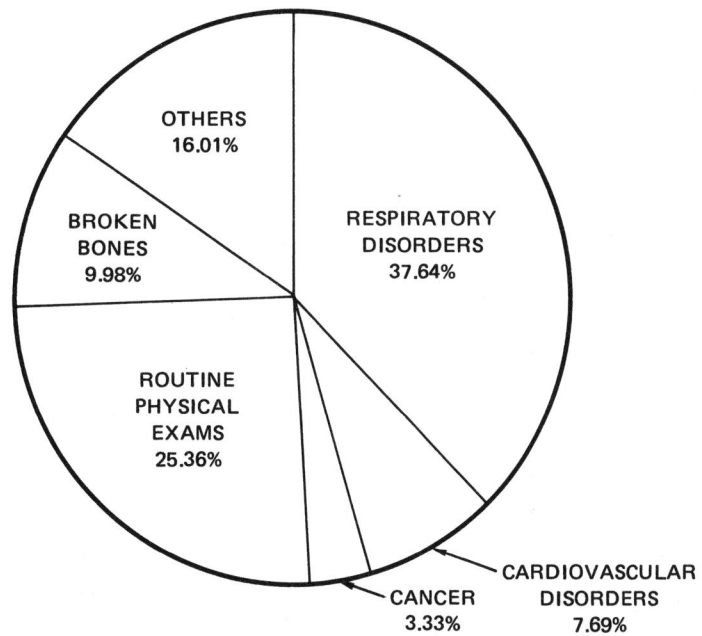

   a. How many people had routine physical exams?
   b. Find the number of people treated for respiratory disorders or cancer.
   c. How many people are treated for broken bones or cardiovascular disorders?
   d. Find the number of people treated for respiratory disorders or cardiovascular disorders or other conditions.

SECTION 5 SYSTEMS OF MEASURE

unit 24 the apothecaries' system of weight

OBJECTIVES

After studying this unit the student should be able to:
- Express Arabic numerals as Roman numerals.
- Express apothecaries' units of weight as equivalent apothecaries' units of weight.
- Express weight measurements in the apothecaries' system as equivalent metric measurements.
- Express weight (mass) measurements in the metric system as equivalent apothecaries' measurements.

THE APOTHECARIES' SYSTEM OF WEIGHT

Doctors use the apothecaries' system when ordering medications. It is an old English system of measure with whole numbers expressed as Roman numerals. Fractions are expressed as fractions, except for one-half which is expressed as 'ss'. It is important that a health worker be able to read, to understand, and to work with this system. The apothecaries' system has equivalent values within the system and in other systems of measure.

When using the apothecaries' system of measure it is customary to use Roman numerals and fractions. The chart shows some Roman numerals and the base ten equivalents.

I = 1	V = 5	X = 10	L = 50	C = 100

- When representing numbers between these values, these principles are used.
  - In a sequence, the letters are never repeated more than three times.
  - When a letter representing a smaller number precedes a larger one, the value of the first is subtracted from the second.

Examples: Subtraction principle in the apothecaries' system.

IV = 5 − 1 *or* 4   XL = 50 − 10 *or* 40

IX = 10 − 1 *or* 9   XC = 100 − 10 *or* 90

- The numerals V and L are not used in a subtractive way.
- When numerals have the same value or when smaller numerals follow larger numerals, the values are added.

Examples: Addition principle in the apothecaries' system.

XVI = 10 + 5 + 1 = 16 XXX = 10 + 10 + 10 = 30

When expressing dosages in the apothecaries' system it is customary to use lower Roman numerals rather than capital letters. This chart illustrates numbers being written using Roman numerals.

NUMBER	ROMAN NUMERAL (capitals)	ROMAN NUMERAL (lower case)	INTERPRETATION
one	I	i	1
two	II	ii	1 + 1 = 2
three	III	iii	1 + 1 + 1 = 3
four	IV	iv	5 - 1 = 4
five	V	v	5
six	VI	vi	5 + 1 = 6
seven	VII	vii	5 + 1 + 1 = 7
eight	VIII	viii	5 + 1 + 1 + 1 = 8
nine	IX	ix	10 - 1 = 9
ten	X	x	10
eleven	XI	xi	10 + 1 = 11
twelve	XII	xii	10 + 1 + 1 = 12
thirteen	XIII	xiii	10 + 1 + 1 + 1 = 13
fourteen	XIV	xiv	10 + (5 - 1) = 14
fifteen	XV	xv	10 + 5 = 15
sixteen	XVI	xvi	10 + 5 + 1 = 16
seventeen	XVII	xvii	10 + 5 + 1 + 1 = 17
eighteen	XVIII	xviii	10 + 5 + 1 + 1 + 1 = 18
nineteen	XIX	xix	10 + (10 - 1) = 19
twenty	XX	xx	10 + 10 = 20

The apothecaries' system of weight has four basic units. The units of weight, the abbreviations or symbol, and an example of the approximate weight of one unit are summarized in this chart.

UNIT	SYMBOL OR ABBREVIATION	EXAMPLE
grain	gr.	one drop of water
dram	ℨ	one teaspoonful of water
ounce	℥	two tablespoons of water
pound	lb.	two teacups of water

When expressing a weight, abbreviations or symbols for the unit may be used. When an abbreviation is used, it appears first followed by the magnitude of the measurement. The magnitude of the measurement is expressed with lower case Roman numerals or fractions. If the unit is not abbreviated, the magnitude of the measurement is written before the unit and is expressed using Arabic numerals.

Example: Express eight grains, one-third dram, four ounces, and one-half pound without and with abbreviations or symbols.

- 8 grains *or* gr. viii
- $\frac{1}{3}$ dram *or* ʒ $\frac{1}{3}$
- 4 ounces *or* ℥ iv
- $\frac{1}{2}$ pound *or* lb. ss

Note: The symbol **ss** is used to express $\frac{1}{2}$.

24.1 EXERCISES

1. Write the numbers 21 through 30 using lower case Roman numerals.
2. Using Roman numerals, write the number corresponding to each of the last five years.

Write the meaning of each measurement.

3. ʒ ss
4. gr. xix
5. ʒ $\frac{1}{4}$
6. lb. xv
7. ℥ xl
8. gr. $\frac{1}{3}$
9. ʒ iv
10. lb. $\frac{3}{4}$
11. ʒ $\frac{5}{6}$

Express each measurement by using abbreviations or symbols.

12. $\frac{1}{4}$ ounce
13. 5 drams
14. 4 pounds
15. $\frac{1}{3}$ grain
16. $4\frac{1}{2}$ ounces
17. 10 grains
18. $\frac{3}{4}$ dram
19. 32 grains
20. $10\frac{1}{2}$ pounds
21. 14 ounces
22. $1\frac{1}{2}$ drams
23. $\frac{1}{2}$ pound

APOTHECARIES' EQUIVALENT MEASUREMENTS OF WEIGHT

In the apothecaries' system these units of weight are equivalent.

60 grains (gr.)	=	1 dram (ʒ)
8 drams (ʒ)	=	1 ounce (℥)
12 ounces (℥)	=	1 pound (lb.)

Expressing equivalence of measurements is accomplished by using proportions.

Example: Express 4 drams as grains.

- Using the proportion: $\dfrac{\text{drams}}{\text{grains}} = \dfrac{\text{drams}}{\text{grains}}$.

$$\dfrac{1 \text{ dram}}{60 \text{ grains}} = \dfrac{4 \text{ drams}}{a \text{ grains}}$$

$$1(a) = 4(60)$$

$$a = \text{gr. ccxl}$$

- Using the proportion: $\dfrac{\text{drams}}{\text{drams}} = \dfrac{\text{grains}}{\text{grains}}$.

$$\dfrac{1 \text{ dram}}{4 \text{ drams}} = \dfrac{60 \text{ grains}}{a \text{ grains}}$$

$$1(a) = 4(60)$$

$$a = \text{gr. ccxl}$$

Example: Express 360 grains as drams.

- $\dfrac{\text{grains}}{\text{drams}} = \dfrac{\text{grains}}{\text{drams}}$

$$\dfrac{360 \text{ grains}}{a \text{ drams}} = \dfrac{60 \text{ grains}}{1 \text{ dram}}$$

$$1(360) = 60(a)$$

$$360 = 60a$$

$$\dfrac{360}{60} = \dfrac{60a}{60}$$

$$ʒ \text{ vi} = a$$

- $\dfrac{\text{grains}}{\text{grains}} = \dfrac{\text{drams}}{\text{drams}}$

$$\dfrac{60 \text{ grains}}{360 \text{ grains}} = \dfrac{1 \text{ dram}}{a \text{ drams}}$$

$$60(a) = 1(360)$$

$$60a = 360$$

$$\dfrac{60a}{60} = \dfrac{360}{60}$$

$$a = ʒ \text{ vi}$$

Example: Express 0.6 ounce as drams.

$$\frac{\text{ounces}}{\text{drams}} = \frac{\text{ounces}}{\text{drams}} \qquad\qquad \frac{\text{ounces}}{\text{ounces}} = \frac{\text{drams}}{\text{drams}}$$

$$\frac{1 \text{ ounce}}{8 \text{ drams}} = \frac{0.6 \text{ ounce}}{b \text{ drams}} \qquad\qquad \frac{1 \text{ ounce}}{0.6 \text{ ounce}} = \frac{8 \text{ drams}}{b \text{ drams}}$$

$$1(b) = 0.6(8) \qquad\qquad 1(b) = 0.6(8)$$

$$b = 4.8 \text{ drams} \qquad\qquad b = 4.8 \text{ drams}$$

Example: Express 32 drams as ounces.

$$\frac{\text{ounces}}{\text{drams}} = \frac{\text{ounces}}{\text{drams}} \qquad\qquad \frac{\text{ounces}}{\text{ounces}} = \frac{\text{drams}}{\text{drams}}$$

$$\frac{1 \text{ ounce}}{8 \text{ drams}} = \frac{y \text{ ounces}}{32 \text{ drams}} \qquad\qquad \frac{1 \text{ ounce}}{y \text{ ounces}} = \frac{8 \text{ drams}}{32 \text{ drams}}$$

$$8(y) = 1(32) \qquad\qquad 8(y) = 1(32)$$

$$8y = 32 \qquad\qquad 8y = 32$$

$$\frac{8y}{8} = \frac{32}{8} \qquad\qquad \frac{8y}{8} = \frac{32}{8}$$

$$y = ℥ \text{ iv} \qquad\qquad y = ℥ \text{ iv}$$

Example: Express 13 pounds as ounces.

$$\frac{\text{ounces}}{\text{pounds}} = \frac{\text{ounces}}{\text{pounds}} \qquad\qquad \frac{\text{ounces}}{\text{ounces}} = \frac{\text{pounds}}{\text{pounds}}$$

$$\frac{12 \text{ ounces}}{1 \text{ pound}} = \frac{z \text{ ounces}}{13 \text{ pounds}} \qquad\qquad \frac{12 \text{ ounces}}{z \text{ ounces}} = \frac{1 \text{ pound}}{13 \text{ pounds}}$$

$$1(z) = 12(13) \qquad\qquad 1(z) = 12(13)$$

$$z = ℥ \text{ clvi} \qquad\qquad z = ℥ \text{ clvi}$$

Example: Express $\frac{3}{8}$ ounce as pounds.

$$\frac{\text{pounds}}{\text{ounces}} = \frac{\text{pounds}}{\text{ounces}} \qquad\qquad \frac{\text{ounces}}{\text{ounces}} = \frac{\text{pounds}}{\text{pounds}}$$

$$\frac{1 \text{ pound}}{12 \text{ ounces}} = \frac{y \text{ pounds}}{\frac{3}{8} \text{ ounce}} \qquad\qquad \frac{12 \text{ ounces}}{\frac{3}{8} \text{ ounce}} = \frac{1 \text{ pound}}{y \text{ pounds}}$$

$$12(y) = 1\left(\frac{3}{8}\right) \qquad\qquad 12(y) = \frac{3}{8}(1)$$

$$12y = \frac{3}{8} \qquad\qquad 12y = \frac{3}{8}$$

$$\frac{12y}{12} = \frac{\frac{3}{8}}{12} \qquad\qquad \frac{12y}{12} = \frac{\frac{3}{8}}{12}$$

$$y = \frac{3}{8} \div 12 \text{ or } \frac{3}{8} \times \frac{1}{12} \qquad\qquad y = \frac{3}{8} \div 12 \text{ or } \frac{3}{8} \times \frac{1}{12}$$

$$y = \text{lb.} \frac{1}{32} \qquad\qquad y = \text{lb.} \frac{1}{32}$$

24.2 EXERCISES

Express each measurement as an equivalent measurement as indicated. Express all answers using the accepted abbreviations.

Grains

1. 0.8 dram
2. ʒ i
3. 0.5 dram
4. ʒ 1¼
5. ℥ iss

Drams

6. gr. xxx
7. gr. ccxl
8. gr. ½
9. gr. lx
10. 12.6 grains
11. ℥ x
12. 16 ounces
13. ℥ xx
14. ℥ ivss
15. ℥ 1¼

Ounces

16. ʒ xii
17. 0.4 dram
18. ʒ clx
19. ʒ 4 4/5
20. ʒ cxx
21. lb. vi
22. 0.5 pound
23. lb. ¼
24. lb. vss
25. lb. v

Pounds

26. ℥ lx
27. ℥ xviii
28. ℥ 4/5
29. 0.6 ounce
30. 600 ounces

APOTHECARIES' — METRIC EQUIVALENT MEASUREMENTS OF WEIGHT

Both the apothecaries' and metric systems are used by doctors and health workers. It is important to be able to rapidly and accurately express equivalences between the two systems. This table provides equivalences that are approximations within the acceptable limits of error. Using slightly different equivalences would produce slightly different answers. The answers, while different, will be very close to each other and within safe limits.

APOTHECARIES' SYSTEM		METRIC SYSTEM
1 grain (gr.)	=	60 milligrams (mg)
15 grains (gr.)	=	1 gram (g)
1 dram (ʒ)	=	4 grams (g)
1 ounce (℥)	=	30 grams (g)
1 pound (lb.)	=	360 grams (g)
32 ounces (℥)	=	1 kilogram (kg)

Expressing equivalences between the two systems is similar to expressing equivalences within the apothecaries' system. Equivalences are found by using proportions.

Example: Express 120 milligrams as grains.

$$\frac{\text{apothecaries'}}{\text{metric}} = \frac{\text{apothecaries'}}{\text{metric}} \qquad \frac{\text{apothecaries'}}{\text{apothecaries'}} = \frac{\text{metric}}{\text{metric}}$$

$$\frac{1 \text{ grain}}{60 \text{ milligrams}} = \frac{z \text{ grains}}{120 \text{ milligrams}} \qquad \frac{1 \text{ grain}}{z \text{ grains}} = \frac{60 \text{ milligrams}}{120 \text{ milligrams}}$$

$$60(z) = 120(1) \qquad\qquad 60(z) = 120(1)$$

$$60z = 120 \qquad\qquad 60z = 120$$

$$\frac{60z}{60} = \frac{120}{60} \qquad\qquad \frac{60z}{60} = \frac{120}{60}$$

$$z = \text{gr. ii} \qquad\qquad z = \text{gr. ii}$$

Example: Express 0.5 dram as grams.

$$\frac{\text{apothecaries'}}{\text{metric}} = \frac{\text{apothecaries'}}{\text{metric}} \qquad \frac{\text{apothecaries'}}{\text{apothecaries'}} = \frac{\text{metric}}{\text{metric}}$$

$$\frac{1 \text{ dram}}{4 \text{ grams}} = \frac{0.5 \text{ dram}}{w \text{ grams}} \qquad \frac{1 \text{ dram}}{0.5 \text{ dram}} = \frac{4 \text{ grams}}{w \text{ grams}}$$

$$1(w) = 0.5(4) \qquad\qquad 1(w) = 0.5(4)$$

$$w = 2.0 \text{ g} \qquad\qquad w = 2.0 \text{ g}$$

Example: Express $\frac{4}{5}$ ounce as kilograms.

$$\frac{\text{apothecaries'}}{\text{metric}} = \frac{\text{apothecaries'}}{\text{metric}} \qquad \frac{\text{apothecaries'}}{\text{apothecaries'}} = \frac{\text{metric}}{\text{metric}}$$

$$\frac{32 \text{ ounces}}{1 \text{ kilogram}} = \frac{\frac{4}{5} \text{ ounce}}{b \text{ kilograms}} \qquad \frac{32 \text{ ounces}}{\frac{4}{5} \text{ ounce}} = \frac{1 \text{ kilogram}}{b \text{ kilograms}}$$

$$32(b) = \frac{4}{5}(1) \qquad\qquad 32(b) = 1\left(\frac{4}{5}\right)$$

$$32b = \frac{4}{5} \qquad\qquad 32b = \frac{4}{5}$$

$$\frac{32b}{32} = \frac{\frac{4}{5}}{32} \qquad\qquad \frac{32b}{32} = \frac{\frac{4}{5}}{32}$$

$$b = \frac{4}{5} \div \frac{32}{1} \text{ or } \frac{4}{5} \times \frac{1}{32} \qquad b = \frac{4}{5} \div \frac{32}{1} \text{ or } \frac{4}{5} \times \frac{1}{32}$$

$$b = \frac{1}{40} \text{ kg} \qquad\qquad b = \frac{1}{40} \text{ kg}$$

24.3 EXERCISES

Express each measurement as an equivalent measurement as indicated.

Grains
1. 150 mg
2. 40 mg
3. 0.6 mg
4. 600 mg
5. 3.6 mg
6. 12 g
7. 6.5 g
8. 0.3 g
9. 2.5 g
10. 5 g

Milligrams
11. gr. x
12. gr. ss
13. gr. ivss
14. 0.25 grain
15. gr. xl

Grams
16. gr. lx
17. gr. ivss
18. gr. xc
19. 0.6 grain
20. gr. lxx
21. ℥ xvi
22. ℥ iiiss
23. ℥ $3\frac{3}{5}$
24. ℥ xiv
25. 8.2 drams
26. ℥ ss
27. ℥ v
28. ℥ iiss
29. ℥ xc
30. 0.1 ounce
31. 10 pounds
32. 0.5 pound
33. 4.3 pounds
34. $\frac{1}{4}$ pound
35. $\frac{1}{9}$ pound

Drams
36. 8.8 g
37. 36 g
38. 0.6 g
39. $4\frac{4}{5}$ g
40. 96 g

Ounces
41. 150 g
42. 4.5 g
43. 6 g
44. 80 g
45. 180 g
46. 0.25 kg
47. 5 kg
48. 3.2 kg
49. $\frac{1}{3}$ kg
50. 15 kg

Pounds
51. 0.360 g
52. 720 g
53. 36 g
54. 540 g
55. 1 800 g

Kilograms
56. ℥ lxiv
57. 9.6 ounces
58. 320 ounces
59. ℥ xlviii
60. 960 ounces

Determine the correct relationship. Use the symbols $<, >, =$.

61. gr. xxv __?__ 2 g
62. 45 g __?__ ℥ ii
63. gr. x __?__ 0.006 g
64. 2.5 g __?__ gr. xxx
65. 0.5 kg __?__ lb. i
66. ℥ iv __?__ 16 g
67. ℥ iiss __?__ 80 g
68. 6 g __?__ ℥ iss
69. 5 mg __?__ gr. $\frac{1}{10}$
70. ℥ v __?__ 120 g

APPLICATIONS

The medical field is involved with the prevention, diagnosis, and the treatment of diseases and illnesses. A physician is responsible for diagnosing the cause of the illness and prescribing the medication. The diagnosis of the illness may require the assistance of laboratory personnel and other health care workers. The prescribed medication is referred to as a *medication order* or a *medicine order.*

A medication order is usually a written document which describes the medicine to be administered to a specific patient. The medication order includes –

- the drug to be used.
- the dose.
- the form of the drug.
- the time to be administered.
- the total number of times to be administered or the dosage.
- the method by which it is to be given.

It may also include directions for checking with the physician in case of complications and/or adverse reactions.

24.4 EXERCISES

1. Prescriptions may be written in either the metric or the apothecaries' system. It is often necessary to express the prescription as an equivalent in the other system. Express the prescriptions in the apothecaries' system as prescriptions in the metric system. Express prescriptions in the metric system as prescriptions in the apothecaries' system.

   a. Atropine gr. $\frac{1}{100}$

   b. Phenobarb gr. $\frac{1}{2}$

   c. Phenobarb gr. ss

   d. Seconal gr. $1\frac{1}{2}$

   e. Potassium Triplex ʒ i

   f. Vasodilan 10 mg

   g. Methadone 7 mg

2. Atropine sulfate is available in gr. $\frac{1}{100}$ tablets. The prescription is for 1 mg of atropine sulfate. How many tablets are required to meet this request?

3. Phenobarbital tablets are available in 5-mg tablets. A patient is given a prescription for gr. ii. How many tablets are required to provide this dosage?

4. Synthroid is available in 0.1-mg tablets. A patient is required to take gr. $\frac{1}{20}$. How many tablets provide this dosage?

unit 25 the apothecaries' system of volume

OBJECTIVES

After studying this unit the student should be able to:
- Express apothecaries' units of volume as equivalent apothecaries' units of volume.
- Express volume measurements in the apothecaries' system as equivalent metric measurements.
- Express volume measurements in the metric system as equivalent apothecaries' measurements.

THE APOTHECARIES' SYSTEM OF VOLUME

As was stated earlier, when expressing doses in the apothecaries' system, lower case Roman numerals rather than capital letters are used. The apothecaries' system of volume has six basic units. The units of volume, the abbreviations or symbols, and an example of the approximate volume of one unit are summarized in this chart.

UNIT	SYMBOL OR ABBREVIATION	EXAMPLE
minim	♏	one drop of water
fluidram	f ʒ	one teaspoon of water
fluidounce	f ℥	two tablespoons of water
pint	pt.	two glassfuls of water
quart	qt.	four glassfuls of water
gallon	gal.	sixteen glassfuls of water

The use of abbreviations or symbols in expressing volume measurements follows the same guidelines as for weight measurements.

Examples: Express these volume measurements without and with abbreviations or symbols: eleven fluid ounces; one-fourth fluidram; four minims; three and one-half pints; five quarts; one-half gallon.

- 11 fluidounces *or* f ℥ xi
- $\frac{1}{4}$ fluidram *or* f ʒ $\frac{1}{4}$
- 4 minims *or* ♏ iv
- $3\frac{1}{2}$ pints *or* pt. iiiss
- 5 quarts *or* qt. v
- $\frac{1}{2}$ gallon *or* gal. ss

25.1 EXERCISES

Write the meaning of each measurement.

1. qt. xxv
2. fʒ viss
3. pt. xl
4. fℨ xix
5. ɱ x
6. gal. xx
7. fʒ lxv
8. ɱ l
9. pt. c
10. fℨ i
11. gal. lxx
12. fℨ ixss
13. pt. xiv
14. ɱ ivss
15. fℨ v
16. ɱ xxvi
17. gal. xlv
18. fℨ xxii
19. fℨ xc
20. qt. xiii

APOTHECARY EQUIVALENT MEASUREMENTS OF VOLUME

In the apothecaries' system, these units of volume are equivalent.

60 minims (ɱ)	=	1 fluidram (fʒ)
8 fluidrams (fʒ)	=	1 fluidounce (fℨ)
16 fluidounces (fℨ)	=	1 pint (pt.)
2 pints (pt.)	=	1 quart (qt.)
4 quarts (qt.)	=	1 gallon (gal.)

Expressing equivalence of measurement is accomplished by using proportions.

Example: Express 4 fluidrams as minims.

$$\frac{1 \text{ fluidram}}{60 \text{ minims}} = \frac{4 \text{ fluidrams}}{q \text{ minims}}$$

$$1(q) = 4(60)$$

$$q = 240 \text{ minims}$$

Example: Express 30 minims as fluidrams.

$$\frac{1 \text{ fluidram}}{60 \text{ minims}} = \frac{y \text{ fluidrams}}{30 \text{ minims}}$$

$$60(y) = 1(30)$$

$$y = \text{fʒ ss}$$

Example: Express 40 fluidrams as fluidounces.

$$\frac{1 \text{ fluidounce}}{8 \text{ fluidrams}} = \frac{a \text{ fluidounces}}{40 \text{ fluidrams}}$$

$$8(a) = 1(40)$$

$$a = \text{fℨ v}$$

Example: Express 8 fluidounces as fluidrams.

$$\frac{1 \text{ fluidounce}}{8 \text{ fluidrams}} = \frac{8 \text{ fluidounces}}{b \text{ fluidrams}}$$

$$1(b) = 8(8)$$

$$b = \text{fʒ lxiv}$$

Example: Express 10 pints as fluidounces.

$$\frac{1 \text{ pint}}{16 \text{ fluidounces}} = \frac{10 \text{ pints}}{r \text{ fluidounces}}$$

$$1(r) = 16(10)$$

$$r = 160 \text{ fluidounces}$$

Example: Express 64 fluidounces as pints.

$$\frac{1 \text{ pint}}{16 \text{ fluidounces}} = \frac{z \text{ pints}}{64 \text{ fluidounces}}$$

$$16(z) = 1(64)$$

$$z = \text{pt. iv}$$

Example: Express 16 pints as quarts.

$$\frac{1 \text{ quart}}{2 \text{ pints}} = \frac{y \text{ quarts}}{16 \text{ pints}}$$

$$2(y) = 1(16)$$

$$y = \text{qt. viii}$$

Example: Express $\frac{1}{4}$ quart as pints.

$$\frac{1 \text{ quart}}{2 \text{ pints}} = \frac{\frac{1}{4} \text{ quart}}{p \text{ pints}}$$

$$1(p) = \frac{1}{4}(2)$$

$$p = \text{pt. ss}$$

Example: Express 10 quarts as gallons.

$$\frac{1 \text{ gallon}}{4 \text{ quarts}} = \frac{d \text{ gallons}}{10 \text{ quarts}}$$

$$4(d) = 1(10)$$

$$d = \text{gal. iiss}$$

Example: Express 20 gallons as quarts.

$$\frac{1 \text{ gallon}}{4 \text{ quarts}} = \frac{20 \text{ gallons}}{y \text{ quarts}}$$

$$1(y) = 20(4)$$

$$y = \text{qt. lxxx}$$

25.2 EXERCISES

Express each measurement as an equivalent measurement as indicated.

Minims

1. f℥ x
2. f℥ ss
3. f℥ $\frac{1}{3}$
4. f℥ vi
5. f℥ xvss

Fluidrams

6. m lxxx
7. 0.6 minim
8. 720 minims
9. 1,200 minims
10. m $\frac{3}{5}$
11. f℥ ss
12. f℥ v
13. f℥ $\frac{1}{8}$
14. 3.1 fluidounces
15. f℥ xx

Fluidounces

16. f℥ xxiv
17. 480 fluidrams
18. f℥ $\frac{4}{5}$
19. 1.6 fluidrams
20. 320 fluidrams
21. pt. iss
22. pt. x
23. pt. $\frac{1}{4}$
24. 0.3 pint
25. pt. xl

Pints

26. f℥ xxxii
27. 6.4 fluidounces
28. 480 fluidounces
29. f℥ xcvi
30. f℥ xxviii
31. qt. lvss
32. 1.8 quarts
33. 120 quarts
34. qt. $\frac{3}{4}$
35. qt. xlv

Quarts

36. pt. xxvi
37. pt. c
38. 14.5 pints
39. pt. $\frac{1}{4}$
40. pt. lx
41. gal. iiss
42. gal. xxxv
43. gal. $\frac{1}{4}$
44. gal. xxi
45. 4.2 gallons

Gallons

46. qt. xvi
47. 3.2 quarts
48. 400 quarts
49. qt. ss
50. qt. lxxxii

Determine each correct relationship (<, >, =).

51. f℥ x ___?___ f℥ ii
52. pt. ss ___?___ f℥ xii
53. qt. iii ___?___ pt. vi
54. f℥ xx ___?___ pt. iss
55. f℥ lxx ___?___ gal. i
56. f℥ ss ___?___ f℥ iv

APOTHECARIES' — METRIC EQUIVALENT MEASUREMENTS OF VOLUME

Expressing equivalences between apothecaries' and metric units of volume follows the same procedure as for units of weight. The equivalences are approximations within the acceptable limits of error.

APOTHECARIES' SYSTEM		METRIC SYSTEM
15 minims (m)	=	1 mL (or 1 cm^3)
1 fluidram (f♷)	=	4 mL (or 4 cm^3)
1 fluidounce (f♶)	=	30 mL (or 30 cm^3)
1 pint (pt.)	=	500 mL (or 500 cm^3)
1 quart (qt.)	=	1 L (or 1 000 cm^3)
1 gallon (gal.)	=	4 L (or 4 000 cm^3)

Expressing equivalences between the two systems utilizes proportions and the table of equivalences.

Example: Express 45 minims as millilitres.

$$\frac{15 \text{ minims}}{1 \text{ mL}} = \frac{45 \text{ minims}}{a \text{ mL}}$$

$$15(a) = 45$$

$$a = 3 \text{ mL}$$

Example: Express 10 fluidrams as millilitres.

$$\frac{1 \text{ fluidram}}{4 \text{ mL}} = \frac{10 \text{ fluidrams}}{b \text{ mL}}$$

$$1(b) = 4(10)$$

$$b = 40 \text{ mL}$$

Example: Express 6 fluidounces as cubic centimetres.

$$\frac{1 \text{ fluidounce}}{30 \text{ cm}^3} = \frac{6 \text{ fluidounces}}{j \text{ cm}^3}$$

$$1(j) = 30(6)$$

$$j = 180 \text{ cm}^3$$

Example: Express 250 cm^3 as pints.

$$\frac{500 \text{ cm}^3}{1 \text{ pint}} = \frac{250 \text{ cm}^3}{y \text{ pint}}$$

$$500(y) = 250(1)$$

$$y = \text{pt. ss}$$

Example: Express 10 quarts as litres.

$$\frac{1 \text{ quart}}{1 \text{ L}} = \frac{10 \text{ quarts}}{z \text{ L}}$$

$$1(z) = 1(10)$$

$$z = 10 \text{ L}$$

Example: Express 2 litres as gallons.

$$\frac{1 \text{ gallon}}{4 \text{ L}} = \frac{r \text{ gallons}}{2 \text{ L}}$$

$$4(r) = 1(2)$$

$$r = \text{gal. ss}$$

25.3 EXERCISES

Express each measurement as an equivalent measurement as indicated.

Millilitres

1. ℥ lx
2. ℥ viiss
3. 0.6 minim
4. ℥ lxxv
5. ℥ xx
6. f℥ $\frac{1}{3}$
7. 0.4 fluidounce
8. f℥ vi
9. f℥ lx
10. f℥ xss

Minims

11. 0.5 cm^3
12. 4 cm^3
13. $\frac{1}{3}$ cm^3
14. 2.3 cm^3
15. 15 cm^3

Cubic Centimetres

16. f℥ iv
17. 0.3 fluidram
18. f℥ vss
19. f℥ $\frac{1}{4}$
20. f℥ l
21. 0.25 pint
22. pt. l
23. pt. ss
24. 0.6 pint
25. 1.1 pints

Fluidrams

26. 8 cm^3
27. 3.2 cm^3
28. 0.48 cm^3
29. 80 cm^3
30. $\frac{1}{2}$ cm^3

Fluidounces

31. 300 cm^3
32. 0.6 cm^3
33. 1.8 cm^3
34. 45 cm^3
35. 50 cm^3

Pints

36. 1 000 mL
37. 3.5 mL
38. 1 200 mL
39. 500 mL
40. 2 500 mL

Litres

41. qt. xxi
42. 5.6 quarts
43. qt. iiss
44. $7\frac{1}{8}$ quarts
45. qt. xlv
46. gal. ss
47. gal. x
48. gal. $\frac{1}{5}$
49. gal. vi
50. 0.6 gallon

Quarts

51. 100 L
52. 18.5 L
53. 27 L
54. $8\frac{1}{3}$ L
55. 0.1 L

Gallons

56. 8 L
57. 0.25 L
58. 3 L
59. 20 L
60. $\frac{1}{8}$ L

APPLICATIONS

When a physician prescribes medication, a prescription is written. The prescription is a means of controlling the sale and use of drugs which can be safely and effectively used only under the supervision of a physician. A prescription consists of the superscription, the inscription, the subscription, and the signature.

▼ The *superscription* includes the patient's name and address, the date, and the symbol ℞ which means "I prescribe" or "take thou."

▼ The *inscription* includes the names and amounts of the drugs that the medication is composed of. In writing the prescription, the most important drug is listed first.

▼ The *subscription* includes the directions to the pharmacist for preparing the prescription.

▼ The *signature* includes the directions to the patient for taking the medicine. It may also include the physician's registration number, if required by state law.

When completing the prescription, the physician uses symbols for the inscription, subscription, and signature. Symbols for the inscription may be in metric units or apothecaries' units. Some common symbols used in the subscription and signature are listed.

SYMBOL	MEANING
$\overline{aa}$	(equal parts) of each
a.c.	before meals
ad lib	if desired, freely
b.i.d.	two times a day
$\overline{c}$	with
comp.	compound
dil.	dilute
elix.	elixir
ext.	extract
h.s.	bedtime
I.M.	intramuscular
I.V.	intravenous
M	mix
p.c.	after meals
p.o.	by mouth
per	through or by
p.r.	by rectum
p.r.n.	when required
q.d.	every day
q.h.	every hour
q.2.h.	every two hours
q.3.h.	every three hours
q.i.d.	four times a day
q.n.	every night
q.n.s.	quantity not sufficient
®	trade name
$\overline{s}$	without
s.c.	subcutaneous (injection)
Sig. or S.	write on label
Sol.	solution
s.o.s.	if necessary
sp.	spirits
s.s.	soap suds
stat.	immediately
syr.	syrup
t.i.d.	three times a day
tr. or tinct.	tincture
ung.	ointment

25.4 EXERCISES

1. A series of medications is prescribed. Find the metric equivalent for each of these amounts.

    a. ♏ xv
    b. f♌ ivss
    c. f♌ iii
    d. ♏ xviii

2. How many cubic centimetres of boric acid are required to prepare f♌ xvi of 4% boric acid?

3. How many cubic centimetres of boric acid are required to prepare f♌ xxx of 1% boric acid?

4. Each millilitre of Decadron contains 0.004 cm^3 of dexamethasome phosphate.

    a. How many minims of dexamethasome phosphate are present in 100 millilitres of Decadron?
    b. How many minims of dexamethasome phosphate are present in 1 litre of Decadron?
    c. How many minims of dexamethasome phosphate are present in 1.5 litres of Decadron?

5. Convert the following to millilitre equivalents.

    a. 23 minims
    b. 6 fluidrams
    c. 14 fluidounces
    d. 1.25 pints
    e. 0.75 quart
    f. 0.75 gallon

6. Convert the following to fluidounce equivalents.

    a. 328 millilitres
    b. 125 millilitres
    c. 15 millilitres
    d. 46 millilitres

unit 26 household-apothecaries' systems of measure

OBJECTIVES

After studying this unit the student should be able to:

- Express household liquid measurements as approximate equivalent measurements.

- Express household measurements as approximate equivalent apothecaries' measurements.

- Express apothecaries' measurements as approximate equivalent household measurements.

THE HOUSEHOLD SYSTEM OF LIQUID MEASURE

The household system can be used, within limits, to safely measure amounts of medicine administered at home. To effectively communicate with a patient in terms the patient can understand, the health worker should be familiar with the household system. The approximate equivalent measures which are given are for water. Other substances may have slightly different equivalents.

Common household measuring articles include droppers, teaspoons, tablespoons, cups, and glasses. In addition, pints and quarts which have been defined in the apothecaries' system of measure, are usually available. This table summarizes some liquid measure equivalents. These equivalents should be used only in those instances when the proper measuring instruments are not available.

APPROXIMATE LIQUID MEASURE EQUIVALENTS		
60 drops	=	1 teaspoonful (t)
4 teaspoonfuls*	=	1 tablespoonful (T)
2 tablespoonfuls	=	1 fluidounce
6 fluidounces	=	1 teacupful
8 fluidounces	=	1 glassful

*In kitchen usage, 3 cooking teaspoonfuls equal one tablespoonful.

Usually equivalent measures can be obtained directly from a table. Using proportions when calculating an equivalent measure can also be helpful.

Example: What part of a teaspoonful is 20 drops?

$$\frac{60 \text{ drops}}{1 \text{ teaspoonful}} = \frac{20 \text{ drops}}{x \text{ teaspoonful}}$$

$$60(x) = 1(20)$$

$$x = \frac{20}{60} \text{ or } \frac{1}{3}$$

20 drops ≈ $\frac{1}{3}$ teaspoonful

Example: Nine ounces are how many teacupfuls?

$$\frac{6 \text{ ounces}}{1 \text{ teacupful}} = \frac{9 \text{ ounces}}{y \text{ teacupfuls}}$$

$$6(y) = 1(9)$$

$$y = \frac{9}{6} \text{ or } 1\frac{1}{2}$$

9 ounces ≈ $1\frac{1}{2}$ teacupfuls

26.1 EXERCISES

Using the table of approximate equivalences, calculate each approximate equivalent measure.

1. ___?___ drops = 1 teaspoonful
2. 30 drops = ___?___ teaspoonfuls
3. ___?___ teaspoonfuls = 15 drops
4. 2 tablespoonfuls = ___?___ teaspoonfuls
5. ___?___ tablespoonfuls = 1 teaspoonful
6. 2 teaspoonfuls = ___?___ tablespoonfuls
7. ___?___ tablespoonfuls = 1 fluidounce
8. 4 fluidounces = ___?___ tablespoonfuls
9. ___?___ fluidounces = 1 tablespoonful
10. 1 teacupful = ___?___ fluidounces
11. ___?___ teacupfuls = 3 fluidounces
12. 12 fluidounces = ___?___ teacupfuls
13. ___?___ glassfuls = 8 fluidounces
14. 4 fluidounces = ___?___ glassfuls
15. ___?___ fluidounces = $1\frac{1}{2}$ glassfuls

Calculate each approximate equivalent measure. Use the table only if necessary.

16. 4 tablespoonfuls = __?__ fluidounces
17. __?__ teaspoonfuls = 40 drops
18. 15 fluidounces = __?__ teacupfuls
19. __?__ fluidounces = 2 glassfuls
20. 9 teaspoonfuls = __?__ tablespoonfuls
21. __?__ drops = $\frac{1}{3}$ tablespoonful
22. 18 fluidounces = __?__ teaspoonfuls
23. __?__ glassfuls = 2 fluidounces
24. 6 teaspoonfuls = __?__ fluidounces
25. __?__ fluidounces = 24 tablespoonfuls

HOUSEHOLD — APOTHECARIES' EQUIVALENT MEASUREMENTS

The household system of measurement, although not as accurate as the apothecaries' system, is frequently used at home by a patient. Using familiar measuring instruments patients can measure drops, teaspoonfuls, tablespoonfuls, ounces, cupfuls, and glassfuls whereas most patients would not know how to measure a quantity given in apothecaries' units. Since measuring instruments such as droppers, cups, teaspoons, and tablespoons are not the same size, the household system and its uses should be avoided.

These tables summarize the approximate weight and liquid measure equivalents for the apothecaries' and household systems.

WEIGHT

APOTHECARIES' SYSTEM		HOUSEHOLD SYSTEM
1 grain (gr.)	=	1 drop
1 dram (ʒ)	=	1 teaspoonful (t)
4 drams	=	1 tablespoonful (T)
1 ounce (℥)	=	2 tablespoonfuls
6 ounces	=	1 teacupful
8 ounces	=	1 glassful

Section 5 Systems of Measure

LIQUID MEASURE

APOTHECARIES' SYSTEM		HOUSEHOLD SYSTEM
1 minim (𝔪)	=	1 drop
1 fluidram (f ℨ)	=	1 teaspoonful (t)
4 fluidrams	=	1 tablespoonful (T)
1 fluidounce (f ℥)	=	2 tablespoonfuls
6 fluidounces	=	1 teacupful
8 fluidounces	=	1 glassful

Proportions using the approximate equivalents are used to express equivalences between the two systems. The equivalences are approximate but are within the limits of error. Keep in mind that drops of different substances vary in size. When minims are ordered, a minim glass or a minim pipette should be used to obtain an accurate measure. When drops are ordered, a medicine dropper may be used.

Example: Two tablespoonfuls will hold approximately how many drams?

$$\frac{1 \text{ tablespoonful}}{4 \text{ drams}} = \frac{2 \text{ tablespoonfuls}}{x \text{ drams}}$$

$$1(x) = 2(4)$$

$$x = 8$$

Two tablespoonfuls hold approximately eight drams.

Example: Approximately how many tablespoonfuls are 5 fluidounces?

$$\frac{1 \text{ fluidounce}}{2 \text{ tablespoonfuls}} = \frac{5 \text{ fluidounces}}{x \text{ tablespoonfuls}}$$

$$1(x) = 2(5)$$

$$x = 10$$

Five fluidounces are approximately ten tablespoonfuls.

26.2 EXERCISES

Using the tables of approximate weight and liquid measure equivalences, find each equivalence.

1. 5 drops = ___?___ grains
2. 2 gr. = ___?___ drops
3. 4 drams = ___?___ teaspoonfuls
4. 2 tablespoonfuls = ___?___ drams
5. ℨ ii = ___?___ T

6. $\frac{1}{2}$ ounce = __?__ tablespoonfuls
7. $\frac{1}{2}$ teacupful = __?__ ounces
8. ℥ vi __?__ teacupfuls
9. 6 ounces = __?__ glassfuls
10. __?__ drops = 3 grains
11. __?__ teaspoonfuls = 2 drams
12. __?__ t = ℥ vi
13. __?__ drams = 1.5 tablespoonfuls
14. __?__ tablespoonfuls = 2 ounces
15. ℥ __?__ = 3 T
16. __?__ ounces = 2 teacupfuls
17. __?__ glassfuls = 4 ounces
18. ℥ __?__ = 1$\frac{1}{2}$ glassfuls
19. __?__ minims = 5 drops
20. __?__ teaspoonfuls = 2 fluidrams
21. f℥ __?__ = $\frac{1}{2}$ t
22. __?__ fluidrams = 1$\frac{1}{2}$ tablespoonfuls
23. __?__ tablespoonfuls = $\frac{1}{2}$ fluidounce
24. f℥ __?__ = 3 T
25. __?__ fluidounces = 1$\frac{1}{2}$ teacupfuls
26. __?__ glassfuls = 4 fluidounces
27. f℥ __?__ = 1$\frac{1}{2}$ glassfuls
28. 3 drops = __?__ minims
29. ℳ ii __?__ drops
30. 1 fluidram = __?__ teaspoonfuls
31. 2 tablespoonfuls = __?__ fluidrams
32. f℥ ss = __?__ t
33. 2 fluidounces = __?__ tablespoonfuls
34. $\frac{1}{2}$ teacupful = __?__ fluidounces
35. f℥ xii = __?__ teacupfuls
36. 2 fluidounces = __?__ glassfuls

Without referring to the tables, complete this chart with the approximate equivalents. Use symbols or abbreviations when possible.

| | HOUSEHOLD SYSTEM | APOTHECARIES' SYSTEM ||
		Weight	Volume (liquid measure)
37.	1 drop	?	1 minim (m)
38.	?	1 dram (ℨ)	1 fluidram (fℨ)
39.	1 tablespoonful (T)	?	4 fluidrams
40.	2 tablespoonfuls	1 ounce (℥)	?
41.	?	6 ounces	6 fluidounces
42.	1 glassful	?	8 fluidounces

HOUSEHOLD — APOTHECARIES' SYMBOLS TRANSLATION

It is important for a health worker to quickly and accurately translate household and apothecaries' symbols. Further understanding of the relationship between the apothecaries' and household systems and additional practice in interpreting and using apothecaries' and household abbreviations and symbols will prove beneficial.

The approximate weight and liquid measure equivalents for the apothecaries' and household systems are summarized in this chart.

| HOUSEHOLD UNITS | APOTHECARIES' UNITS ||
	Weight	Volume (liquid measure)
1 drop	gr. i	m i
1 t	ℨ i	fℨ i
1 T	ℨ iv	fℨ iv
2 T	℥ i	f℥ i
1 teacupful	℥ vi	f℥ vi
1 glassful	℥ viii	f℥ viii

Example: Nine ounces are how many teacupfuls?

$$\frac{1 \text{ teacupful}}{℥ \text{ vi}} = \frac{x \text{ teacupfuls}}{℥ \text{ ix}}$$

$$6(x) = 9$$

$$x = \frac{9}{6} \text{ or } 1\frac{1}{2}$$

Nine ounces are approximately $1\frac{1}{2}$ teacupfuls.

Example: How many fluidounces are contained in $2\frac{1}{2}$ glassfuls?

$$\frac{1 \text{ glassful}}{\text{f}\mathfrak{z} \text{ viii}} = \frac{2\frac{1}{2} \text{ glassfuls}}{y}$$

$$1(y) = 2\frac{1}{2}(8)$$

$$y = \frac{5}{2}\left(\frac{8}{1}\right) \text{ or } 20$$

Two and one-half glassfuls contains f$\mathfrak{z}$ xx.

26.3 EXERCISES

Express each measurement as an equivalent measurement as indicated. Use abbreviations or symbols when possible.

Apothecaries' Weight

1. 4 T
2. 2 teacupfuls
3. 2 glassfuls
4. 6 drops
5. $\frac{1}{2}$ t
6. 3 drops
7. 2 t
8. $\frac{1}{2}$ T
9. $\frac{1}{3}$ teacupful
10. $\frac{1}{2}$ glassful

Apothecaries' Liquid Measure

11. $\frac{1}{2}$ teacupful
12. 4 t
13. 5 drops
14. $\frac{1}{4}$ T
15. 1 glassful
16. 3 T
17. $1\frac{1}{2}$ teacupfuls
18. $\frac{1}{4}$ glassful
19. 2 drops
20. 1 t

Household

21. gr. v
22. f$\mathfrak{z}$ vi
23. ṃ ix
24. lb. i
25. qt. ss
26. f$\mathfrak{z}$ xii
27. $\mathfrak{z}$ viii
28. gr. xiv
29. $\mathfrak{z}$ iv
30. f$\mathfrak{z}$ xxiv
31. $\mathfrak{z}$ iv
32. qt. i
33. gr. iiss
34. f$\mathfrak{z}$ xii
35. ṃ vi
36. f$\mathfrak{z}$ ii
37. qt. iss
38. f$\mathfrak{z}$ ix
39. lb. $\frac{1}{4}$
40. ṃ xx

Section 5 Systems of Measure

Determine the correct relationship (<, >, =).

41. 3 T ___?___ ʒ ii
42. fʒ v ___?___ 6 T
43. ɱ iv ___?___ 6 drops
44. ʒ vi ___?___ 1 teacupful
45. fʒ vi ___?___ 12 T
46. fʒ xx ___?___ 2½ glassfuls
47. 2 T ___?___ ʒ viii
48. 1 t ___?___ ʒ iiss
49. 1.5 glassfuls ___?___ fʒ x
50. gr. vii ___?___ 7 drops
51. ʒ iss ___?___ 6 t
52. fʒ vi ___?___ 1⅓ T
53. 1⅓ teacupfuls ___?___ ʒ vi
54. 17 drops ___?___ ɱ xvii

Each dosage is given in apothecaries' units. Determine the most reasonable household equivalent.

55. fʒ v
    a. 7 t
    b. 1 teacupful
    c. 2½ T

56. ʒ ii
    a. 2 T
    b. 2 t
    c. 1 t

57. ʒ vi
    a. 5 t
    b. 1½ T
    c. 7 t

58. fʒ xxxii
    a. 5 glassfuls
    b. 1 quart
    c. 3 glassfuls

59. lb. i
    a. 10 T
    b. 1 glassful
    c. 2 teacupfuls

60. gr. xv
    a. ½ t
    b. ⅓ t
    c. 15 drops

61. qt. i
    a. 5 teacupfuls
    b. 4 glassfuls
    c. 6 teacupfuls

62. ʒ x
    a. 10 T
    b. 1⅔ teacupfuls
    c. 1½ teacupfuls

63. ʒ xviii
    a. 2½ glassfuls
    b. 2 glassfuls
    c. 3 teacupfuls

64. ɱ vi
    a. ⅛ t
    b. 6 drops
    c. ¼ t

APPLICATIONS

Household units of measure are found in every home and are used during everyday activities such as cooking, cleaning, or shopping. When purchasing nonprescription drugs such as aspirin, cough medicine, or liquid vitamins, the directions are given in household units of measure. For example, the directions for taking cough medicine may read: "two tablespoons four times a day." Unfortunately, every person's tablespoon is not the same size. This means that the amount of medication that is taken may vary from person to person.

The health care worker must be aware of the inaccuracy of the measuring instruments in the household system. This awareness should lead the health care worker away from using the household system unless in an emergency or in situations where the system can be used safely; preparing a salt solution for gargle may be done safely with household units. If the household system is to be used, the conscientious health care worker uses caution and forethought.

26.4 EXERCISES

1. Two cough medicines are compared. Brand A contains a 5% concentration of cough inhibitor. Brand B contains an 8% concentration of cough inhibitor. The recommended dosage for both brands is one tablespoon every four hours.

    a. After three doses of Brand A, how much cough inhibitor will be consumed?
    b. After three doses of Brand B, how much cough inhibitor will be consumed?

2. A patient is required to drink 4 glassfuls of water in two hours. How many fluidounces does this represent?

3. A total of 4 drams of medication are added to a glassful of water. What is the percent of medication in the glassful of water? Round the answer to the nearer tenth percent.

4. A patient on a soft diet is allowed to consume:

    1 teacupful of tea
    1 teacupful of soup (broth)
    10 teaspoonfuls of pudding

    Approximately how many fluidounces does this represent?

5. Cough medicine is sold in a variety of bottle sizes. Brand A sells for $1.45 in the 8-fluidounce size and for $1.95 in the 12-fluidounce size. Brand B sells for $1.55 in the 10-fluidounce size and for $2.25 in the 16-fluidounce size. To provide the same dose as Brand A, $\frac{1}{8}$ as much of Brand B must be given.

    a. Which brand and size is the best purchase?
    b. How many teaspoons of medication can be obtained from the size and brand representing the best purchase?

unit 27 household-metric systems of measure

OBJECTIVES

After studying this unit the student should be able to:

- Express household measurements as approximate equivalent metric measurements.

- Express metric measurements as approximate equivalent household measurements.

HOUSEHOLD — METRIC EQUIVALENT MEASUREMENTS

As indicated earlier, the household system is not an accurate system of measurement. At present, it is still the more familiar system for patients. It is the responsibility of the health worker to make the approximate equivalents between the household and metric systems and to communicate these equivalences to the patient.

These tables summarize the approximate weight and liquid measure equivalents for the metric and household systems.

WEIGHT (MASS)

METRIC SYSTEM		HOUSEHOLD SYSTEM
0.06 gram (g) or 60 milligrams (mg)	=	1 drop
5 grams	=	1 teaspoonful (t)
15 grams	=	1 tablespoonful (T)
180 grams	=	1 teacupful
240 grams	=	1 glassful

LIQUID MEASURE

METRIC SYSTEM		HOUSEHOLD SYSTEM
0.06 millilitres (mL)	=	1 drop
5 millilitres	=	1 teaspoonful (t)
15 millilitres	=	1 tablespoonful (T)
180 millilitres	=	1 teacupful
240 millilitres	=	1 glassful

Note: 1 scant teaspoon = 4 millilitres

Proportions using the approximate equivalents are used to express equivalences between the two systems. The equivalences are within the limits of error.

Example: Approximately how many millilitres are 2 teaspoonfuls?

$$\frac{5 \text{ millilitres}}{1 \text{ teaspoonful}} = \frac{x \text{ millilitres}}{2 \text{ teaspoonfuls}}$$

$$1(x) = 5(2)$$
$$x = 10$$

Two teaspoonfuls are approximately ten millilitres.

Example: One and one-half teacupfuls contain approximately how many grams?

$$\frac{1 \text{ teacupful}}{180 \text{ g}} = \frac{1\frac{1}{2} \text{ teacupfuls}}{y \text{ g}}$$

$$1(y) = 1\frac{1}{2}(180)$$
$$y = \frac{3}{2}\left(\frac{180}{1}\right)$$
$$y = 270$$

One and one-half teacupfuls contain approximately 270 grams.

27.1 EXERCISES

Using the tables of approximate weight and liquid measure equivalences, find each equivalence.

1. 2 drops = __?__ milligrams
2. 5 drops = __?__ mg
3. 2.5 grams = __?__ teaspoonfuls
4. $\frac{1}{3}$ tablespoonful = __?__ grams
5. 37.5 g = __?__ T
6. 120 grams = __?__ teacupfuls
7. $1\frac{1}{3}$ glassfuls = __?__ grams
8. 360 g = __?__ glassfuls
9. __?__ drops = 1.2 grams
10. __?__ teaspoonfuls = 20 grams
11. __?__ t = 12.5 g
12. __?__ grams = 4 tablespoonfuls
13. __?__ teacupfuls = 180 grams
14. __?__ g = $\frac{1}{2}$ teacupful
15. __?__ grams = $\frac{5}{6}$ glassfuls
16. 10 drops = __?__ millilitres
17. 1.8 mL = __?__ drops
18. 7.5 millilitres = __?__ teaspoonfuls
19. $2\frac{1}{2}$ tablespoonfuls = __?__ millilitres
20. 75 mL = __?__ T
21. $\frac{1}{5}$ teacupful = __?__ millilitres
22. 300 millilitres = __?__ glassfuls
23. $\frac{3}{4}$ glassful = __?__ mL
24. __?__ millilitres = 45 drops
25. __?__ teaspoonfuls = 20 millilitres
26. __?__ mL = 3.5 t
27. __?__ millilitres = $1\frac{1}{3}$ tablespoonfuls
28. __?__ teacupfuls = 90 millilitres
29. __?__ mL = $1\frac{1}{2}$ teacupfuls
30. __?__ glassfuls = 80 millilitres

Without referring to the tables, complete this chart with the approximate equivalents. Use abbreviations or symbols when possible.

	HOUSEHOLD SYSTEM	METRIC SYSTEM	
		Weight (mass)	Volume (liquid measure)
31.	1 drop	0.06 grams (g)	?
32.	?	5 grams	5 millilitres (mL)
33.	1 tablespoonful (T)	?	15 millilitres
34.	1 teacupful	180 grams	?
35.	?	240 grams	240 millilitres

HOUSEHOLD – METRIC SYMBOLS TRANSLATION

It is important for a health worker to be able to quickly and accurately translate household and metric symbols. Further understanding of the relationship between the metric and household systems and additional practice in interpreting and using the metric and household abbreviations and symbols will prove beneficial.

The approximate weight and liquid measure equivalents for the metric and household systems are summarized in this chart.

	METRIC UNITS	
HOUSEHOLD UNITS	Weight (mass)	Volume (liquid measure)
1 drop	0.06 g	0.06 mL
1 t	5 g	5 mL
1 T	15 g	15 mL
1 teacupful	180 g	180 mL
1 glassful	240 g	240 mL

Example: Approximately how many tablespoonfuls will hold 40 grams?

$$\frac{1\,T}{15\,g} = \frac{x\,T}{40\,g}$$

$$15(x) = 40$$

$$x = \frac{40}{15} \text{ or } 2\frac{2}{3}$$

Two and two-thirds tablespoonfuls will hold approximately 40 grams.

Example: Two-thirds teacupful contains approximately how many millilitres?

$$\frac{1 \text{ teacupful}}{180 \text{ mL}} = \frac{\frac{2}{3} \text{ teacupful}}{x \text{ mL}}$$

$$1(x) = \frac{2}{3}(180)$$

$$x = \frac{2}{\cancel{3}}(\frac{\cancel{180}^{60}}{1}) \text{ or } 120$$

Two-thirds teacupful contains approximately 120 millilitres.

Unit 27 Household — Metric Systems of Measure   237

27.2 EXERCISES

Express each measurement as an equivalent measurement as indicated. Use abbreviations or symbols when possible.

Metric Weight (Mass)

1. $\frac{1}{2}$ glassful
2. $\frac{1}{3}$ teacupful
3. $\frac{1}{2}$ t
4. 6 drops
5. $\frac{1}{2}$ T
6. 2 t
7. 4 drops
8. 2 glassfuls
9. 2 teacupfuls
10. 4 T

Metric Liquid Measure

11. 3 T
12. $\frac{1}{4}$ glassful
13. 1 t
14. $\frac{1}{2}$ teacupful
15. 5 drops
16. $1\frac{1}{2}$ teacupfuls
17. 2 drops
18. 4 t
19. 1 glassful
20. $\frac{1}{5}$ T

Household

21. 30 g
22. 0.007 5 L
23. $2\frac{1}{2}$ mL
24. 0.48 kg
25. 0.015 L
26. 60 mg
27. 60 mL
28. 0.960 L
29. 0.6 mL
30. 30 mL
31. 90 mL
32. 1 g
33. 0.06 g
34. 45 g
35. 360 mL
36. 0.72 kg
37. 0.011 25 L
38. 1.5 g
39. 120 mg
40. 0.18 kg

Determine the correct relationship ($<, >, =$).

41. $\frac{1}{2}$ t ___?___ 2 mL
42. 12 g ___?___ 1 T
43. $1\frac{1}{2}$ mL ___?___ $\frac{2}{3}$ t
44. 360 g ___?___ 2 teacupfuls
45. 1.5 t ___?___ 0.008 L
46. 4 500 mg ___?___ 2 t
47. 150 mL ___?___ $\frac{2}{3}$ teacupful
48. 5 glassfuls ___?___ 1 kg
49. $2\frac{1}{2}$ teacupfuls ___?___ $\frac{1}{2}$ L
50. $1\frac{1}{2}$ T ___?___ 0.025 kg
51. 0.080 L ___?___ $\frac{1}{4}$ glassful
52. $\frac{1}{3}$ T ___?___ 1 000 mg

Each dosage is given in metric units. Determine the most reasonable household equivalent.

53. 6 mL
    a. 1 T
    b. 5 T
    c. $1\frac{1}{5}$ t

54. 120 mL
    a. 5 T
    b. $\frac{2}{3}$ teacupful
    c. $\frac{3}{4}$ teacupful

55. 10 g
    a. 2 t
    b. 1 T
    c. $\frac{1}{2}$ T

56. 3 g
    a. $\frac{1}{8}$ T
    b. $\frac{3}{5}$ t
    c. $\frac{1}{4}$ t

57. 5 mL
    a. $\frac{1}{4}$ t
    b. $\frac{1}{2}$ t
    c. 1 t

58. 30 mL
    a. $\frac{1}{4}$ teacupful
    b. 5 t
    c. 2 T

59. 2 500 mg
    a. $\frac{1}{2}$ t
    b. $\frac{1}{2}$ T
    c. $\frac{1}{4}$ T

60. 120 g
    a. 1 teacupful
    b. $\frac{1}{2}$ glassful
    c. $\frac{1}{3}$ glassful

61. $\frac{1}{2}$ L
    a. 3 teacupfuls
    b. $1\frac{1}{2}$ glassfuls
    c. 2 glassfuls

62. 0.007 5 kg
    a. 1.5 t
    b. $\frac{1}{2}$ T
    c. $1\frac{3}{4}$ t

63. 0.240 kg
    a. 12 tablespoonful
    b. 72 teaspoonful
    c. 1 glassful

64. 0.750 kg
    a. $4\frac{1}{2}$ glassfull
    b. $4\frac{1}{5}$ teacupful
    c. 12 teaspoonful

APPLICATIONS

Household measures are not accurate and should not be used when administering medication in medical treatment facilities. The lack of accuracy is partly due to the many designs and capacities for teaspoons, tablespoons, teacups and glasses. Even the size of a drop can vary according to the size of the opening in the pipette. Gradually, with the passage of time, household measures will be replaced with more refined measures. In the interim, the health care worker should understand and be able to administer medication in the household system.

Nonprescription liquid medication is usually prescribed by the teaspoon or the tablespoon. Drops for eyes and ear treatments are not uncommon. Dietary requirements have been indicated in teacup or glass sizes. Today, more pharmaceutical companies are supplying graduated plastic cups and pipettes for more accurate measurement of medication. Most frequently these instruments are graduated in metric units.

27.3 EXERCISES

1. Several brands of eye drops are on the market. Three brands are compared. It is determined that 15 mL of each contains similar medication but in different amounts.

    Brand A contains 5 mg of medication per 15 mL.
    Brand B contains 7 mg of medication per 15 mL.
    Brand C contains 10 mg of medication per 15 mL.

    a. How much medication will a patient receive if one drop of Brand A is placed in each eye?

    b. How much medication will a patient receive if one drop of Brand B is placed in each eye?

    c. How much medication will a patient receive if one drop of Brand C is placed in each eye?

    d. The recommended dose for each treatment is 0.04 mg per eye. Brand A is dispensed in a 15-mL container and costs $1.59. Brand C is dispensed in a 10-mL container and costs $1.79. To achieve the recommended dose, which brand is the better buy?

2. A child receives a prescription for medication for relieving an upset stomach. The recommended dose is one teaspoon every three hours.

    a. Express, in metric units, the total amount of medication that is consumed within a 24-hour period.

    b. Express, in apothecaries' units, the total amount of medication that is consumed within a 24-hour period.

3. A pharmacist dispenses a prescription for 50 mL of medication.

    a. How many drops can be obtained from this prescription?

    b. How many scant teaspoonfuls can be obtained from this prescription?

    c. How many tablespoonfuls can be obtained from this prescription?

4. Once a day, vitamins are added to a baby's formula. If ten drops are added to each amount of formula, what percent vitamins is present in a formula containing —

   a. 250 millilitres?

   b. 30 millilitres?

   c. 500 millilitres?

5. A prescription for 20 mL of medication is requested. Each time the medication is administered, two drops of medication are added to one glassful of milk.

   a. If all the medication is to be used, how many fluidounces of milk are needed?

   b. How many millilitres of milk are needed if all the medication is to be used?

6. A patient is to receive 16 mL of cough medicine in a 24-hour period.

   a. How many scant teaspoonfuls of cough medicine does this represent?

   b. How many fluidrams of cough medicine does this represent?

7. A patient is given a prescription and directed to take one tablespoonful each hour for six hours.

   a. What is the total millilitres taken?

   b. How many drops are taken?

8. Eight glassful of water are to be taken during an 8-hour period.

   a. How many kilograms are taken?

   b. How many grams are taken?

9. A patient is directed to put four drops of medication into each ear every three hours. How many millilitres must the doctor prescribe to provide the patient enough for five treatments over a 12-hour period?

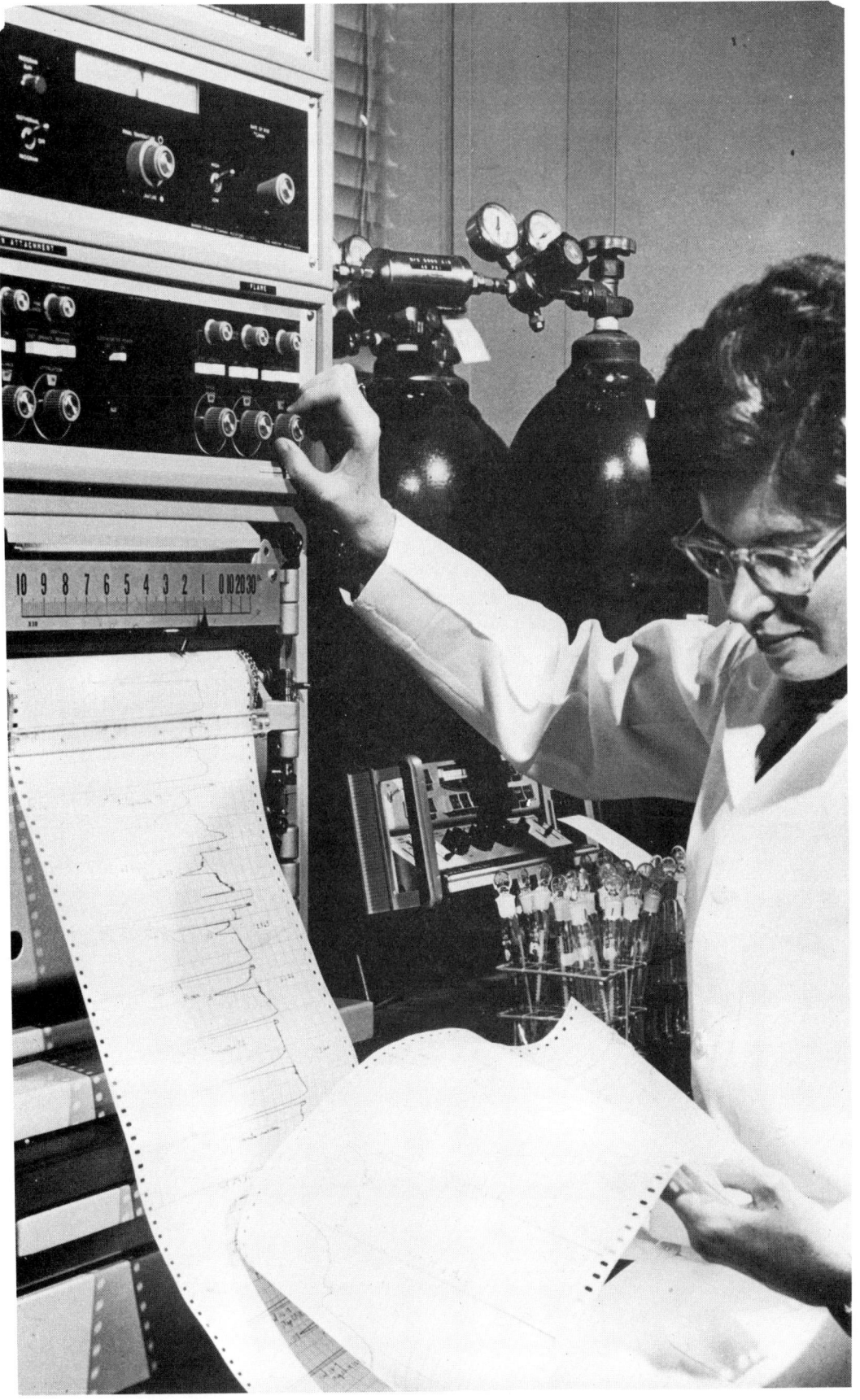

SECTION 6 ORGANIZING AND REPORTING DATA

unit 28 interpreting charts and graphs

OBJECTIVES

After studying this unit the student should be able to:

- Collect and arrange data in a table.

- Analyze data displayed on bar graphs, broken-line graphs, circle graphs, and pictographs.

- Determine the mean, median and mode of a set of data.

COLLECTING AND ARRANGING DATA

Every day the health worker handles numerical information. It is important that the health worker is able to understand, analyze, and interpret this information. At times it is necessary to use a variety of sources when collecting information about a particular topic. The information that is collected is referred to as data. *Data* represents a group of facts about a specific topic. The science of analyzing and interpreting data is *statistics*. Analyzing and interpreting data depends on the data collected. If different sets of data are collected, the statistics may vary.

Example: Janet gathers data about the hospitals in a state. Based on the number of beds available, she determines the five largest hospitals.

St. Anne 325	Proctor 200	Mennonite 450
General 1,500	Brokaw 775	

This data is arranged for easier reading and interpretation. It is arranged from the largest hospital to the fifth largest hospital.

HOSPITAL	NUMBER OF BEDS AVAILABLE
General	1,500
Brokaw	775
Mennonite	450
St. Anne	325
Proctor	200

Example: In a community, find the number of deaths in each age group during a three-week period: 0-10 yr.; 11-25 yr.; 26-35 yr.; 36-50 yr.; 51-64 yr.; 65+ yr.

Jeff researches this question, gathers data, and records it in the table.

DEATHS IN WILLIAMSVILLE BETWEEN AUGUST 14 and SEPTEMBER 5	
Age Group	Number
0-10 yr.	1
11-25 yr.	0
26-35 yr.	2
36-50 yr.	10
51-64 yr.	3
65+ yr.	6

Note: The information could be arranged in order according to the number of deaths instead of by age groups.

28.1 EXERCISES

1. The boiling point in degrees Celsius for some substances are: acetone 57 °C; camphor 205 °C; ethyl alcohol 78.3 °C; methyl alcohol 64.7 °C; chloroform 61.2 °C; ether 34.6 °C; glycerine 291 °C.

    a. Arrange the data in a table.

    b. Which substance has the highest boiling point?

    c. Which substance has the lowest boiling point?

    d. Which substance has a boiling point about five times higher than acetone?

    e. Which two substances have the closest boiling point temperatures?

2. Find the population for the five largest cities in the country.

   a. Arrange the data in a table.

   b. What is the difference in population between the largest and smallest cities?

   c. The largest city is ___?___ % larger than the smallest city.

   d. The largest city is ___?___ % larger than the second smallest city.

   e. The largest city is ___?___ % larger than the second largest city.

3. Collect and arrange data about these topics.

   a. The six most common communicable diseases in the Western Hemisphere.

   b. The six most common causes of death in a country, state, or province.

   c. The doctor-patient ratio in six cities or regions in a country, state, or province.

INTERPRETING CHARTS AND GRAPHS

Statistical data can be displayed in many ways. The most common method is with a chart or graph. Charts and graphs are visual representations of data. Among the many types of graphs are the bar graph, the broken-line graph, the circle graph, and the pictograph.

Example: The occurrence of influenza in Williamsville is documented for 1984 through 1989. The number of reported cases per thousand population are recorded as:

1984 – 10	1986 – 18	1988 – 6
1985 – 27	1987 – 9	1989 – 47

This data is represented with different types of graphs.

BAR GRAPH   BROKEN-LINE GRAPH

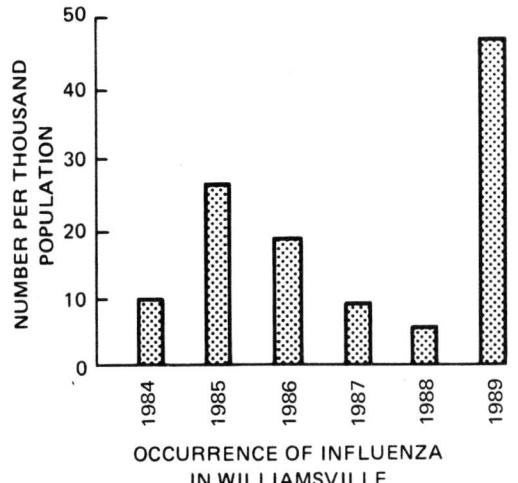
OCCURRENCE OF INFLUENZA IN WILLIAMSVILLE

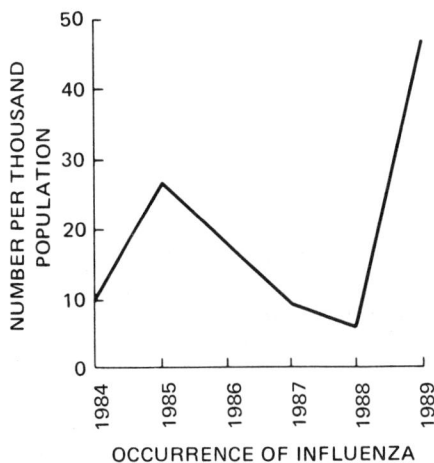
OCCURRENCE OF INFLUENZA IN WILLIAMSVILLE

CIRCLE GRAPH

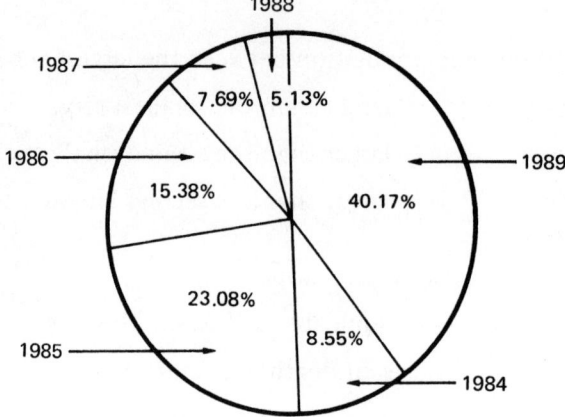

Percent distribution of 117 influenza cases in Williamsville during a five-year period.

PICTOGRAPH

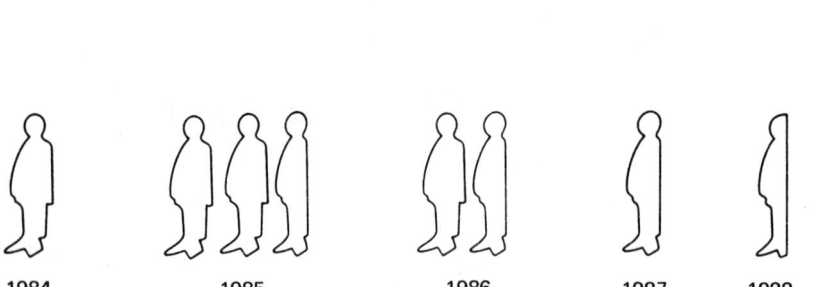

When interpreting charts and graphs it is important to analyze the method used. Data that is displayed incorrectly can lead to errors in interpreting the chart or graph. It is also important to understand the relationships or comparisons that a graph is displaying. Analyzing the subject and graphic scales should precede analyzing the data.

- In analyzing a graph:
  - Read the title of a graph.
  - Determine what information is given.
  - Determine the value of each major unit on the vertical and horizontal scales.

INTERPRETING BAR GRAPHS

Bar graphs visually represent quantities by comparing bars of varying lengths and uniform widths. Bar graphs are best used in showing the size or the amount of different items at the same time, or the size or the amount of the same item at different times.

Example: This bar graph shows the occurrences of influenza in Williamsville during the years 1984 through 1989.

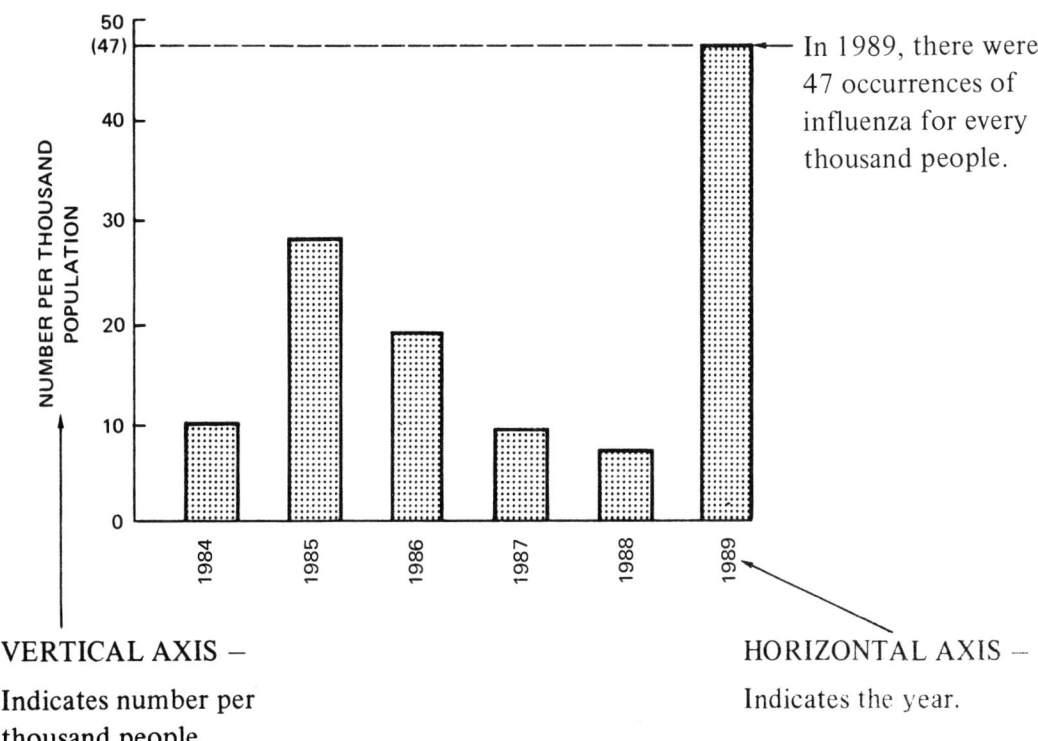

In this bar graph, the number of occurrences of influenza (same item) is shown for different times. This bar graph can compare the number of occurrences for each year. For example, there were three times more occurrences of influenza in 1986 than in 1988. Notice that additional computation is needed to find this comparison. It could not be read directly from the graph.

INTERPRETING LINE GRAPHS

There are three basic types of line graphs. The straight-line graph and the curved-line graph are used for related facts where there is regularity in changes. The broken-line graph is used for related data where the changes are irregular. The advantage of using a line graph is that other values may be determined without additional computations.

Example: Temperature is measured every hour and displayed in a broken-line graph.

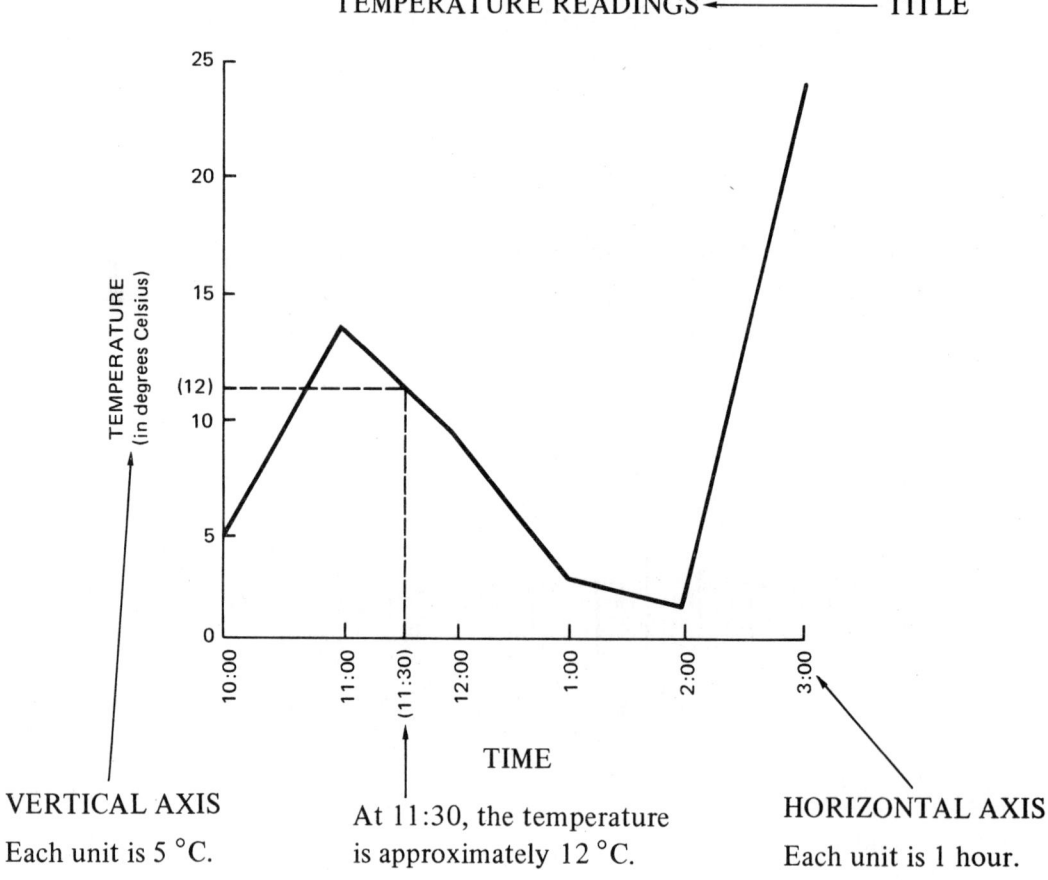

VERTICAL AXIS
Each unit is 5 °C.

At 11:30, the temperature is approximately 12 °C.

HORIZONTAL AXIS
Each unit is 1 hour.

This broken-line graph shows the relationship of the temperature and the time of day. Readings for values not on the axis can be found without additional computations; for example, the temperature reading at 11:30 is approximately 12 °C. Reading values not on the axis is possible because the temperature constantly changed.

When data is accumulated over a period of time and then recorded, as in the occurrences of influenza, the broken-line graph only shows a trend or pattern. In such cases, the broken-line graph is not useful for computations.

Example: This broken-line graph shows the number of automobile accidents in a community during selected months of a year.

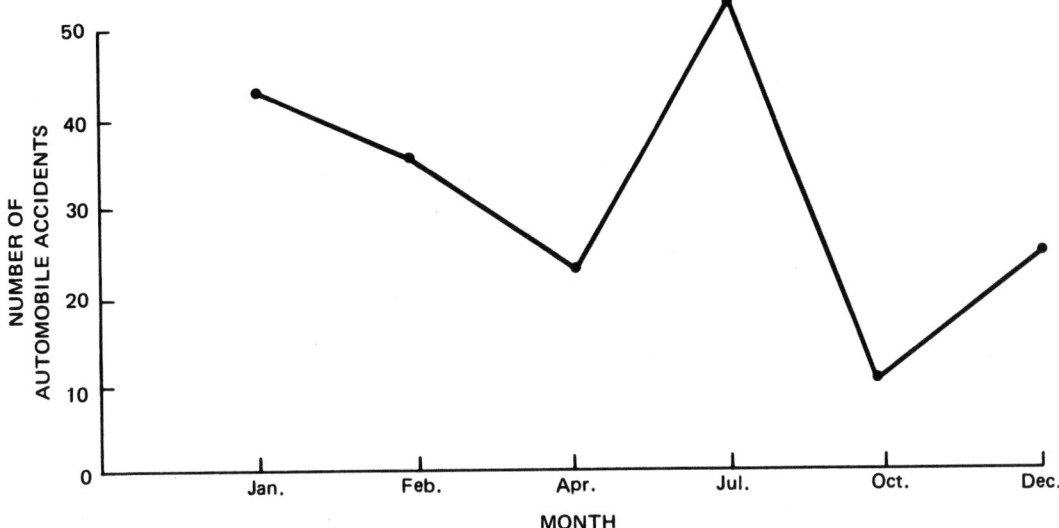

This graph only shows a trend or pattern for the given months. It does not represent the months in sequential order or all the months of the year. No information or trend can be determined for the months of March, May, June, August, September, or November.

The same data can be represented differently.

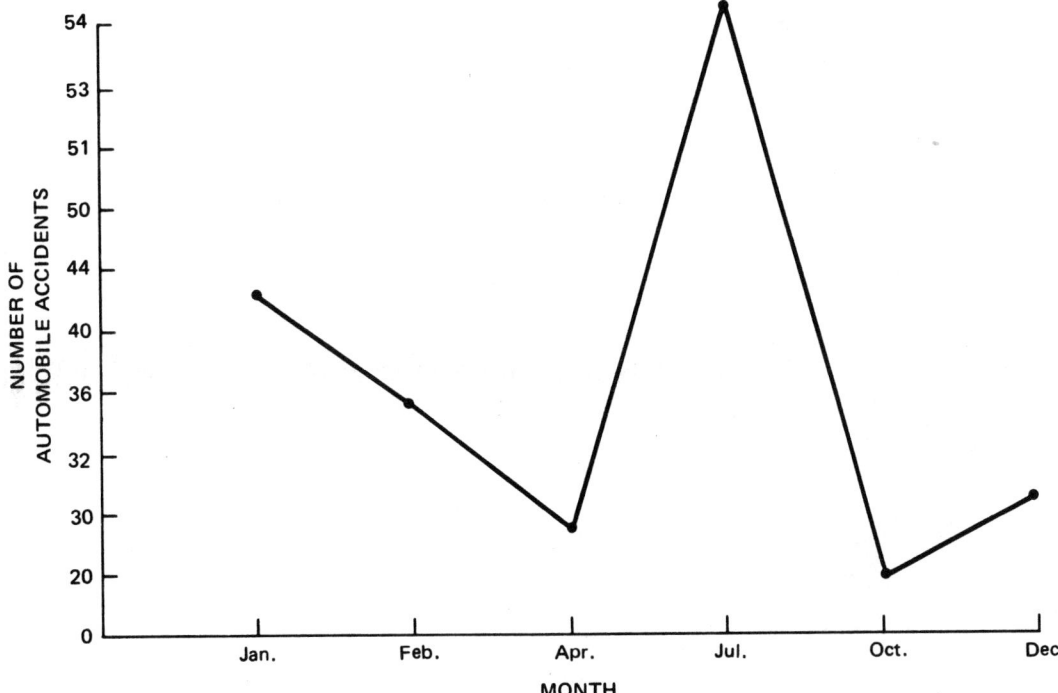

Notice the lack of uniform value intervals along the vertical axis. The same data gives a totally different visual presentation.

28.2 EXERCISES

Analyze each graph and supply the requested information.

1. A survey is conducted in a community of 5,000. The occurrence of common communicable diseases from January 1 through June 30 is determined. This bar graph shows the accumulated data.

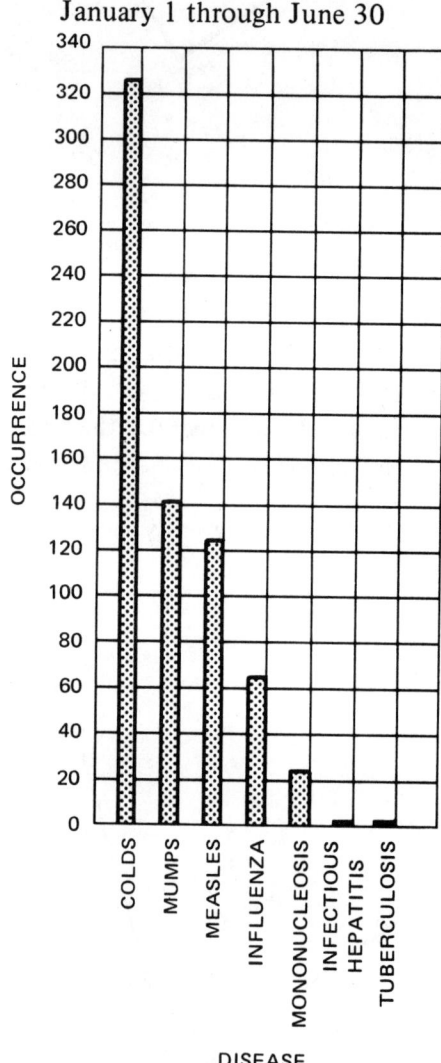

a. What is the subject of the graph?

b. What information is given on the vertical scale?

c. Which disease occurs most often?

d. How many cases of measles are reported?

e. What disease occurs about five times as often as mononucleosis?

f. How effective would a broken-line graph be in representing this data?

2. A community study is conducted to discover the relationship between persons 35 years or older with smoking and/or drinking habits and common forms of cancer. The survey reveals that approximately 60% of the community in this age group has smoking and/or drinking habits. The total population of the community is 37,495 with 15,962 males and 21,533 females. In the age group 35 and over, 9,483 are males and 10,986 are females.

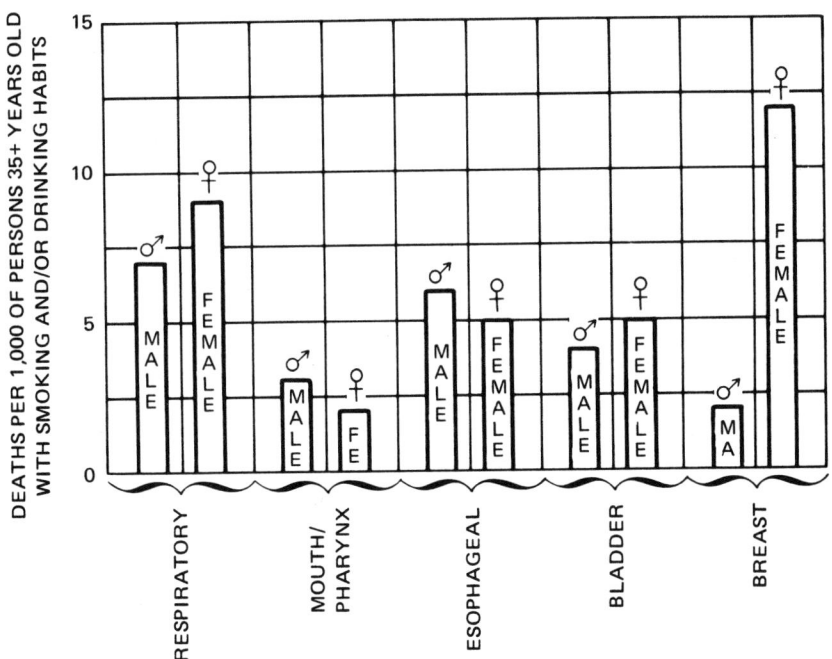

a. How many males involved in this study have smoking and/or drinking habits?

b. How many females involved in this study have smoking and/or drinking habits?

How many persons in this community, age 35+, with smoking and/or drinking habits actually died from —

	MALES	FEMALES
c. respiratory cancer?	?	?
d. mouth/pharynx cancer?	?	?
e. esophageal cancer?	?	?
f. bladder cancer?	?	?
g. breast cancer?	?	?

h. What can be concluded from this study about smoking and/or drinking habits and the relationship with cancer?

3. Liquids, when heated to temperatures above room temperature, tend to cool over a period of time. A 125-mL beaker is filled with 100 mL of water and heated to 60 °C. It is then allowed to cool and the temperature is recorded in ten-minute intervals. The temperatures are recorded on a broken-line graph.

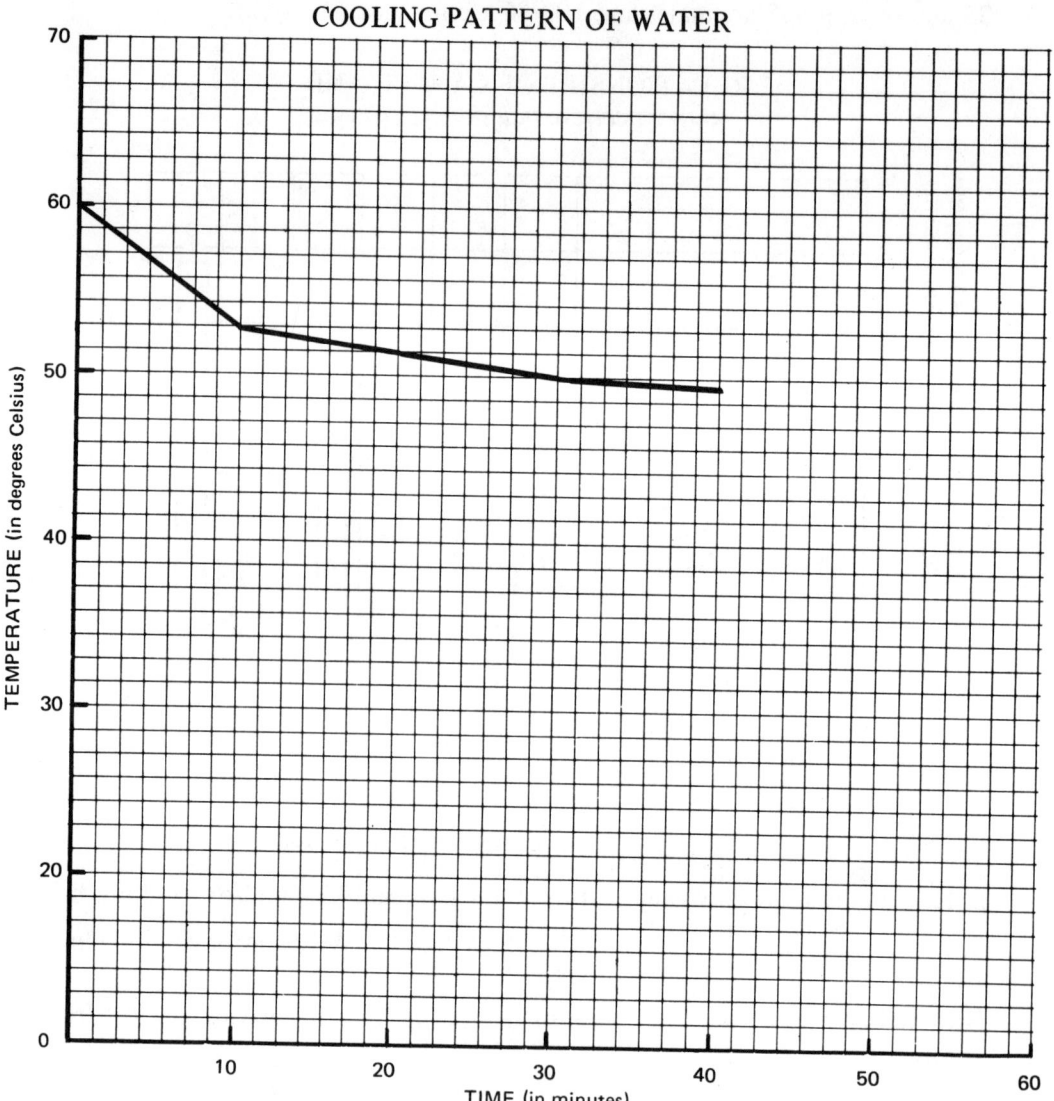

a. What is the temperature at 20 minutes?

b. In which time period is the decrease in temperature the greatest?

c. How many degrees does the temperature decline in 30 minutes?

d. Assuming that the room temperature is 23 °C, is it possible to project the pattern of cooling over a longer period of time without actually making the measurements?

e. What variables must be considered when projecting the cooling pattern of a liquid?

INTERPRETING CIRCLE GRAPHS

Circle graphs illustrate how one part is related to another part or to the whole. The circle graph is used primarily for comparison purposes and is impractical when determining other numerical values.

Example: A circle graph is prepared to show the percent distribution of influenza cases in a school.

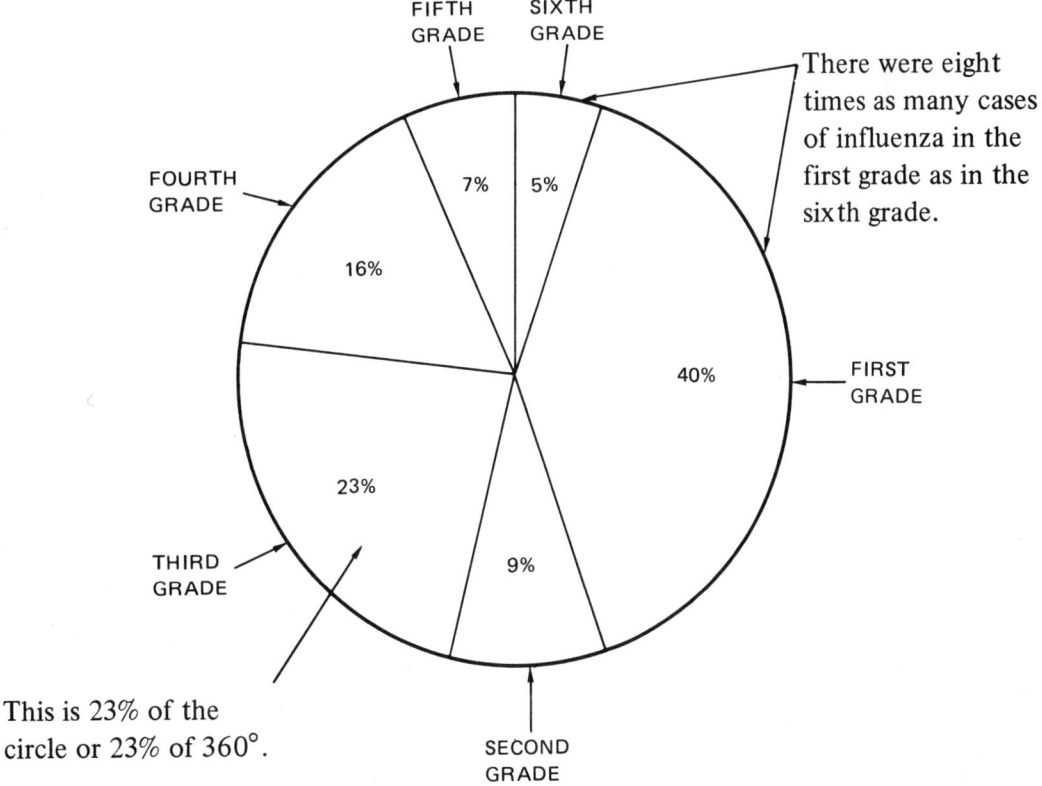

This graph compares the influenza cases in each grade to the total influenza cases. The fourth grade students had 16% of the influenza cases. This does <u>not</u> mean that 16% of the fourth grade students had influenza, but rather that 16% of all students having influenza were fourth grade students. Comparisons can also be made between different grades. For example, there were eight times as many cases of influenza in the first grade as in the sixth grade. In order to find the actual number of cases for each grade, the percent is multiplied by the total number of cases.

INTERPRETING PICTOGRAPHS

Pictographs are probably the easiest graphs to read but are the most difficult to draw. The pictograph shows approximations and is used for comparisons. Accurate numerical values usually cannot be obtained from pictographs.

Example: A pictograph is designed to display the influenza cases in Williamsville during a 5-year period.

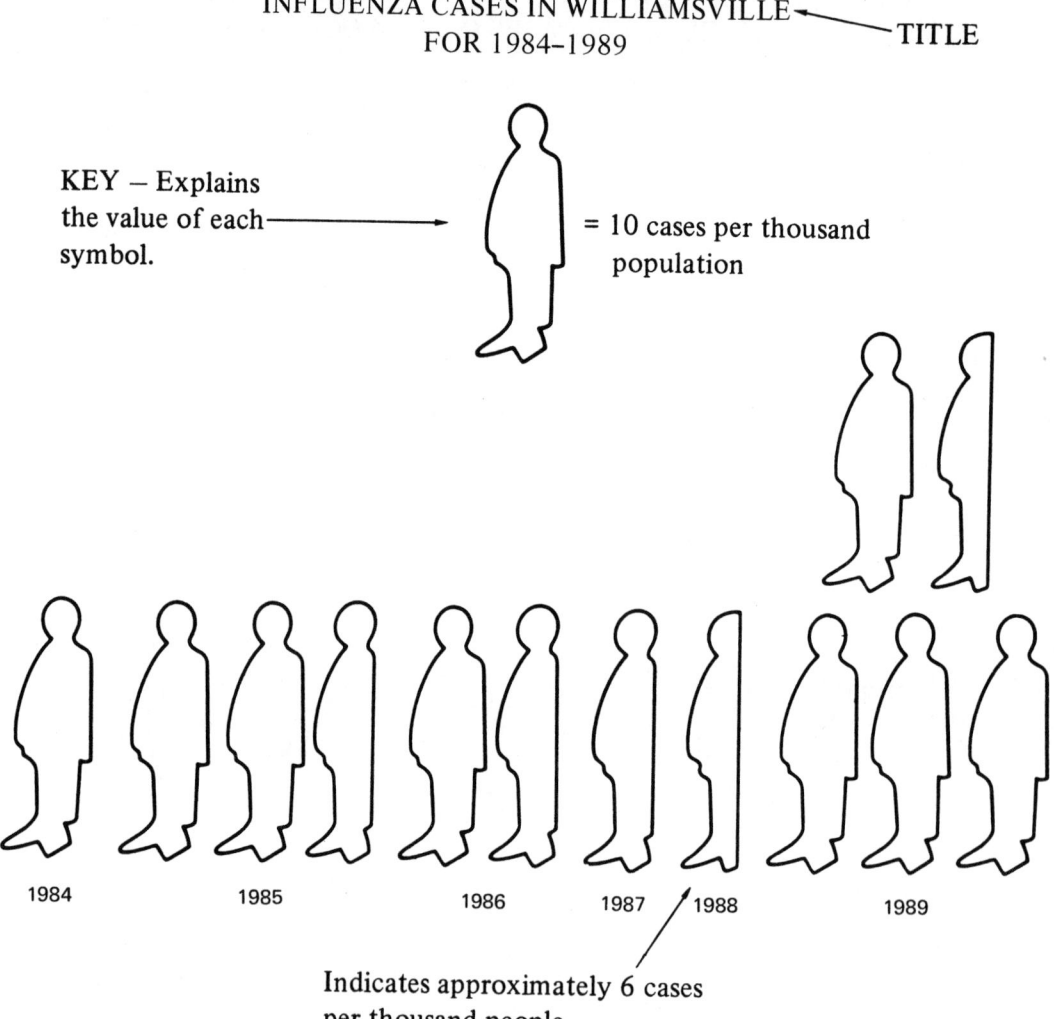

Notice the difficulty in distinguishing between the actual numbers of cases. Five cases looks like six cases or even seven cases. The graph is best used to determine years in which the most or least number of cases occurred or years in which the greatest change occurred.

Displaying statistical data with pictographs can be misleading. The comparisons may be misrepresented or the presentation may be inaccurate.

Example: This pictograph is supposed to show that three times as many people live in City *B* as in City *A*.

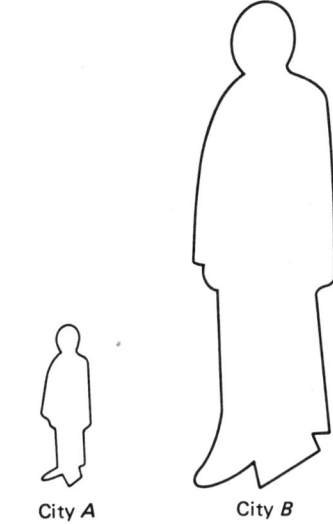

COMPARATIVE POPULATIONS OF TWO CITIES

The figure representing City *B* is actually nine times larger than the one representing City *A*. As the figure was increased in height it was also increased in width.

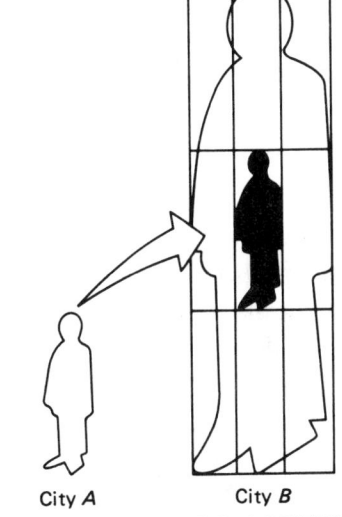

COMPARATIVE POPULATIONS OF TWO CITIES

A better method of comparison would be to assign each figure a value. If each figure represents a population of 25,000, the pictograph is then a valid comparison.

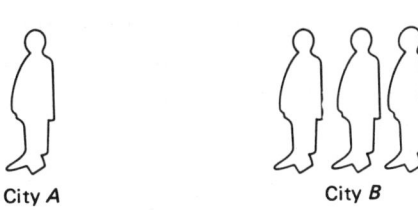

COMPARATIVE POPULATIONS OF TWO CITIES

28.3 EXERCISES

Analyze each graph and supply the requested information.

1. Within one portion of the current hospital budget, funds are allocated as presented in this circle graph.

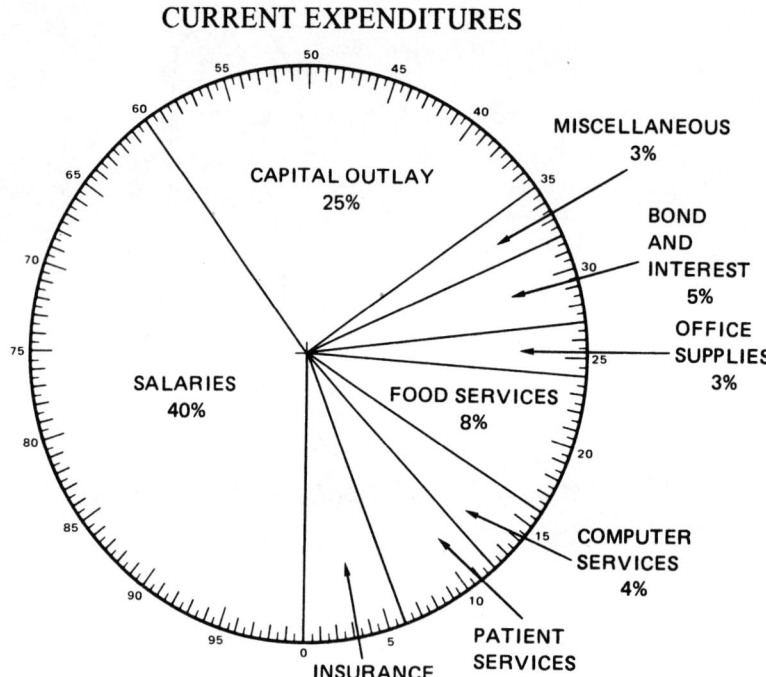

CURRENT EXPENDITURES

This portion of the budget contains $1,462,983. How many actual dollars exist in each area?

a. Salaries
b. Capital Outlay
c. Miscellaneous
d. Bond and Interest
e. Office Supplies
f. Food Services
g. Computer Services
h. Patient Services
i. Insurance

There are 360° in a circle. How many degrees are allowed for each category in the circle graph? Round the answer to the nearer tenth if necessary.

j. Salaries
k. Capital Outlay
l. Food Services
m. Patient Services

2. The emergency room deals with a variety of patients. The data from the monthly report is displayed in a circle graph. The number of patients that are admitted is 130.

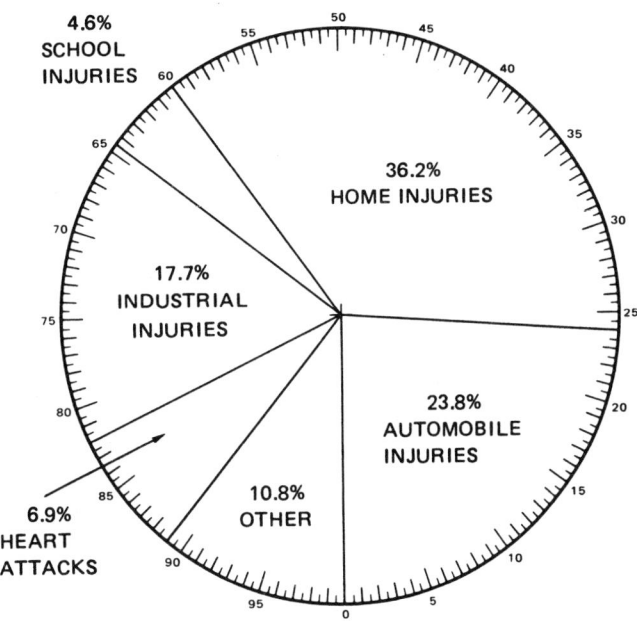

EMERGENCY ROOM INJURIES

Find the number of cases in each category.

a. Automobile Injuries
b. Home Injuries
c. School Injuries
d. Industrial Injuries
e. Heart Attacks
f. Other

Commercially prepared circle graph paper is available and is divided into increments of 0.5%. It is sometimes necessary to construct graphs with the aid of a compass and protractor. Assuming this approach must be followed, how many degrees must be allotted for each of the categories? Round each answer to the nearer tenth.

Note: There are 360° in a circle.

g. Automobile Injuries
h. Home Injuries
i. School Injuries
j. Industrial Injuries
k. Heart Attacks
l. Other

3. The county health department records the number of babies born during a year. This data is used to construct a pictograph.

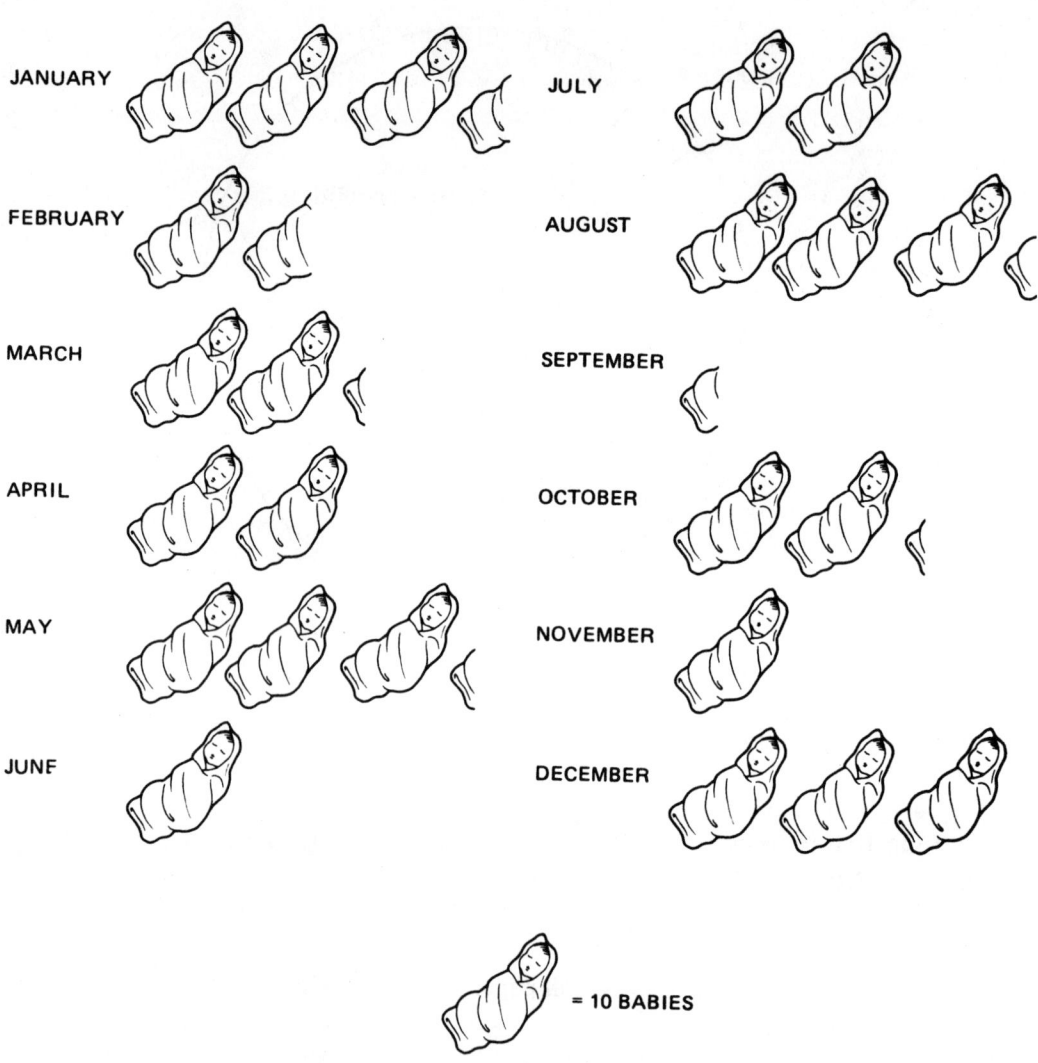

BIRTHS FOR A TWELVE-MONTH PERIOD

= 10 BABIES

a. What does each symbol represent?
b. Approximately how many babies are born in September?
c. Approximately how many babies are born in the last quarter of the year?
d. Approximately how many more babies are born in May than in November?
e. In which month are the most babies born?
f. Approximately how many times as many babies are born in December as in November?

MEAN, MEDIAN, AND MODE

When data is analyzed and presented, it is useful to make a comparative descriptive measure. In statistics, there are four descriptive measures that are useful to the health worker. These measures are the range, the mean, the median, and the mode. When calculating these measures, it is convenient to arrange the data from the smallest value to the largest value.

- ▼ The *range* is the difference between the largest and smallest numbers.
- ▼ The *mean* is the arithmetic average of a set of numbers. It is the sum of the numbers divided by the number of items in the set. In a set of numbers, the mean need not be one of the numbers in the set.
- ▼ The *median* is a positional average. If there is an odd number of items in a set, the median is the middle number. If there is an even number of items in the set, the median is the mean of the two middle numbers. Since the median is a positional average, an extremely large or small number does not affect it.
- ▼ The *mode* is the number (or numbers) that occurs most frequently in a set of numbers. A set of data with more than one mode is termed *bimodal*.

Example: A study is made to determine the effects that a mother's diet has on the birth weight of her child. To undertake the study two groups of mothers are established, the control group and the experimental group. Each group of mothers has the same general characteristics in terms of height, weight prior to pregnancy, and physical condition. Each mother in the control group continues with the diet of her choice. Each mother in the experimental group receives a carefully planned diet designed to encourage proper development of the child. At birth, the weights, in kilograms are recorded and arranged from smallest to largest. The range, mean, median, and mode are then calculated.

CONTROL GROUP				EXPERIMENTAL GROUP			
2.2	2.7	3.1	3.6	2.5	2.9	3.3	3.7
2.3	2.7	3.3	3.7	2.6	2.9	3.3	3.7
2.4	2.8	3.3	3.8	2.6	2.9	3.3	3.9
2.4	2.9	3.3	3.9	2.6	3.0	3.7	4.0
2.5	2.9	3.3	4.2	2.7	3.0	3.7	4.1
2.5	3.0	3.5	4.4	2.9	3.1	3.7	4.1
2.6	3.1			2.9			

- RANGE − The difference between the smallest and largest weight
  Control Group: $4.4 - 2.2 = 2.2$
  Experimental Group: $4.1 - 2.5 = 1.6$

- MEAN − The average weight
  Control Group: $\frac{80.3}{26} = 3.09$
  Experimental Group: $\frac{81.1}{25} = 3.24$

- MEDIAN – The weight of the baby in the middle of the set
  Control Group: $\frac{3.0 + 3.1}{2} = 3.05$
  Experimental Group: 3.1
- MODE – The weight that occurs most often
  Control Group: 3.3
  Experimental Group: 2.9 and 3.7

These descriptive measures indicate that:
- There is less difference in the range of weight for the experimental group.
- The average weight of the babies as determined by the mean and median is higher for the experimental group.

Note: Care must be taken when drawing conclusions. A heavier baby does not always indicate a healthier baby.

28.4 EXERCISES

1. Arrange the data from smallest to largest and find the range, mean, median, and mode or modes.
   a. 8, 1, 2, 4, 5, 3, 9, 4, 5, 4
   b. 13, 10, 4, 5, 1, 5, 10, 5, 10

2. Multiply each number in this set by ten.
   $$8, 1, 2, 4, 5, 3, 9, 4, 5, 4$$
   How does the mean of the new set of numbers compare with the original set?

3. Replace one of the numbers in this set so the mean of the numbers in the new set is 10.
   $$8, 4, 10, 8, 40$$

4. Replace one of the numbers in this set so the median of the new set is 6.
   $$5, 6, 8, 12$$

5. Is the mode always a member of the set of data?

6. Is the median always a member of the set of data?

7. A laboratory coat manufacturer has equipment to make only one size coat — small, medium, or large. The equipment cannot make all three. To sell the most coats, the manufacturer must properly determine the market needs. Which measure (mean, median, mode) should the manufacturer use to determine production?

8. In a junior college, the average age of a group of ten people is 20 years. Nine of the people are students and the other person is the teacher. Which measure best typifies the age of the group: mean, median, mode?

9. The president of an institution proposes that the minimum annual salary for a specific class of employees with at least 5 years of experience be set at $12,000. An assistant calculates how this minimum salary would effect the payroll. The assistant reports that the institution employs 250 persons with at least 5 years experience and that their average salary is $11,000. The conclusion is that the cost is 250 times $1,000 per year. The actual cost is $450,000. Explain how the assistant obtained $250,000 and give some reasons for the difference between the estimated and actual costs.

10. The Laboratory Electronic Technicians' Union is striking for higher wages. The union announces that the average worker receives a salary of only $9,000 while management claims the average wage is $22,636. Both sides use this data: $9,000; $9,000; $9,000; $10,500; $12,000; $13,500; $18,000; $18,000; $45,000; $45,000; $60,000.

   a. Which measure (mean, median, mode) is each side using?
   b. Which measure is the more appropriate?

APPLICATIONS

When performing laboratory tests or experiments, or when taking any measurement, there is some error. The error may be due to many factors including lack of accuracy in the measuring instrument or in the laboratory procedure. The amount of error is therefore taken into account and limits within which an error may be tolerated are established.

The allowable limits of error in a procedure may be determined for the normal range of values. This calculation uses the mean and the range of the normal biological range. The percent of allowable limits of error is:

$$\text{PERCENT OF ALLOWABLE LIMITS OF ERROR} = \frac{\frac{\text{range}}{4}}{\text{mean}} \times 100$$

Example: The normal range for hematocrit for adult males is 42 mL/100 mL to 52 mL/100 mL. Find the percent of allowable limits of error, to the nearer tenth percent.

$$\text{PERCENT OF ALLOWABLE LIMITS OF ERROR} = \frac{\frac{\text{range}}{4}}{\text{mean}} \times 100$$

$$\text{PERCENT OF ALLOWABLE LIMITS OF ERROR} = \frac{\frac{10}{4}}{47} \times 100 \qquad \text{range} = 52 - 42 \text{ or } 10$$

$$\text{mean} = \frac{42 + 52}{2} \text{ or } 47$$

$$\text{PERCENT OF ALLOWABLE LIMITS OF ERROR} = \frac{2.5}{47} \times 100$$

$$\text{PERCENT OF ALLOWABLE LIMITS OF ERROR} = 5.3\%$$

The percent of allowable limits of error is used to determine how a derived measurement compares with an accepted value. It may also be used to determine if a second or "follow-up" test or procedure shows a significant difference or is an allowable difference. The accepted limit is found by multiplying the accepted value by the percent of allowable limits of error. If the derived measurement falls within these limits, the measurement is acceptable.

Example: A sample of blood has a hemotocrit value (derived measurement) of 45 mL/100 mL. The known concentration (accepted measurement) of the original sample is 47 mL/100mL. Is the derived measurement within the allowable limits of error? (The percent of allowable limits of error is 5.3%.)

47 × 5.3% = 47 × 0.053 *or* 2.4
UPPER LIMIT = 47 + 2.4 *or* 49.4 mL/100 mL
LOWER LIMIT = 47 − 2.4 *or* 44.6 mL/100 mL

Since 45 mL/100 mL falls within the limits, it is an allowable value.

Note: This information gains importance when interpreting laboratory data. For example, in monitoring the progress of a patient, a change from 47 mL/100 mL to 45 mL/100 mL may not be a significant difference since the 45 mL/100 mL is within the allowable limits. The percent of allowable limits of error is used to determine values that fall within the normal range and also the significance of differences that fall in the abnormal range.

28.5 EXCERCISES

1. In order to determine the normal range for calcium content in the blood, 235 specimens of serum are tested. The results are illustrated in this bar graph.

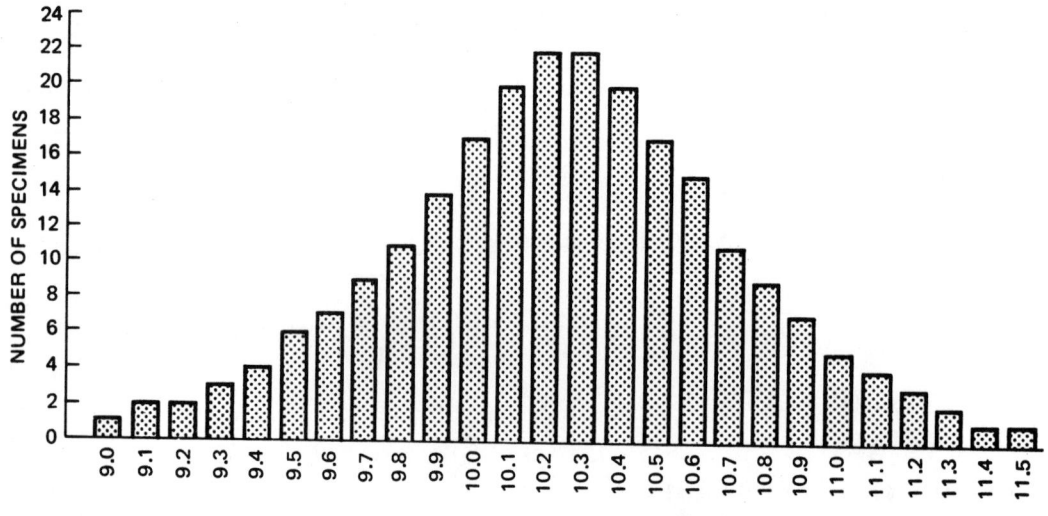

CALCIUM CONTENT OF THE BLOOD

a. What is the normal range of values as indicated by this graph?

b. Find the range of the data items.

c. Find the mode(s).

d. Find the median.

e. The mean of the data items is calculated to be 10.25 mg/100 cm^3 of serum. Using this value, find the percent of allowable limits of error to the nearer tenth percent.

f. Using the mean as the accepted measurement, determine the allowable limits of error.

g. Is a derived reading of 9.8 within the allowable limits of error?

h. Is a derived reading of 11.1 within the allowable limits of error?

2. A serum specimen indicates that the chloride in the body is 98 milliequivalents per litre of serum (derived measurement). The known concentration is 103 milliequivalents per litre and the normal range is 100 to 106 milliequivalents per litre.

a. Find the percent of allowable limits of error to the nearer tenth percent.

b. Find the allowable limits of error to the nearer tenth.

c. Is the derived measurement within the allowable limits of error?

3. The degree of acidity or alkalinity of the urine is expressed by pH values. The pH values for ten specimens are:

4.8	6.4
5.2	6.4
5.3	7.8
5.9	7.8
6.4	8.0

a. Find the range of the pH values.

b. Find the mode(s).

c. Find the median value.

d. Determine the mean.

e. Using the mean and the range, calculate the percent of allowable limits of error to the nearer tenth.

unit 29 computers—tools of the 21st century

OBJECTIVES

After studying this unit the student should be able to:

- Describe some of the essential values of the computer.
- Apply skills in mathematics to create interactive tables for data management.
- Develop confidence in the use of computers to solve mathematical problems.

THE COMPUTER AS A TOOL

Computers are the tools of the 21st century. Their ability to store, organize, and retrieve information greatly increases the speed at which we can complete our work. Computers are not new! They have been with us for a number of years. Since the early 1980s however and the development of the personal computer, they have become more available to students and workers on the job.

It was during the early 1980s that many educators thought it was necessary for every student to become knowledgeable about the total operation of the computer. Detailed courses on the operation and programming of computers were taught. One of the reasons for teaching programming in the early years was because few programs existed for use on the computers being developed.

Even if you have never used a computer, it is possible to understand their usefulness to your work. Computers consist of the hardware which includes the computer itself and some type of printer. Some computers may also have a modem that allows the computer to send or receive information over a telephone line. The interacting computers and printers may be in the same building or thousands of miles apart.

Each computer contains information that allows it to understand further information it is given. This is considered the permanent memory of the computer. Additional information, known as software, is also required. Software is the set of instructions written to control the operation of the computer. The information is stored on disks that may be inserted into the computer at the time of use. This software is generally called "the program" and may be specific to the type of computer you are using or in some cases may be compatible to other brands of computers.

WORD PROCESSING, DATA MANAGEMENT, AND SPREADSHEETING

The three most common applications of the computer are word processing, data management, and spreadsheeting.

In its simplest form, word processing allows the computer operator to enter information just as they would on a typewriter. The information appears on the screen of the computer as it is typed. The information can be saved to a storage disk at anytime the operator desires. As a matter of fact, if the electricity should fail anytime prior to saving the information, it is lost and must be re-entered. Once all of the information has been entered and saved to the storage disk, the disk can be removed and stored in a file box for later use. At some future date, the stored data can be loaded back into the computer for entry of more information or revision made of the original material that was entered. When revised and stored, it will replace all of the previous information that was entered with the new version.

Word processing makes it possible to type and store an entire handbook. From this small storage disk, the handbook may be printed on one of several types of printers. In the future, if changes occur, the original handbook can be retrieved on the computer, changed, stored and the new version printed. This saves many hours of retyping. Newer programs and printers allow variations in page layout and type style.

Data management allows the entry of information by various categories. Each category can be sorted by either numerical or alphabetical order, depending on how it was entered. A simple example would be entry of a person's name, address, city, state, zip code, and telephone. This would represent six different categories or fields and allow you to organize the data in any one or a combination of categories. The collection of six fields represents one record. Most data management programs will also allow some mathematical calculations.

Example: A prescription drug has been sold to a number of individuals.

You can enter the name of the patient, the code assigned to the patient, the number of pills sold, and the price paid by the patient. Once each three months you may be asked to print reports showing the total number of pills purchased by each patient, the total number of pills sold to all patients, and the total number of dollars collected. The data therefore, once entered, can be used to generate a series of different reports, each with the data presented in a different way. Prior to the application of the computer, this would have required lengthy handwritten or typed reports that were prepared manually. Now, in the blink of an eye, the data can be sorted and ready for printing.

SPREADSHEETING—A POWERFUL TOOL FOR MATHEMATICAL CALCULATIONS

A spreadsheet is really quite simple. It consists of a grid on a screen as shown in Figure 29-1. Letters are used across the top of the grid. Each of these letters represent a column that extends below. Along the left hand side of the grid is a series of numbers in ascend-order. Each number represents a row of information extending to the right. If you follow column C down to row 10 you will find a box. This box is known as the coordi-

	A	B	C	D	E
1					
2					
3					
4					
5					
6					
7					
8					
9					
10					

FIGURE 29-1

nate of column C, row 10 and is termed a cell. Information can be entered into each cell. This information may be either a label or a value.

This grid of cells allows you to set up a table for the purpose of doing a wide variety of mathematical calculations. The remainder of Unit 29 will introduce sample applications of the spreadsheet and ask you to try your skill at setting up a table. The single mathematics function of multiplication will be used in both the examples and problems. It is possible to use multiplication (*), division (/), addition (+), and subtraction (-) all within the same formula if the problem requires this type of calculation. The formula is not limited to the size of the cell. If you are actually working with a computer, consult the manual relative to the spreadsheet program you are using. All spreadsheet programs are similar in how they operate but may have some unique characteristics for entering the data.

Example: Patients entering the clinic are provided a medical service. It has been determined that there are two levels of services that may be provided with the staff and equipment available. Additionally, the cost of the service is also determined by the length of time the patient must remain in the treatment process. Periodically, due to increased staff, materials, and equipment costs, it is necessary to adjust the cost of the treatment. To determine exact cost quickly and accurately, a chart must be established for staff use during billing.

The first step is to create the basic table layout. We know, through study, that the cost must fall into two levels. We also know the cost should increase for each 15 minutes of service. Further, it has been determined that the basic cost for the service is $45.00. From this it is possible to determine the percent of increase for each 15 minutes of service at each level of service. Figure 29-2A shows the creation of the basic table including the labels and values.

Once the basic table has been created it is possible to enter the formulae necessary to make the table do the automatic calculations. Figure 29-2B shows the formulae entered under each cost column. Notice that, in this case, the calculations are

	A	B	C	D	E
1		PHYSICAL MEDICAL SERVICES - OUT PATIENT			
2					
3		LEVEL I		LEVEL II	
4	TIME	%	COST	%	COST
5					
6	90 MIN	1.25		2.00	
7	75 MIN	1.20		1.90	
8	60 MIN	1.15		1.80	
9	45 MIN	1.10		1.70	
10	30 MIN	1.05		1.60	
11	15 MIN	1.00		1.50	
12					
13					
14		BASE COST:	45.00		
15					

FIGURE 29-2A

simply the coordinate found in the B and C columns times the basic cost found in coordinate C14. The method used to enter the formula may vary slightly from one spreadsheet program to another. In this case the = sign tells the computer a value is being entered rather than a label. The full formula such as =B6*C14 is really telling the computer to take the percent shown in B6 (1.25) times the base cost shown in C14 (45.00).

	A	B	C	D	E
1		PHYSICAL MEDICAL SERVICES - OUT PATIENT			
2					
3		LEVEL I		LEVEL II	
4	TIME	%	COST	%	COST
5					
6	90 MIN	1.25	=B6*C14	2.00	=D6*C14
7	75 MIN	1.20	=B7*C14	1.90	=D7*C14
8	60 MIN	1.15	=B8*C14	1.80	=D8*C14
9	45 MIN	1.10	=B9*C14	1.70	=D9*C14
10	30 MIN	1.05	=B10*C14	1.60	=D10*C14
11	15 MIN	1.00	=B11*C14	1.50	=D11*C14
12					
13					
14		BASE COST:	45.00		
15					

FIGURE 29-2B

Figure 29-2C indicates the actual costs after entry of these formulae.

	A	B	C	D	E
1		PHYSICAL MEDICAL SERVICES - OUT PATIENT			
2					
3		LEVEL I		LEVEL II	
4	TIME	%	COST	%	COST
5					
6	90 MIN	1.25	56.25	2.00	90.00
7	75 MIN	1.20	54.00	1.90	85.50
8	60 MIN	1.15	51.75	1.80	81.00
9	45 MIN	1.10	49.50	1.70	76.50
10	30 MIN	1.05	47.25	1.60	72.00
11	15 MIN	1.00	45.00	1.50	67.50
12					
13					
14		BASE COST:	45.00		
15					

FIGURE 29-2C

Now let's assume the cost of the service must be increased. The cost of staff and materials indicate the new base rate must be $60.00. The new base cost would be entered into coordinate C14 and instantly the entire chart will change to reveal what is indicated in Figure 29-2D.

	A	B	C	D	E
1		PHYSICAL MEDICAL SERVICES - OUT PATIENT			
2					
3		LEVEL I		LEVEL II	
4	TIME	%	COST	%	COST
5					
6	90 MIN	1.25	75.00	2.00	120.00
7	75 MIN	1.20	72.00	1.90	114.00
8	60 MIN	1.15	69.00	1.80	108.00
9	45 MIN	1.10	66.00	1.70	102.00
10	30 MIN	1.05	63.00	1.60	96.00
11	15 MIN	1.00	60.00	1.50	90.00
12					
13					
14		BASE COST:	60.00		
15					

FIGURE 29-2D

After a period of several months it is noted that increased costs must once again require a change in the level of charges to the patient. This time is it not necessary to change the base cost but the percent of charge beyond 15 minutes at LEVEL I must be increased. Figure 29-2E reveals the new charges after the percents have been changed in columns B and D. Note that it is not necessary to change any of the original formulae and that the calculations on a computer are automatic.

	A	B	C	D	E
1		PHYSICAL MEDICAL SERVICES - OUT PATIENT			
2					
3		LEVEL I		LEVEL II	
4	TIME	%	COST	%	COST
5					
6	90 MIN	1.75	105.00	3.15	189.00
7	75 MIN	1.60	96.00	2.95	177.00
8	60 MIN	1.45	87.00	2.75	165.00
9	45 MIN	1.30	78.00	2.55	153.00
10	30 MIN	1.15	69.00	2.35	141.00
11	15 MIN	1.00	60.00	2.15	129.00
12					
13					
14		BASE COST:	60.00		
15					

FIGURE 29-2E

29.1 EXERCISES

1. It is found that one of the medical supplies is sometimes distributed in different amounts to each patient, depending on the nature of their treatment. The most frequent pattern of distribution is packages of 10, 50, and 100. Furthermore, there is a base cost of $16.00 for the first 10 but after that the cost per unit is $1.45 for 11 through 50 and then 1.30 for units 51 through 100. Create a spreadsheet to show the formulae to automatically calculate the cost.

	A	B	C	D	E
1					
2					
3					
4					
5					
6					
7					
8					
9					
10					
11					
12					
13					
14					
15					

2. A salary schedule is established for a classification of clinical workers based on their years of experience and their level of training. It is determined that the base salary for beginners with no experience and LEVEL I training will be $15,000 for 12 months of work. The workers would receive a salary increase of 2.00% for each additional year of experience up to five years at which time they would not receive additional increases without further training. LEVEL II workers, with more training, would receive 5.00% more than a LEVEL I worker at the beginning step and a 3.00% increase each year up to the tenth year and they too would need additional training to move to the next level. LEVEL III workers would receive 5.00% more than a LEVEL II worker at the beginning step and a 5.00% increase for each additional year of experience up to the fifteenth year of service. At this point, a LEVEL III worker at the fifteenth year would represent the top of the salary schedule. The only way the pay at any step could be increased would be to increase the base step for the LEVEL I worker. This would therefore affect all other salaries since they are a function of the first step for a LEVEL I worker. It would also be possible to increase salaries by changing the percent differences between the various levels and years of experience. Create your table to allow automatic calculations of the entire schedule simply by changing the amount paid to a LEVEL I worker with no experience.

APPENDIX

SECTION I

DENOMINATE NUMBERS

Denominate numbers are numbers that include units of measurement. The units of measurement are arranged from the largest units at the left to the smallest unit at the right. For example: 6 yd. 2 ft. 4 in.

All basic operations of arithmetic can be performed on denominate numbers.

I EQUIVALENT MEASURES

Measurements that are equal can be expressed in different terms. For example, 12 in. = 1 ft. If these equivalents are divided, the answer is 1.

$$\frac{1 \text{ ft.}}{12 \text{ in.}} = 1 \qquad \frac{12 \text{ in.}}{1 \text{ ft.}} = 1$$

To express one measurement as another equal measurement, multiply by the equivalent in the form of 1.

To express 6 inches in equivalent foot measurement, multiply 6 inches by one in the form of $\frac{1 \text{ ft.}}{12 \text{ in.}}$. In the numerator and denominator, divide by a common factor.

$$6 \text{ in.} = \frac{\cancel{6 \text{ in.}}^{1}}{1} \times \frac{1 \text{ ft.}}{\cancel{12 \text{ in.}}_{2}} = \frac{1}{2} \text{ ft. or } 0.5 \text{ ft.}$$

To express 4 feet in equivalent inch measurement, multiply 4 feet by one in the form of $\frac{12 \text{ in.}}{1 \text{ ft.}}$.

$$4 \text{ ft.} = \cancel{4 \text{ ft.}}^{4} \times \frac{12 \text{ in.}}{\cancel{1 \text{ ft.}}_{1}} = \frac{48 \text{ in.}}{1} = 48 \text{ in.}$$

Per means division, as with a fraction bar. For example, 50 miles per hour can be written $\frac{50 \text{ miles}}{1 \text{ hour}}$.

II. BASIC OPERATIONS

A. ADDITION

SAMPLE: 2 yd. 1 ft. 5 in. + 1 ft. 8 in. + 5 yd. 2 ft.

1. Write the denominate numbers in a column with like units in the same column.

2. Add the denominate numbers in each column.

3. Express the answer using the largest possible units.

```
      2 yd.   1 ft.   5 in.
              1 ft.   8 in.
   +  5 yd.   2 ft.
      7 yd.   4 ft.  13 in.

      7 yd.                  =   7 yd.
              4 ft.          =   1 yd.   1 ft.
                     13 in.  = +         1 ft.   1 in.
      7 yd.   4 ft.  13 in.  =   8 yd.   2 ft.   1 in.
```

B. SUBTRACTION

SAMPLE: 4 yd. 3 ft. 5 in. − 2 yd. 1 ft. 7 in.

1. Write the denominate numbers in columns with like units in the same column.

2. Starting at the right, examine each column to compare the numbers. If the bottom number is larger, exchange one unit from the column at the left for its equivalent. Combine like units.

3. Subtract the denominate numbers

4. Express the answer using the largest possible units.

```
      4 yd.   3 ft.   5 in.
   −  2 yd.   1 ft.   7 in.

                7 in. is larger than 5 in.
                3 ft. = 2 ft. 12 in.
                12 in. + 5 in. = 17 in.

      4 yd.   2 ft.  17 in.
   −  2 yd.   1 ft.   7 in.
      2 yd.   1 ft.  10 in.

      2 yd.   1 ft.  10 in.
```

C. MULTIPLICATION

− By a constant

SAMPLE: 1 hr. 24 min. × 3

1. Multiply the denominate number by the constant.

2. Express the answer using the largest possible units.

```
         1 hr.  24 min.
      ×            3
         3 hr.  72 min.

         3 hr.           =   3 hr.
                72 min.  =   1 hr. 12 min.
         3 hr.  72 min.  =   4 hr. 12 min.
```

— By a denominate number expressing linear measurement

SAMPLE: 9 ft. 6 in. × 10 ft.

1. Express all denominate numbers in the same unit.

   9 ft. 6 in. = $9\frac{1}{2}$ ft.

2. Multiply the denominate numbers. (This includes the units of measure, such as ft. × ft. = sq. ft.)

   $9\frac{1}{2}$ ft. × 10 ft. =

   $\frac{19}{2}$ ft. × 10 ft. =

   95 sq. ft.

— By a denominate number expressing square measurement

SAMPLE: 3 ft. × 6 sq. ft.

1. Multiply the denominate numbers. (This includes the units of measure, such as ft. × ft. = sq. ft. and sq. ft. × ft. = cu. ft.)

   3 ft. × 6 sq. ft. = 18 cu. ft.

— By a denominate number expressing rate

SAMPLE: 50 miles per hour × 3 hours

1. Express the rate as a fraction using the fraction bar for *per*.

   $\frac{50 \text{ miles}}{1 \text{ hour}} \times \frac{3 \text{ hours}}{1} =$

2. Divide the numerator and denominator by any common factors, including units of measure.

   $\frac{50 \text{ miles}}{1 \text{ hour}} \times \frac{3 \text{ hours}}{1} =$

3. Multiply numerators. Multiply denominators.

   $\frac{150 \text{ miles}}{1} =$

4. Express the answer in the remaining unit.

   150 miles

D. DIVISION

— By a constant

SAMPLE: 8 gal. 3 qt. ÷ 5

1. Express all denominate numbers in the same unit.

   8 gal. 3 qt. = 35 qt.

2. Divide the denominate number by the constant.

   35 qt. ÷ 5 = 7 qt.

3. Express the answer using the largest possible units.

   7 qt. = 1 gal. 3 qt.

— By a denominate number expressing linear measurement

SAMPLE: 11 ft. 4 in. ÷ 8 in.

1. Express all denominate numbers in the same unit.
2. Divide the denominate numbers by a common factor. (This includes the units of measure, such as inches ÷ inches = 1.)

11 ft. 4 in. = 136 in.
136 in. ÷ 8 in. =
$$\frac{\cancel{136 \text{ in.}}^{17}}{\cancel{8 \text{ in.}}_{1}} = \frac{17}{1} = 17$$

— By a linear measure with a square measurement as the dividend

SAMPLE: 20 sq. ft. ÷ 4 ft.

1. Divide the denominate numbers. (This includes the units of measure, such as sq. ft. ÷ ft. = ft.)
2. Express the answer in the remaining unit.

20 sq. ft. ÷ 4 ft.
$$\frac{\cancel{20 \text{ sq. ft.}}^{5 \text{ ft.}}}{\cancel{4 \text{ ft.}}_{1}} = \frac{5 \text{ ft.}}{1}$$
5 ft.

— By denominate numbers used to find rate

SAMPLE: 200 mi. ÷ 10 gal.

1. Divide the denominate numbers
2. Express the units with the fraction bar meaning *per*.

$$\frac{\cancel{200 \text{ mi.}}^{20 \text{ mi.}}}{\cancel{10 \text{ gal.}}_{1 \text{ gal.}}} = \frac{20 \text{ mi.}}{1 \text{ gal.}}$$

$$\frac{20 \text{ mi.}}{1 \text{ gal.}} = 20 \text{ miles per gallon}$$

Note: Alterate methods of performing the basic operations will produce the same result. The choice of method is determined by the individual.

SECTION II

TABLE I
SQUARES AND SQUARE ROOTS

n	n^2	$\sqrt{n}$	n	n^2	$\sqrt{n}$	n	n^2	$\sqrt{n}$
1	1	1.000	51	2,601	7.141	101	10,201	10.050
2	4	1.414	52	2,704	7.211	102	10,404	10.100
3	9	1.732	53	2,809	7.280	103	10,609	10.149
4	16	2.000	54	2,916	7.348	104	10,816	10.198
5	25	2.236	55	3,025	7.416	105	11,025	10.247
6	36	2.449	56	3,136	7.483	106	11,236	10.296
7	49	2.646	57	3,249	7.550	107	11,449	10.344
8	64	2.828	58	3,364	7.616	108	11,664	10.392
9	81	3.000	59	3,481	7.681	109	11,881	10.440
10	100	3.162	60	3,600	7.746	110	12,100	10.488
11	121	3.317	61	3,721	7.810	111	12,321	10.536
12	144	3.464	62	3,844	7.874	112	12,544	10.583
13	169	3.606	63	3,969	7.937	113	12,769	10.630
14	196	3.742	64	4,096	8.000	114	12,996	10.677
15	225	3.873	65	4,225	8.062	115	13,225	10.724
16	256	4.000	66	4,356	8.124	116	13,456	10.770
17	289	4.123	67	4,489	8.185	117	13,689	10.817
18	324	4.243	68	4,624	8.246	118	13,924	10.863
19	361	4.359	69	4,761	8.307	119	14,161	10.909
20	400	4.472	70	4,900	8.367	120	14,400	10.954
21	441	4.583	71	5,041	8.426	121	14,641	11.000
22	484	4.690	72	5,184	8.485	122	14,884	11.045
23	529	4.796	73	5,329	8.544	123	15,129	11.091
24	576	4.899	74	5,476	8.602	124	15,376	11.136
25	625	5.000	75	5,625	8.660	125	15,625	11.180
26	676	5.099	76	5,776	8.718	126	15,876	11.225
27	729	5.196	77	5,929	8.775	127	16,129	11.269
28	784	5.292	78	6,084	8.832	128	16,384	11.314
29	841	5.385	79	6,241	8.888	129	16,641	11.358
30	900	5.477	80	6,400	8.944	130	16,900	11.402
31	961	5.568	81	6,561	9.000	131	17,161	11.446
32	1,024	5.657	82	6,724	9.055	132	17,424	11.489
33	1,089	5.745	83	6,889	9.110	133	17,689	11.533
34	1,156	5.831	84	7,056	9.165	134	17,956	11.576
35	1,225	5.916	85	7,225	9.220	135	18,225	11.619
36	1,296	6.000	86	7,396	9.274	136	18,496	11.662
37	1,369	6.083	87	7,569	9.327	137	18,769	11.705
38	1,444	6.164	88	7,744	9.381	138	19,044	11.747
39	1,521	6.245	89	7,921	9.434	139	19,321	11.790
40	1,600	6.325	90	8,100	9.487	140	19,600	11.832
41	1,681	6.403	91	8,281	9.539	141	19,881	11.874
42	1,764	6.481	92	8,464	9.592	142	20,164	11.916
43	1,849	6.557	93	8,649	9.644	143	20,449	11.958
44	1,936	6.633	94	8,836	9.695	144	20,736	12.000
45	2,025	6.708	95	9,025	9.747	145	21,025	12.042
46	2,116	6.782	96	9,216	9.798	146	21,316	12.083
47	2,209	6.856	97	9,409	9.849	147	21,609	12.124
48	2,304	6.928	98	9,604	9.899	148	21,904	12.166
49	2,401	7.000	99	9,801	9.950	149	22,201	12.207
50	2,500	7.071	100	10,000	10.000	150	22,500	12.247

TABLE II
METRIC RELATIONSHIPS

The base units in SI metrics include the metre and the gram. Other units of measure are related to these units. The relationship between the units is based on powers of ten and uses these prefixes:
   kilo (1 000)   deci (0.1)   hecto (100)   centi (0.01)   deka (10)   milli (0.001)
These tables show the most frequently used units with an asterisk (*).

METRIC LENGTH MEASURE

10 millimetres (mm)*	=	1 centimetre (cm)*
10 centimetres (cm)	=	1 decimetre (dm)
10 decimetres (dm)	=	1 metre (m)*
10 metres (m)	=	1 dekametre (dam)
10 dekametres (dam)	=	1 hectometre (hm)
10 hectometres (hm)	=	1 kilometre (km)*

METRIC AREA MEASURE

100 square millimetres (mm^2)	=	1 square centimetre (cm^2)*
100 square centimetres (cm^2)	=	1 square decimetre (dm^2)
100 square decimetres (dm^2)	=	1 square metre (m^2)*
100 square metres (m^2)	=	1 square dekametre (dam^2)
100 square dekametres (dam^2)	=	1 square hectometre (hm^2)*
100 square hectometres (hm^2)	=	1 square kilometre (km^2)

METRIC VOLUME MEASURE FOR SOLIDS

1 000 cubic millimetres (mm^3)	=	1 cubic centimetre (cm^3)*
1 000 cubic centimetres (cm^3)	=	1 cubic decimetre (dm^3)*
1 000 cubic decimetres (dm^3)	=	1 cubic metre (m^3)*
1 000 cubic metres (m^3)	=	1 cubic dekametre (dam^3)
1 000 cubic dekametres (dam^3)	=	1 cubic hectometre (hm^3)
1 000 cubic hectometres (hm^3)	=	1 cubic kilometre (km^3)

METRIC VOLUME MEASURE FOR FLUIDS

10 millilitres (mL)*	=	1 centilitre (cL)
10 centilitres (cL)	=	1 decilitre (dL)
10 decilitres (dL)	=	1 litre (L)*
10 litres (L)	=	1 dekalitre (daL)
10 dekalitres (daL)	=	1 hectolitre (hL)
10 hectolitres (hL)	=	1 kilolitre (kL)

METRIC VOLUME MEASURE EQUIVALENTS

1 cubic decimetre (dm^3)	=	1 litre (L)
1 000 cubic centimetres (cm^3)	=	1 litre (L)
1 cubic centimetre (cm^3)	=	1 millilitre (mL)

METRIC MASS MEASURE

10 milligrams (mg)*	=	1 centigram (cg)
10 centigrams (cg)	=	1 decigram (dg)
10 decigrams (dg)	=	1 gram (g)*
10 grams (g)	=	1 dekagram (dag)
10 dekagrams (dag)	=	1 hectogram (hg)
10 hectograms (hg)	=	1 kilogram (kg)*
1 000 kilograms (kg)	=	1 megagram (Mg)*

▲ To express a metric length unit as a smaller metric length unit, multiply by a positive power of ten such as 10, 100, 1 000, 10 000, etc.

▲ To express a metric length unit as a larger metric length unit, multiply by a negative power of ten such as 0.1, 0.01, 0.001, 0.000 1, etc.

▲ To express a metric area unit as a smaller metric area unit, multiply by 100, 10 000, 1 000 000, etc.

▲ To express a metric area unit as a larger metric area unit, multiply by 0.01, 0.000 1, 0.000 001, etc.

▲ To express a metric volume unit for solids as a smaller metric volume unit for solids, multiply by 1 000, 1 000 000, 1 000 000 000, etc.

▲ To express a metric volume unit for solids as a larger metric volume unit for solids, multiply by 0.001, 0.000 001, 0.000 000 001, etc.

▲ To express a metric volume unit for fluids as a smaller metric volume unit for fluids, multiply by 10, 100, 1 000, 10 000, etc.

▲ To express a metric volume unit for fluids as a larger metric volume unit for fluids, multiply by 0.1, 0.01, 0.001, 0.000 1, etc.

▲ To express a metric mass unit as a smaller metric mass unit, multiply by 10, 100, 1 000, 10 000, etc.

▲ To express a metric mass unit as a larger metric mass unit, multiply by 0.1, 0.01, 0.001, 0.000 1, etc.

Metric measurements are expressed in decimal parts of a whole number. For example, one-half millimetre is written as 0.5 mm.

In calculating with the metric system, all measurements are expressed using the same prefixes. If answers are needed in millimetres, all parts of the problem should be expressed in millimetres before the final solution is attempted. Diagrams that give dimensions in different prefixes must first be expressed using the same unit.

Appendix 277

TABLE III

HOUSEHOLD EQUIVALENTS

APPROXIMATE LIQUID MEASURE EQUIVALENTS

60 drops	=	1 teaspoonful (t)
3 teaspoonfuls	=	1 tablespoonful (T)
2 tablespoonfuls	=	1 fluidounce
6 fluidounces	=	1 teacupful
8 fluidounces	=	1 glassful

TABLE IV

APOTHECARIES EQUIVALENTS

EQUIVALENT MEASUREMENTS OF VOLUME

60 minims (m)	=	1 fluidram (f℈)
8 fluidrams (f℈)	=	1 fluidounce (f℥)
16 fluidounces (f℥)	=	1 pint (pt.)
2 pints (pt.)	=	1 quart (qt.)
4 quarts (qt.)	=	1 gallon (gal.)

EQUIVALENT MEASUREMENTS OF WEIGHT

60 grains (gr.)	=	1 dram (℈)
8 drams (℈)	=	1 ounce (℥)
12 ounces (℥)	=	1 pound (lb.)

TABLE V

METRIC SYSTEM			APOTHECARIES' SYSTEM				HOUSEHOLD SYSTEM
	Volume						
Weight (mass)	Solid	Fluid	Weight (mass)	Symbol	Volume (liquid)	Symbol	
0.06 g or 60 mg	60 mm^3	0.06 mL	1 grain (gr.)	gr. i	1 minim	m i	1 drop
1 g	1 cm^3	1 mL	15 grains	gr. xv	15 minims	m xv	
4 g	4 cm^3	4 mL	1 dram	℈ i	1 fluidram	f℈ i	1 scant teaspoonful
5 g	5 cm^3	5 mL					1 teaspoonful (t)
15 g	15 cm^3	15 mL	4 drams	℈ iv	4 fluidrams	f℈ iv	1 tablespoonful (T)
30 g	30 cm^3	30 mL	1 ounce	℥ i	1 fluidounce	f℥ i	2 tablespoonfuls
180 g	180 cm^3	180 mL	6 ounces	℥ vi	6 fluidounces	f℥ vi	1 teacupful
240 g	240 cm^3	240 mL	8 ounces	℥ viii	8 fluidounces	f℥ viii	1 glassful
360 g	360 cm^3		12 ounces	℥ xii			2 teacupfuls
			1 pound	lb. i			
500 g	500 cm^3	500 mL			1 pint	pt. i	2 glassfuls
1 000 g or 1 kg	1 dm^3	1 L	32 ounces	℥ xxxii	1 quart	qt. i	4 glassfuls
4 kg	4 dm^3	4 L			1 gallon	gal. i	16 glassfuls

SECTION III

MATHEMATICAL AND HEALTH RELATED FORMULAS

AREAS

square: $A = s^2$

rectangle: $A = lw$

triangle: $A = \frac{1}{2} bh$

circle: $A = \pi r^2$

CIRCUMFERENCE

$r = \frac{1}{2} d$

$C = \pi d$

$C = 2\pi r$

DOSES AND DOSAGES

Young's rule: CHILD'S DOSE $= \dfrac{\text{Child's Age (in years)}}{\text{Child's Age (in years)} + 12} \times$ Adult Dose

Fried's rule: INFANT'S DOSE $= \dfrac{\text{Age (in months)}}{150 \text{ pounds}} \times$ Adult Dose

Clark's rule: CHILD'S DOSE $= \dfrac{\text{Weight of Child (in pounds)}}{150 \text{ pounds}} \times$ Adult Dose

or

CHILD'S DOSE $= \dfrac{\text{Weight of Child (in kilograms)}}{68 \text{ kilograms}} \times$ Adult Dose

SOLUTIONS

$$\text{ratio strength of solutions} = \frac{\text{amount of drug}}{\text{amount of solution}}$$

$$\text{percent strength by volume} = \frac{\text{volume of solute}}{\text{volume of solution}} \times 100$$

$$\text{percent strength by weight (mass)} = \frac{\text{mass of solute}}{\text{volume of solution}} \times 100$$

$$\frac{\text{amount of solute}}{\text{amount of first solution}} = \frac{\text{amount of solute}}{\text{amount of second solution}}$$

smaller % strength : larger % strength = smaller volume : larger volume

or

weaker : stronger - solute : solvent

desired solution : solution on hand = amount of solute : amount of solution

$$D \quad : \quad H \quad = \quad q \quad : \quad Q$$

or

$$\frac{D}{H} = \frac{q}{Q}$$

VOLUMES

rectangular solid: $V = lwh$

cylindrical solid: $V = \pi r^2 h$

equivalences: $1 \text{ cm}^3 = 0.002 \text{ L}$ *or* $1 \text{ cm}^3 = 1 \text{ mL}$
$1\,000 \text{ cm}^3 = 1 \text{ L}$

At 4 °C and standard pressure (760 millimetres), the volume and mass of water are equivalent relationships.

$$1\,000 \text{ cm}^3 = 1\,000 \text{ mL} = 1\,000 \text{ g}$$

or

$$1 \text{ dm}^3 = 1 \text{ L} = 1 \text{ kg}$$

GLOSSARY

Agar — A dried gelatine-like product obtained from certain species of algae, especially Gelideum. Since it is unaffected by bacterial enzymes, it is widely used as a solidifying agent for bacterial culture media.

Agar-agar — A bacterial culture medium made from certain species of seaweed, not specific in nature.

Autotrophic — Self-nourishing or capable of growing in the absence of organic compounds.

Bacteria — Any of the class Schizomycetes of microscopic plants having round, rod-like, spiral, or filamentous single-celled or noncellular bodies. Bacterial often aggregate into colonies or move by means of flagella; live in soil, water, organic matter, or in the bodies of plants and animals; are autotrophic, saprophytic, or parasitic in nutrition; are important to humans because of the chemical effects. Pathogenic bacteria are commonly called germs.

Bacteria culture — A cultivation of bacteria in a prepared nutrient medium.

Bacteriology — The science that deals with bacteria and the relationships to medicine, industry, and agriculture.

Cell — The basic unit in the human body. It consists of a nucleus, a cytoplasm, and a membrane.

Chromatography — The separation of various organic chemical compounds, such as carotene and chlorophyll, by differential or selective absorption.

Compound — A substance that consists of two or more elements chemically united in a definite proportion so that the elements lose individual characteristics.

Cresols — A yellowish-brown liquid obtained from coal tar and not containing more than 5% phenol. It is used as a disinfectant for inanimate articles and areas which do not come into contact with food.

Czapek solution agar — A culture medium for various fungi consisting essentially of a balanced and buffered mixture of inorganic salts, a sugar, and water being used with added agar as a solid.

Dosage — The total quantity of a drug that is to be administered during a given period of time.

Dose — The portion of the drug that is to be administered at one time.

Drug — A substance or a mixture of substances that have been found to have a definite value in the detection, prevention, or treatment of disease.

Enzyme — A substance that initiates and accelerates a chemical reaction.

Erlenmeyer flask — A flask with a conical body, broad base, and narrow neck.

Fehling's solution — A solution used for detecting the presence of sugar in urine.

Flask — A laboratory vessel usually made of glass and having a constricted neck.

Glossary

Gram's iodine solution — A solution containing iodine, potassium iodine, and water which is used in the straining of bacteria.

Hayem's solution — A solution used to dilute the blood prior to counting the blood cells.

Hemacytometer — A piece of apparatus used in counting blood cells.

Hematocrit — The volume of red blood cells (erythrocytes) packed by centrifugation in a given volume of cells.

Intracellular water — The body water that is within the cells. It comprises about 2/3 of the total body water.

Lugol's solution — Strong iodine solution used in iodine therapy.

Lysol solution — A proprietary preparation of a mixture of cresols used for disinfection of inanimate objects.

Manometer — A device used to determine the rate at which oxygen is used by a bacteria culture.

Medicine glass — A graduated container. It may be graduated in millilitres, ounces, or drams.

Medium — A substance used for the cultivation of microorganisms or cellular tissue.

Microbiology — The study of simple forms of living matter which cannot be seen by the naked eye.

Microorganism — Minute living body not visible to the naked eye, especially a bacterium or a protozoon.

Minim glass — A graduated container used to measure small portions. It is graduated in minims and drams.

Milliequivalences per litre (mEq/L) — A measure of electrolyte concentration which refers to the amount of electrolytes in each litre of body fluid.

Mycology — The science of fungi.

Nutrient — Food that supplies the body with its necessary elements. Carbohydrates, fats, proteins, and alcohol provide energy; water electrolytes, minerals, and vitamins are essential to the metabolic processes.

Pathogenic — Disease producing.

Petri dish — Shallow dish with cover that is used to hold solid media for culturing bacteria.

Physiological saline solution — An isotonic sterile solution containing sodium chloride in distilled water; 0.85% salt solution. This solution may be used for dehydration, shock or hemorrhaging.

Physiological solution — A solution which matches a person's body chemistry.

Pipette — A narrow glass tube with both ends open. It is used for transferring and measuring liquids.

Protozoa — A phylum of the animal kingdom which includes all of the unicellular forms. Most consist of a single cell or of an aggregation of nondifferentiated cells but not forming a tissue.

Pure drug — A medical substance which is not mixed, combined, or diluted; having a strength of 100%.

Ratio strength of a solution — The ratio of the amount of solute (drug) to the amount of solution. This ratio may also be expressed as a percent or a fraction.

Ringer's solution — A solution resembling the blood serum in its salt constituents. For topical use on burns and wounds.

Saline — Containing or pertaining to salt.

Solute — The substance that is dissolved in the liquid to form a solution.

Solution — A liquid containing one or more dissolved substances.

Solvent — The liquid in which the substance or substances are dissolved to form a solution.

Stock solution — A solution which is kept on hand. It has a strength of less than 100% and is usually diluted further.

Substrate — The substance that an enzyme acts upon.

Viable — Capable of living.

Vial — A small bottle.

Virus — Minute organisms that are not visible with ordinary light microscopy. Parasitic in nature and dependent upon the nutrients inside the cells for metabolic and reproductive needs.

Yeast — Any of the spherical-shaped or oval-shaped fungi which reproduce by budding. Plant cells which are capable of fermenting carbohydrates.

HEALTH OCCUPATION INFORMATION

Health occupations involve the categories of physicians, nurses, dentists, and therapists as well as the all-important behind the scenes categories of technologists, technicians, administrators, and assistants. Each category of health occupations is related to another category and no occupation stands alone.

Health occupations are classified as dental occupations; medical professions; medical technologist, technician, and assistant occupations; nursing occupations; therapy and rehabilitation occupations; and other health occupations. Brief descriptions of job titles in each classification will be presented. For further information consult governmental publications such as the *Dictionary of Occupational Titles* and the *Occupational Outlook Handbook* or consult private organizations. The *Occupational Outlook Handbook* lists some such organizations and also lists sources of additional information for each particular occupation.

DENTAL OCCUPATIONS

Dental care—preventative and corrective— is an integral part of a person's overall health. There are four key health occupations involving dental care.

Dentists examine teeth and tissues of the mouth to diagnose disease or abnormalities. They also concentrate on preventative medicine through properly educating their patients.

Dental hygienists maintain medical and dental records for each patient. They also scale, clean, and polish the teeth as well as advise the patient on certain prophylaxis procedures. They are often responsible for preparing x-rays of the teeth.

Dental assistants work with the dentists during the treatment of patients. This involvement includes providing the many pieces of equipment and supplies necessary for the treatment. Dental assistants also play a major role in preparing the patient for treatment and providing pretreatment and post-treatment instructions.

Dental laboratory technicians make dentures, fabricate crowns to restore teeth, construct bridges to replace missing teeth, and make other dental orthodontic appliances. The field of dental technology involves many areas of specialty, but the main concern of all dental laboratory technicians is to provide the patient with a natural appearance.

MEDICAL PROFESSIONS

Medical professionals prevent, cure, and alleviate disease. The group of medical professions is composed of physicians, osteopaths, chiropractors, optometrists, podiatrists, and veterinarians.

Physicians, osteopaths, and chiropractors treat diseases that affect the entire body; chiropractors and osteopaths specialize in the manipulation of muscles and bones. Optometrists specialize in care for the eyes, and podiatrists care for foot disease and deformities. Veterinarians provide care for animals.

All of these medical professionals complete from six to nine years of postsecondary education. Within each category there are assistants and/or technicians and technologists whose occupation usually requires less postsecondary education.

MEDICAL TECHNOLOGIST, TECHNICIAN, AND ASSISTANT OCCUPATIONS

The development of sophisticated diagnostic tools and techniques for treatment of diseases, along with the advances in medical sciences and technology, have produced the need for medical technologists, technicians, and assistants.

Electrocardiograph (EKG) technicians are responsible for correctly setting up the equipment and preparing the patient for an electrocardiogram. They also manipulate the switches of the electrocardiograph and move electrodes across the patient's chest. Electrocardiograph technicians sometimes conduct other tests such as vectorcardiograms and phonocardiograms.

Electroencephalographic (EEG) technicians have the primary responsibility of conducting EEG examinations of a patient. The EEG examination is involved with the gathering of information about the electrical impulses given off by the patient's brain. This information is vital in diagnosing and treating certain types of disorders associated with the nervous system.

Medical assistants aid the doctor in the care and treatment of patients. Their duties may range from making appointments to carrying out various laboratory procedures. They will prepare patients for examination and may gather preliminary data.

Medical laboratory workers are on three different levels: medical laboratory assistants, technicians, and technologists. The duties at each level increase as does the amount of postsecondary education needed. In general medical laboratory workers perform tests under the direction of pathologists, physicians, or scientists who specialize in clinical chemistry, microbiology, or other biological sciences. They also analyze the blood, tissue, and fluids from the human body.

Medical record technicians are responsible for maintaining up-to-date records for each patient. This requires a system for recording and retrieving data. Much of the record keeping is now carried out with the aid of a computer. The records are important for prompt, efficient, and complete treatment of the patient and also serve as a historical record of the patient.

Operating room technicians may be involved in preoperative, operative, and postoperative activities. This requires them to prepare the operating room and patient for surgery. During the operation, they must supply the necessary equipment for the surgery. Following the surgery, they may be required to assist in patient and operating room cleanup.

Optometric assistants may serve both as secretaries and technicians. They may be responsible for conducting preliminary tests for the optometrist. They may also aid patients in the selection of eye glasses and provide supervision in certain exercises recommended by the optometrist. In some offices, highly trained optometric technicians may cut and polish eye glass lenses or contact lenses.

Radiologic (x-ray) technologists, working with radiologists, apply x-rays and radioactive substances to patients for diagnostic and therapeutic purposes. The findings of this team may be used by the physician in further treatment of the patients.

Respiratory therapy workers, sometimes called inhalation therapy workers, treat patients who have cardiorespiratory problems. The treatment they provide ranges from giving temporary relief to asthma or emphysema patients to giving emergency care in case of stroke, heart failure, shock, or drowning. This treatment is given by therapists, technicians, or assistants depending on the severity of the problem and the complexity of the treatment. Therapists have the highest level of expertise, followed by technicians, then followed by assistants who are in the process of training.

NURSING OCCUPATIONS

The nursing field consists of registered nurses (RN); licensed practical nurses (LPN); nurse aides or nursing assistants; orderlies; and attendants. The nursing field accounts for one-half of the total employment in the health occupations.

Nurses assume the role of caring for the sick, aiding in the prevention of disease and promoting good health. Nursing assignments may entail a variety of duties and there are many variations in the nursing assignments.

Nurse aides or nursing assistants, orderlies and attendants care for sick and injured people in various ways. They are the all-essential "back-up" team and aid in the efficiency and effectiveness of health care facilities.

THERAPY AND REHABILITATION OCCUPATIONS

Therapy allows handicapped persons to learn to build satisfying and productive lives. People involved in therapy and rehabilitation occupations aid the handicapped in this therapy.

Rehabilitation occupations can be divided into three areas: occupational therapy, physical therapy, and speech therapy and audiology.

Occupational therapists help mentally and physically disabled patients by planning and directing educational, vocational, and recreational activities. They teach manual and creative skills; business and industrial skills, and daily routines such as eating, dressing, and writing. Occupational therapists may design special equipment and adaptive devices.

Occupational therapy assistants may work with both physically and mentally handicapped patients. They assist the therapist in helping the patients adjust to their physical and/or mental limitations. They may serve as a teacher of arts and crafts as well as provide vocational training.

Physical therapists aid people who have muscle, nerve, joint, and bone diseases or injuries in overcoming their disabilities. They perform and interpret tests, prescribe and evaluate treatment, and aid the disabled person in accepting and adjusting to handicaps.

Physical therapy assistants and aides work with patients who are recovering from physical disorders which may be the result of disease, surgery, or accident. Supervised by physical therapists, the assistants help in conducting both physical exercises and educational programs for the patients.

Prosthetists and orthotists work with the physical therapists and the doctors in the development of mechanical aids that allow patients to regain some degree of normal function. This involves the use of many kinds of materials to recreate lost limbs or to prepare braces that strengthen weakened limbs.

Speech pathologists diagnose and treat speech and language problems of children and adults. The speech problems may be the result of hearing loss, brain injury, mental retardation, or emotional problems. Speech pathologists may also conduct research to develop diagnostic and treatment techniques or apparatus. *Speech therapists* work under the supervision of speech pathologists.

Audiologists perform diagnostic evaluations of hearing, prescribe and execute habilitation and rehabilitation treatment, and conduct research. They may design and develop clinical and research procedures and apparatus. Since speech and hearing are so interrelated, competence in one field mandates having a working knowledge in the other field and sometimes performing the same duties.

OTHER HEALTH OCCUPATIONS

The cure and prevention of diseases and illnesses together with proper nutrition and wellbeing unite technology, science, and medicine. There are many occupations in technology and science that contribute to the prevention of disease and the goal to cure and prevent illnesses has encouraged the development of many technological and scientific occupations.

Biomedical equipment technicians serve as a valuable link between the field of medicine and the world of technology. Their assignments include the operation and maintenance of many complex pieces of equipment used in the field of health services. The technicians also play a significant role in the development of new equipment to better serve the patients.

Cytotechnologists assist the pathologist in preparing living or dead cells for detailed examination. Special dyes are used to prepare and stain the cells. The staining allows for detailed identification of specific structures within the cell. A wide variety of medical disorders requires this type of examination.

Dietitians are involved with the careful planning of nutritious and appetizing meals which will aid in maintaining or recovering good health. Dietitians often specialize in a certain area such as administrative, clinical, research, or nutrition. Dietitians are aided by *dietetic technicians* who are responsible for the nutritional care of patients. Dietetic technicians may be involved directly with the patient as they gather information relating to nutritional needs. Some technicians may work in food service administration, research, or with health agencies.

Environmental health technicians work to identify various environmental factors that may influence the continued good health of the community, nation, or world. Water and air pollution are only two of the many areas of concern. These technicians also take an active role in the safety of recreational areas and water-processing systems.

Histologic technicians work closely with the surgeon to determine the cause of numerous disorders. They may prepare frozen sections of tissue removed from the patient. These small sections are then examined with a microscope. The ability to carry out this study while the patient is still on the operating table is vital to the patient's health. This information then becomes useful to the surgeon in determining the extent of surgery to be conducted.

Medical or dental secretaries must have many of the skills common to an executive secretary. Further, they must have a knowledge of medical terminology. The duties may vary but they must be able to type, take shorthand, arrange meetings, and maintain certain financial records. They handle the clerical duties essential to the efficient schedule of a physician.

Mental health technicians may conduct interviews or even serve as teachers for patients. They may provide assistance to mentally ill or mentally retarded patients who need to adjust to the surrounding community.

Index

A
Addition, defined, 1
Allowable limits of error, 261
Apothecaries' system of volume, 216–222
  basic units, 216
  equivalent measurements, 217–219
  metric equivalent measurements, 220–222
Apothecaries' system of weight, 207–215
  basic units, 208
  equivalent measurements, 210–212
  metric equivalent, 212–214
  uses, 207–209
Area
  of a circle, 112
  defined, 109
  of a rectangle, 110
  of a square, 110
  of a triangle, 111
Area measure, metric units of, 109–118
Attitudes, of health care workers, 89

B
Bacteria
  defined, 80
Bar graph(s), 245
  interpreting, 247
Base
  number used as factor, 71
  of triangle, 111
Base units, metric system and, 97
Broken-line graph, 245

C
Cancellation, defined, 32
Celsius scale, 142
Center, defined, 104
Charts, interpreting, 245–246
Chiropractors, role of, 52
Circle, finding the area of, 112–113
Circle graph(s), 246
  interpreting, 253
Circumference, defined, 104
Common denominator(s)
  and comparison of fractions, 27–28
  defined, 20
  finding, 21–22
Common factors, defined, 4
Common fractions, 1–45
  addition, 20–29
  division, 35–41
  expressed as decimal fractions, 55–56
  multiplication, 30–35
  subtraction, 20–29
Common multiple, defined, 4

Components
  defined, 151
  fractional, 159–160
  implied, 158–159
Computations
  proportional, 154
  rate pair, 156–158
Computers, using, 264–269
Cylindrical solid, finding the volume of, 121–123

D
Data
  collecting and arranging, 243–269
  defined, 243
  organizing and reporting, 243–269
Decimal fractions, 49–88
  addition of, 61
  basic operations with, 61–70
  common fractions expressed as, 55–56
  comparison of, 51–52
  division of, 66–69
  expressed as common fractions, 49
  multiplication of, 63–65
  in place-value systems, 50–51
  repeating, 57–59
  subtraction of, 62
Decimal(s)
  equivalent, expressing percent as, 169–170
  misplaced, 52, 89
  repeating, 57–58
  terminating, 57–58
Decimal numbers, 53–60
  rounding, 53–55
Denominators
  common, 20–22, 27–28
  defined, 7
  like, 20–21
  unlike, 23–24
Derived units, metric system and, 97
Diameter, defined, 104
Difference, defined, 1
Divisibility, defined, 2
Division
  defined, 1
  involving zero, 3
Dosage
  defined, 29
  factors determining, 42
  terms used in calculating, 43
Dose
  average, 43
  defined, 29, 42
  initial, 43
  lethal, 43
  maximum, 43

  terms used in calculating, 43
Drug(s)
  administration of, 42
  defined, 42

E
Equality symbol, 2
Equations
  involving percents, 175–183
Equipment, checking for accuracy, 89
Equivalent decimals, expressing percents as, 169–170
Equivalent fractions, 8
  defined, 8
  expressing percents as, 168–169
  and number line, 14
Equivalent percents
  expressing decimals as, 170
  expressing fractions as, 170–171
Error of measurement, defined, 105
Estimating, with percents, 190–191
Estimation, 81–83
Exponent(s), 71–73
  defined, 71
  in multiplication and division, 73–75
  negative, 72
Extremes, defined, 152

F
Factor(s)
  common, 4
  defined, 1, 4
  greatest common (GCF), 8, 12
  prime, 4
Factorization
  defined, 4
  prime, 4, 12, 21
Fahrenheit scale, 142
Flask, defined, 18
Fluids
  finding the volume of, 126–132
Fraction bar, 169
Fraction(s)
  common, 1–45, 55–56
  comparison of, 15–16
    using common denominators, 27–28
  decimal, 49–88
  defined, 7, 12
  division of, 35–38
  equivalent, 8–11, 14
    expressing percents as, 168–169
  expressed, 12–13
  as equivalent percents, 170–171
  with like denominators, 20–21
  lowest-term, 8, 12–13, 168
  and number line, 12–13
  multiplication of, 30–33

Index 287

with unlike denominators, 23–24
Fractional components, of proportions, 159–160
Fractional parts, 7–8

G

Glass containers
  minim, 18
  medicine, 18
Graphs
  bar, 245, 247
  circle, 246, 253
  interpreting, 245–246
  line, 245, 248–249
Greatest common factor (GCF), 12
  defined, 8

H

Health care assistants, 41
Health care work principles, 89
Health work metric measurements frequently used, 146
Health work problems
  and metric measure to solve, 146
  and ratios, proportions and percents, 196
Height, defined, 111
Household-apothecaries' systems of measure, 225–233
  equivalent measurements, 227–230
  of liquid measure, 225–227
  symbols translation, 230–232
Household measuring articles, 225
Household-metric systems of measure, 234–240
  equivalent measurements, 234–236
  symbols translation, 236–238

I

Implied components, of proportions, 158–159
Inequality symbol, 2
Inscription, defined, 223

L

Larger % of strength (stronger), defined, 193
Larger volume (solvent), defined, 193
Le Systeme International d'Unites, 93
Least common multiple (LCM), 21
Length measure, 97
  applications of, 107
  metric units of, 101–108
Line graphs, interpreting, 248–249
Lowest-term fraction, defined, 8
Lowest terms, defined, 8

M

Manometer, use of, 91
Mass, defined, 133
Mass measure, 97
  metric units of, 133–141

Mathematical system, 1–6
Mathematics
  basis of, 1
  English system of, 93
Mean
  defined, 259
Means, defined, 152
Measurement systems
  Apothecaries' volume, 216–224
  Apothecaries' weight, 207–215
  household-Apothecaries', 225–233
  household-metric, 234–240
Measuring process, 95–96
Median, defined, 259
Medical assistant, role of, 29, 41
Medical laboratory assistant, role of, 41
Medical records clerks, role of, 41
Medication(s)
  administration of, 69
  measuring, 28–29
  order, 215
  preparing and administering, 43–45
  use of decimals in preparing, 52, 59, 87–88
Medication containers, use of common fractions and, 18–19
Metric area measure, 109–118
  units of, 115
Metric length measure, 101–108
  of a circle, 104–105
  error of measurement and, 105
  units of, 101
Metric mass measure, 133–141
  units of, 133
Metric measure, 95–149
  area, 109–118
  Greek and Latin prefixes, and, 98
  length, 101–108
  mass, 133–141
  place-value system and, 96–97
  standard units of, 100
  temperature, 142–145
  volume, 119–132
    of fluids, 126–132
    of solids, 120–125
Metric system
  based upon powers of ten, 96
  kinds of units and, 97–98
  relationship between, 136–139
Microbiologist, role of, 79
Microbiology, defined, 79
Microorganisms, measurement of, 79
Midpoint, defined, 296
Mixed numbers, 16–19
  addition and subtraction of, 25–29
  defined, 8, 16
  division, 35–41
  expressed as fraction, 17
  multiplication, 30–35
  subtraction, 20–29
Mode, defined, 259
Multiple, defined, 4

Multiplication, defined, 1

N

Negative exponent, 72
Number, mixed, 8
Number line
  and fractions, 13–14
Numbers
  decimal, 53–60
  mixed, 16–19, 25–27, 30–41
  prime, 21
  whole, 1–3
Numerator, defined, 7

O

Object, process of measuring an, 95
Occupational therapists, role of, 52
Operating room technician, role of, 29

P

Percent(s), 166–174
  combining, 186
  computations with, 184–193
  of decrease, 184–186
  defined, 168
  equations involving, 175–183
  equivalent
    expressing decimals as, 170
    expressing fractions as, 170–171
  estimating with, 190–191
  expressing as equivalent decimals, 169–170
  expressing as equivalent fractions, 168–169
  of increase, 184–186
  other methods of calculating, 179–181
Percent by volume, defined, 173
Percent of decrease, 184–186
Percent of increase, 184–186
Percent problems
  and proportional rate pairs to solve, 175–178
  types of, 175–178
Period, of repeating decimal, 58
Pi (π), defined, 104
Pictograph(s), 246
  interpreting, 254–255
Place-value system
  decimal fractions in, 50–51
  metric measure and, 96–97
  and powers of ten in, 72
Power, defined, 71
Prescription
  inscription, 222
  signature, 222
  subscription, 222
  superscription, 222
  symbols used in, 223
Prime factor, defined, 4
Prime factorization, 12, 21
  defined, 4

Prime number, defined, 4
Product, defined, 1
Proportion(s), 152–153
  computations with, 156–163
  defined, 152
  fractional components of, 159–160
  implied components of, 158–159
Proportional computations, 154
Protozoa, 79
Pure drugs, defined, 196
Pure solution, defined, 173

Q

Quality control
  defined, 89
Quotient, defined, 1

R

Radius, defined, 104
Range
  defined, 259
Rate, defined, 153
Rate pair(s)
  computations, 156–158
  defined, 153
Ratio(s), 151–152
  defined, 151
  percent notation for, 166
  simplest-term, 152
Ratio strength of the solution, 155
Rectangle, finding the area of, 110
Rectangular solid, finding the volume of, 120
Repeating decimal, period of, 58
Roman numerals
  use in Apothecaries' system of measure, 207–208
  of volume, 216–222
Rounding
  defined, 53
  in estimation, 81–83

S

Scientific notation, 75–78
SI metrics style guide, 93
Signature, defined, 223
Significant digits
  defined, 83
  retention of, 85–87
    in addition and subtraction, 86
    in multiplication and division, 86–87
  rules for determining, 84
Simplest-term ratio, 152
Smaller % strength (weaker), defined, 193
Smaller volume (solute), defined, 193
Solids, finding the volume of, 120–125
Solute, defined, 155
Solution(s)
  defined, 155, 196
  preparing, 196–197
  pure, 173
  stock, 173–196
Solvent, defined, 155
Spreadsheeting, 265–269
Square, finding the area of, 110
Standards, setting, 89
Statistics
  defined, 243
Stock solution(s)
  defined, 173, 196
Subscription, defined, 223
Subtraction, 1
Sum, defined, 1
Superscription, defined, 222
Supplementary units, metric system and, 97
Symbol(s)
  approximately equal to, 53
  equal numbers, 2
  greater than, 2
  household-apothecaries, 1, 230
  less than, 2–3
  multiplication, 71
  percent, 167
  for prescription writing, 223
  unequal numbers, 2
Systems of measure, 207–240

T

Temperature measure, metric units of, 142–145
Terminating decimal, 57–58
Terms
  defined, 151
Triangle
  finding the area of, 111
  parts of a, 111

V

Vertex, defined, 111
Vial, defined, 18
Viruses, 79
Volume
  Apothecaries' system of, 207–215
  of a cylindrical solid, 121
  defined, 119
  of a rectangular solid, 120
Volume measure, 97
  metric units of, 119–132

W

Water
  boiling point of, 142
  freezing point of, 142
Weight
  Apothecaries' system of, 207–215
  defined, 133
Whole numbers
  basic of mathematics, 1
  comparison of, 2–3
Word processing, 265

Y

Yeast, defined, 79

Z

Zero
  in division, 3
  as placeholders, 84
Zero power, 72

COUNTY COLLEGE OF MORRIS LIBRARY

COUNTY COLLEGE OF MORRIS
SHERMAN H. MASTEN
LEARNING RESOURCE CENTER
RANDOLPH, NJ   07869